ISSUES IN PHYSICIAN SATISFACTION

New Perspectives

ISSUES IN PHYSICIAN SATISFACTION

New Perspectives

Paula L. Stamps
and
N. Tess Boley Cruz

Health Administration Press
Ann Arbor, Michigan 1994

AHSR

98 97 96 95 94   5 4 3 2 1

Library of Congress Cataloging-in-Publication Data

Stamps, Paula L.
  Issues in physician satisfaction : new perspectives / Paula L. Stamps, N. Tess Boley Cruz.
      p.   cm.
  Includes bibliographical references and index.
  ISBN 1-56793-010-7 (softbound : alk. paper)
  1. Physicians—Job satisfaction—Massachusetts. 2. Physicians—Massachusetts—Attitudes. 3. Health care reform—United States.
4. Surveys—Methodology. I. Cruz, N. Tess Boley. II. Title.
  [DNLM: 1. Physicians—Massachusetts. 2. Job Satisfaction. 3. Professional Practice. W 62 S783i 1994]
  R690.S725   1994   610.69'52'09744—dc20
  DNLM/DLC for Library of Congress   93-49787 CIP

The paper used in this publication meets the minimum requirements of American National Standard for Information Sciences—Permanence of Paper for Printed Library Materials, ANSI Z39.48-1984. ∞™

Health Administration Press
A division of the Foundation of the
  American College of Healthcare
  Executives
1021 East Huron Street
Ann Arbor, Michigan 48104-9990
(313) 764-1380

The Association for Health
  Services Research
1350 Connecticut Avenue, NW
Suite 1100
Washington, DC 20036
(202) 223-2477

To C.C.R.D.—its members, friends, and associates.
You all kept me focused on the important issues.
—P.S.

To Jon and Jesse.
For their encouragement and humor.
—N.T.B.C.

Contents

Preface

The purpose of this book is to contribute to the development of a new conceptual focus around which to organize research into physicians' behaviors, attitudes, and motivations. We think it important that this focus be clarified in order to increase the chance that *any* particular health care reform will have a greater likelihood of success. The idea of "reforming the American health care system" is far from new; rather, the urge to change it has been virtually the most constant theme expressed over a 40-year span; only the details have differed. The next most common theme has been dissatisfaction with the various alterations that have been made. Although the reasons for dissatisfaction are diverse, one problem—and the primary rationale of this book—is that it is far too easy to rush into reform (usually through regulation) without the appropriate research that accurately identifies the problem and predicts the consequences. Although none would disagree that restructuring the health care system is inherently a political process, there seems to be a general unwillingness to conduct research to help identify the perceptions of the various players.

We focus on developing such an understanding about one set of players: physicians. Devoting ourselves to this does not commit us to a position of advocacy, but rather to a position of clarity. It is our contention that a better understanding of physicians is central to the development of successful health policy. To develop an improved knowledge base requires an understanding of four broad content areas: supply of physicians, income determinants of physicians, the role of gender in medical practice patterns, and identification of those factors that provide satisfaction and dissatisfaction to physicians. For each of these topics, we provide a review and critique of previous research, national empirical data, and the data collected from physician respondents in four counties of western Massachusetts. The book is organized so that each major topic—supply, income determinants, women in medicine, and physician satisfaction—is a separate chapter.

The first chapter provides a general background, including a specific description of the political climate of Massachusetts that helps set the context for the study. This chapter presents the need for conceptualizing research on physicians in a slightly different manner, one that more appropriately addresses the concerns of the health care system of the 1990s.

The focus of the second chapter is methodological, including the questionnaire development phase and actual formatting of the survey, as well as the plans made for aggressive, targeted follow-up efforts that were a key to obtaining a 70 percent response rate. This chapter also identifies and compares the validity and reliability of the various lists and registries available to those who are doing research on physicians.

The third chapter describes the first of the four major topics: physician supply. It is ironic that in this age of highly developed technology the struggle continues with the seemingly simple concept of enumerating physicians. We describe several definitions that might be used and show the effect on the ubiquitous physician/population ratios that are so intricately a part of current health policy analysis. We also compare our results to those obtained by others, including the American Medical Association (AMA) and the Graduate Medical Education National Advisory Committee (GMENAC). This chapter presents a new way of enumerating physicians. We propose that using what we term the direct care–equivalent physician estimate will provide more precise enumeration of the physician supply.

Three chapters of what might be called "hard results" are included here. The first (Chapter 4) focuses on an important aspect of physician practice: the amount of money physicians make, factors that affect physician income, and physician thoughts and opinions about their income. Just enough economics theory is included in this chapter to explain the several unexpected findings.

Chapter 5 uses gender as the important analytic focus. This chapter provides a critique of previous research on women in medicine and concludes with suggestions concerning new ways of doing research on the subject.

One of the major themes of this book is the need to be able to understand the "world view" of physicians, to be more knowledgeable about perceptions of physicians about themselves, their profession, and the medical care system. Chapter 6 provides a mechanism by which this notion of physician perceptions might be more quantified by focusing on those factors that satisfy and dissatisfy physicians.

The final chapter addresses the general concern about the type of research that is done on physicians, including philosophical and political issues as well as methodological. This chapter raises what we consider to be some of the more important issues confronted in moving from research to health care reform.

Two additional words about the structure of the book are appropriate. Because of the massive data base, we have literally thousands of tables. We have chosen to include in the text only the most relevant of the data tables, so the more casual reader will not be overwhelmed. However, since one of the objectives of writing this book is to provide researchers with a new model for research about physicians, it is important to include as much technical information as possible. We have chosen to include this material in the four technical appendixes provided especially for those who are interested in replicating our work in other parts of the country. In some cases, we have also placed in an appendix data specifically relevant to Massachusetts.

Finally, although we have concentrated on the empirical findings, we do not wish to ignore another very important aspect of this research: the voices of the respondents. A great many physicians who responded to our questionnaire took the time to write additional comments on medicine and on being a physician. Some of these comments were short, but many were very lengthy; in some cases physicians wrote separate letters. These comments provided an important perspective and enabled us to understand much better what physicians "out in the frontlines" are thinking. We have chosen to incorporate their comments where appropriate to give breadth and context to the more quantitative findings.

Throughout this volume, three overall themes provide a common denominator for each of the content areas addressed. The first is that a necessary link exists between research and reform; when that link is broken, the result is frequently the kind of "reform" and regulations that do not work—that may create worse situations. The second broad theme is that the ability to understand the perceptions of physicians is necessary, since physicians do constitute one of the major interest groups in the health care system. This understanding needs to be based on information gathered directly from physicians, not on suppositions inferred from other sources. The third theme is that much of the previous research on each of the four major topics in this book has been limited by methodological problems. Little agreement has been reached on basic terminology (for example, on specialty designations, as discussed in Chapter 3); there is little agreement on either conceptual or operational definitions. Frequently, previous research is of limited usefulness because the earlier medical-social environment is very different from the current one.

Although the original impetus for this research project arose from some particular interests in one state, the results have wide-ranging implications for others. We hope that this volume contributes to the beginning of new methods of conducting research on physicians—both conceptually and operationally.

April 1994

Paula L. Stamps
Amherst, Massachusetts

N. Tess Boley Cruz
Goleta, California

Acknowledgments

The project that resulted in this book involved a great many people over its four-year history. The initial vision for this whole effort came from Henry Drinker, M.D., who at the time was president of the Hampshire County Medical Society. It was his dedication to the need for developing an accurate data base to describe the physician supply in western Massachusetts, and the importance he attached to assessing the concerns of his colleagues, that gave life to the overall project. Additionally, his comments on various drafts of Chapter 3 had a significant influence on our thought process about the perplexing problem of supply as we worked to improve the final version of that chapter.

Funding for this project was provided by the Massachusetts Medical Society in the form of an unrestricted grant to the principal investigator (Paula Stamps). The Massachusetts Medical Society provided encouragement and support throughout all phases of the research, while allowing the researchers independence. There were no strings attached to the money that was provided. Dr. Will Lybrand and Mr. David Pomeranz of the Massachusetts Medical Society were particularly helpful and supportive. The School of Public Health at the University of Massachusetts/ Amherst also provided support in terms of departmental services and faculty time.

The design of the questionnaire itself was much assisted by the Massachusetts Medical Society, which brought together representatives from several organizations, including the Health Data Consortium, ABT Associates, and faculty and staff from Boston University School of Public Health. Several faculty and students at the University of Massachusetts School of Public Health also reviewed the questionnaire, and this led to significant improvements. Ed Stanek, Ph.D., Associate Professor of

Biostatistics/Epidemiology was particularly helpful in both the design of the questionnaire and the later data analysis.

Several students contributed significantly to this work while pursuing their graduate degrees at the School of Public Health. Allison Nichols-Dunismuir, M.S. was involved in the original phase of the development of the project. She contributed significantly to the development of the literature that provided the background for Chapter 1. She is currently a program evaluation specialist in Christchurch, New Zealand. Amy Sandridge, M.S. was instrumental in the development and coding of the multiple lists of physicians as well as in the data analysis. She is now working for the Centers for Disease Control and is based in Costa Rica. Colette Orzulak, M.P.H. developed the background literature relating to physician supply, with a particular focus on location choice and practice patterns of physicians. She is now a primary care specialist in Hartford, Connecticut. Scott Evans, a doctoral student in Biostatistics, and Abhijit Sanyat, a doctoral student in the School of Management, both provided valuable assistance in the statistical analysis of the data. Abhijit was particularly helpful in the analysis related to creating the six indexes to measure physician satisfaction in Chapter 6.

The preparation of this manuscript involved innumerable revisions as well as endless "playing with tables," where the phrase "let's just see what this looks like" was all too common. A particular problem was that much of this manuscript was actually handwritten, and the writing of Paula Stamps is notoriously awful. Nancy Perwak did a wonderful job of deciphering this handwriting, as well as providing the necessary technical expertise at getting the computer to do what it was supposed to do. Her enthusiasm, support, and friendship are much appreciated. The manuscript preparation was completed in a calm and competent manner by Elizabeth Samit who—in addition to typing—filled in missing words, edited, and significantly improved the manuscript. Her proficiency with the various software is much appreciated.

The manuscript was also significantly improved by the reviewers for Health Administration Press, as well as by suggestions made by Ed Kobrinski, acquisitions editor for Health Administration Press during our early preparation phase. His patience with our always too optimistic deadlines made the manuscript preparation process easier.

At the more personal level, our husbands provided emotional support as well as technical assistance from their respective fields. Tom Duston, Ph.D., provided Paula Stamps with valuable insights and extensive technical expertise in economics, which was particularly helpful in analyzing the various parameters related to income, especially when addressing the differences based on gender. He also provided the emotional support for her to be able to finish this book, whose scope and time commitment turned out to be much larger than original estimates. The value she places on his personal and professional support cannot be easily summarized here or anywhere else. A special note of thanks goes to Jessie and Christopher, both of whom understood the need to "go upstairs and work." Jon Cruz, Ph.D. supplied many important questions and insights related to the antecedents and implications of our results. At the same time, he provided N. Tess Cruz with the encouragement and support to bring this work to completion. Thanks also go to Jesse Cruz for rescuing Tess at critical moments in the editing process.

Finally, we are particularly indebted to the many physicians who participated in this entire project. The two dozen or so we consulted for information and help in the pretest phase contributed significantly to the integrity of the questionnaire. We are especially grateful to the 908 physicians in western Massachusetts who took the time to respond to our questionnaire. We hope that this volume rewards their interest.

Of course the final responsibility for content, interpretation, and decisions about what to include rests with us. We hope that this volume is helpful to others who wish to better understand the physicians who are such an important resource for the health care delivery system.

Chapter 1

Introduction and Overview

The primary focus of this book is on one of the many human resources on which the health care system depends: the physician. Physicians are not a particularly popular focus today, since most research of the 1980s–early 1990s has been emphasizing the organizational structure within which physicians and health care providers work, with a secondary concentration on other direct care providers. We do not mean to imply that organizational structure and the numerous other health professionals are unimportant. This focus on comprehensiveness has provided uniquely helpful ways of analyzing medical care services. However, in our opinion, the pendulum has swung a bit too far. Into the 1990s, the physician's role in the delivery of medical care has changed, and very little is known about how physicians now perceive their role in contemporary society, or what they perceive to be satisfying or dissatisfying about the practice of their profession.

Some might argue that the physician perspective is not relevant, but we would strongly disagree for three basic reasons. First, physicians are an important human resource for the medical care system: they require years of intense education and hands-on training, and a fair amount of societal resources. Second, unhappy or dissatisfied doctors are not good for the nation's consumers or patients. Nobody wants to be cared for by a burned-out, alienated physician. The third reason is more pressing in terms of the health policy agenda of the 1990s. Not only has the profession of medicine changed remarkably in the last twenty years, but it seems quite likely that the next ten years may see even more dramatic changes. For perhaps the first time since the Truman presidency, enough special interest groups have converged to make some sort of organizational restructuring of the medical care system more likely than before. Many previous changes have been in health care financing, and none of them has accomplished what has been desired. Before more drastic changes occur in the medical care system—whether structural, organizational, financial, or some combination of these—the effect of the changes on physicians should be determined. This task cannot be accomplished given the current knowledge base of physician opinion about their professional duties and the health care system itself.

Most changes in financing medical care services have rested on the assumption that physician behavior is primarily responsive to economic incentives. When one particular set of economic incentives has not worked, the most common policy response has been to create another, usually slightly different, set of financial incentives. An alternative approach is to reconsider an underlying assumption: perhaps physician behavior is *not* as deeply rooted in economics as has been thought. There are many assumptions concerning the relationship between money, productivity, and professional satisfaction, but very little understanding. The "us-them" mentality pervades almost all health policy; the interests of society are pitted against what are primarily viewed as the economic desires of physicians. In the health care industry of the 1990s, there is actually a clearer understanding of the needs of society than of the professional needs of physicians.

This book is concerned primarily with creating a conceptual basis around which to organize research into physician attitudes and behavior. This conceptualization relies heavily on identifying what motivates physicians, as well as what satisfies and dissatisfies them. This framework rests on the assumption that the professional perceptions of physicians are important. By understanding the world view of this professional group, any specific restructuring of the American medical care system will have a far greater chance of success.

This first chapter sets the stage for the empirical research project, the results of which will be used to identify important areas that need to be addressed in developing an adequate knowledge base about physicians. This chapter starts with a very brief overview of historical and current perceptions about the role of the physician in American society, providing a backdrop for a better understanding of the physician in Massachusetts, the setting of this particular research. Some of the specific political and medical practice issues within the state of Massachusetts are described. These two background descriptive sections—one national and the other specific to one particular state—are used to identify the themes around which this book is organized.

The World View of Physicians

This short section cannot provide a comprehensive view of the role of physicians in either the medical system or in American society. Several authors have written thought-provoking articles and books, the most comprehensive of which is probably by Paul Starr (1982), although his work was made possible by the earlier analysis of American medicine by Rosemary Stevens (1971).

Partly because of technological advances, and partly because of increased communication through the media, expectations of medicine and doctors are currently quite high, but these expectations originated much earlier, during the efforts to professionalize medicine (Starr 1982). Before the Flexner Report came out early in this century, multiple "healers" were available. It took a concentrated action—occasioned by Flexner's observations—to obtain societal legitimation of only one degree as *the* acceptable medical degree. Since this 1910–1920 effort, the ability of the American Medical Association (AMA) to speak on behalf of all physicians has been remarkable. The current breakdown in this ability is probably due as much to the increase in specialty and subspecialty group identification as to anything else: specialists and subspecialists have established a stronger identity among themselves than with the generalist practitioners at the base of the medical profession pyramid. The development of many subspecialties, each with its own professional identity, has effectively destroyed the educational concept on which medicine was based (Starr 1982; Stevens 1971). One obvious consequence is the vast, and continually increasing, income differentials between the diagnostic and the procedure-intensive specialties.

The historical development of medicine as a profession was such that this group was viewed as the "ideal" profession—the one against which all others were measured, and the one that Friedson (1972) used to originally define a profession. Of the several criteria put forward by Friedson, professional autonomy has perhaps been the most important, undoubtedly because of the recognition that a profession having the right to control educational and training standards, as well as licensure and certification, is a significant social control. Many physicians in the 1990s would argue that medicine no longer meets the criterion of professional autonomy, and they are particularly sensitive to this loss. Those who are not physicians but who are involved in the regulation of physician behavior would argue either that physicians have clinical autonomy (that only the money is controlled), or that physicians have misused their professional autonomy to such an extent that external regulation is now imperative. The latter argument is the more common of the two, and is based on the recognition that control of the reimbursement patterns for a profession with expensive services means control of the distribution of the services themselves. So the primary argument is that, since physicians have failed to control or regulate themselves, people external to the profession now must do so. No one would argue with the observation that external controls and regulations on physician behavior have slowly and steadily increased in the 1980s and early 1990s.

Most of the regulations exist in the financial areas and have been based on certain assumptions about the sensitivity of physician behavior to economic incentives. Cost control regulations of the 1980s have been based on a three-part policy: an emphasis on segmentation of the insured population, an encouragement of competition in the hopes of lowering costs, and an increasing utilization review by the third party payers (Fuchs 1987). Many examples of specific regulations and actions related to each of these concepts can be shown, but none has been as effective as originally desired, and some now are identified as intensifying the perceived cost problem. For example, the segmentation of the insured population, with more and more specific policies related to certain targeted groups, is viewed today as a major source of the unacceptably high administrative costs of the U.S. medical care system. Competition seems to have fostered the growth of increasingly "corporatized" organizations with which there is some ideological discomfort. Efforts to control costs by using the private sector model are made more difficult by the nature of health services—a commodity characterized by unlimited demand. Of course, utilization controls are ubiquitous today, and physicians are accustomed to them as well as to a variety of methods of reimbursement; but it is the increasing use of the so-called third generation of utilization review, in which nonphysicians make determinations of appropriate care over the telephone, that has signaled to physicians that a significant change has taken place in their professional autonomy.

An alternative to the question of how well—or poorly—these economic controls have worked is to address an even more basic issue: what do financial constraints imply about society's view of physicians? Hafferty (1986) has argued that physicians are viewed today not so much as a way to obtain needed health services, but more likely as the key to spending money on health services. This view, of course, puts the physician in the proverbial hard place, since patients are demanding increasing services while society is demanding fewer, or at least more careful justification of the resources expanded. It is hard to argue that increased review and external regulation is related to anything but a lower level of trust in physicians to regulate themselves, and Starr (1982) has discussed this extensively, appropriately describing the "transformation" of the medical profession.

Physicians are not very often asked about their perceptions of issues related to increasing external regulation of their profession; rather, physicians' attitudes are inferred from three general sources of information. The first source is truly inferential: assumptions about physicians' attitudes are deduced from observations of physician behavior. For example, since physicians are usually opposed to cost-containment regulations, it is concluded that physicians are opposed to all regulations that restrict their income. This inference is consistent with the assumption that physician behavior is primarily dependent on economic incentives. Generalizing from reactions to one particular regulation to reactions about all regulations is obviously ill advised.

The second source is slightly more direct: much information is gleaned from physicians writing about the medical field as well as about various regulatory efforts. When physicians do discuss the effect of regulations on their practices, they are most likely to describe it in terms of professional—and particularly clinical—autonomy; they no longer view themselves as the sole clinical decision makers. Reed and Evans have noted that the current environment "amplifies the sacrifices of being a physician with no apparent compensatory increase in satisfactions" (1987, 3279). Other physicians have written about the lack of trust that they perceive as responsible for increasing regulations: the term "deprofessionalized medicine" is used to express the fear that physicians will become "protocol-oriented medical automatons" (Reed and Evans 1987, 3279). Of course, it is equally ill advised to generalize from such anecdotal evidence offered by a single or small group of physicians, especially since physicians have been writing such opinions for a long while. For example, R. B. Scott started a 1955 *Lancet* article with the following statement: "It is commonly said that the esteem in which the public holds the medical profession has fallen" (p. 341).

The third source of information about physician perceptions comes from physicians themselves, primarily through national surveys. Two such examples are a survey done by the Equitable Life Assurance Company and a series of physician surveys done by the American Medical Association (Harvey and Shubat 1989). These national surveys are usually conducted by one of the polling companies (Harris or Gallup). Often the attitudes of those defined as "physician leaders" are contrasted to practicing physicians, or the attitudes of the public on similar issues are compared with physician responses. Sometimes the survey has a particular focus; for example, the 1984 Equitable survey focused on cost-containment issues (Taylor and Paranjpe 1984).

Not surprisingly, the results of these surveys demonstrate the diversity of physician opinion, usually along specialty distinctions or age. For example, younger physicians seem more receptive to major health care system changes than older physicians, and practicing physicians as a group seem more receptive to a variety of proposed changes in the health care system than are their physician leaders, who include the heads of state, local, and specialty medical societies (Taylor and Paranjpe 1984).

Although the Equitable survey and the various surveys done by the AMA do show generally negative views of physicians toward what are commonly called "government price controls," unanimity of opinion is remarkably absent when a particular cost-containment policy is specified. For example, in a recent survey of physician attitudes on cost-containment, about half of the physicians felt most strongly that what they needed was a course in cost-containment measures so they would be able to understand the various new rules under which they are now practicing (Greene et al. 1989).

When these three sources of information are combined, it is clear that the existing knowledge base about physicians' perceptions of their job, their role in the medical care system, and the place of the medical care system in American society is woefully inadequate. Very little is known about what motivates physicians; equally little is known about what satisfies physicians about medical practice or what determines their behavior. This inadequate knowledge base leads to health policy based on anecdotal evidence or on corporate self-interest. It seems important to develop a more comprehensive understanding of how physicians perceive the health care world of the 1990s: to make any significant—or nonsignificant—changes in the fabric of health care without understanding how it would affect physicians will no doubt lead to repetitions of previous half-successes.

Because of a unique political environment in Massachusetts, we were able to conduct an in-depth survey of a large group of the state's practicing physicians; the major focus was physician perceptions of the state's medical practice climate. The issues that were of primary concern in Massachusetts are many of the same ones summarized here, although some other issues were unique to this one state.

The Political Environment in Massachusetts

The medical practice climate in each state is obviously influenced by national legislation, but there is also a fair amount of state level influence, so that there are important differences in the regulatory environment for physicians. During the mid- to late 1980s, the medical practice environment in Massachusetts had become acrimonious. In October 1987 the president of the Massachusetts Medical Society referred to Massachusetts as the "Beirut of Medicine," while he introduced a resolution to the annual meeting of the state medical society warning medical colleagues to avoid practicing in Massachusetts because it was "an undesirable location in which to practice" (Knox 1990, 31). Many viewed the passage of this resolution as representing a grass roots movement of physicians who felt powerless to change what the medical establishment viewed as extremely strict regulations on practicing physicians. The major issues creating such dissatisfaction included various restrictions on fees, malpractice premiums, and Medicare and Medicaid reimbursements.

Blue Shield

The major focus of complaints about income restrictions centers on Blue Shield of Massachusetts, primarily because this insurer is able to create severe financial penalties for those who do not participate and also because it enjoys some unique specific advantages over other insurers in the state. Blue Shield was created in 1941 in order to provide "a means whereby persons of low and average income could obtain otherwise unobtainable medical care insurance" (Massachusetts Medical Society 1987, 12). This legislation contained an agreement that prohibited a physician from billing patients for over and above whatever reimbursement Blue Shield paid, with only very limited exceptions. This ban on balance billing was agreed to by physicians with the understanding that reimbursements would be based on regularly updated "usual and customary charges" and that payment would be prompt. The system ran into trouble in 1976 when financial concerns prompted Blue Shield to freeze reimbursements at 1975 levels. Then, at Blue Shield's request, the insurance commissioner agreed to allow the insurer control of the timing and levels of reimbursement updates, and to limit the annual increases to a fixed percentage of Boston's consumer price index (excluding medical care). The resulting "discount" between the physician submitted charges and Blue Shield payments increased so that by 1981, physicians were reimbursed about 70 percent of what they charged. Physicians could not bill above the fixed charge and could not bill patients for the remainder. This difference persisted throughout the 1980s.

Legal action was brought against Blue Shield by the Massachusetts Medical Society based on charges of violating the Sherman Anti-Trust Act, since the regulations served to "lock in" participating physicians and "lock out" those who chose not to participate. The medical society charged that these features led to a 74 percent market share, and the 30 percent discount meant that Blue Shield could offer lower premiums than competing private insurers (Massachusetts Medical Society 1987). The court struck down the ban on balance billing as illegal restraint on trade, but Blue Shield and consumers lobbied intensely, and in July 1984 state legislation was passed banning balance billing. This enabled Blue Shield to become immune to federal antitrust laws.

Many physicians have resented the favored position enjoyed by Blue Shield, which alone among the "private" insurers has a ban on balance billing (Haddad 1988), and the Massachusetts Medical Society (1987) has termed it to be "uniquely restrictive" legislation, providing a mechanism that cuts Blue Shield's expenses and allows the insurer to offer its products at prices lower than commercial insurers' prices. The ban on balance billing was negotiated originally in exchange for an agreement by Blue Shield to offer three Medicare supplements and never refuse to sell insurance to anyone, even if the person was unemployed. Blue Shield recently lost its tax-exempt status (which was also part of the original legislation), and discussions have been under way for some time concerning other aspects of Blue Shield's favored status.

Many physicians view the ban on balance billing as an example of an unfair income restriction. For example, one physician respondent in our study noted the following: "I have become a nonparticipating M.D. because of Blue Cross/Blue Shield. Because of the escalating malpractice premiums and the fixed reimbursement from Blue Cross/Blue Shield, my partner and I decided that to remain solvent, we would drop out of Blue Cross/Blue Shield, and later re-open our doors to new patients." Some physicians in the western part of the state took an even more serious course of action in response to their dissatisfaction with Blue Shield. In the largest city in western Massachusetts, 110 physicians resigned from Blue Shield between early 1986 and mid-1987. In the next four years, a few dozen other physicians joined them, including six obstetricians/gynecologists in one other mid-sized city (Haddad 1988). This defection has thus far been limited to the western part of the state, perhaps because with a lower proportion of Blue Shield subscribers the economic effect on the physicians of leaving the insurer is less than in the rest of the state. The physicians, who must act "independently" for fear of antitrust charges, hope that this drastic action will get the attention of Blue Shield administrators. In response to this, Blue Shield has arranged for subscribers to be reimbursed for care from these physicians through a subsidiary based in Chicago, as Massachusetts regulations technically prohibit such payment (Haddad 1988).

Medicare and Medicaid

As a result of the 1984 legislation, organized advocacy groups for the elderly were also able to extend the ban on balance billing to Medicare beneficiaries. It is not required for physicians to participate in Medicare, and only about half of Massachusetts physicians do so. This low level of participation is partly because Blue Shield is the Medicare carrier in the state. However, another historical fact contributes to the low participation and the relatively negative feelings of physicians toward Medicare. Most primary care physicians in Massachusetts had responded to the

AMA's voluntary price control effort of 1983 and thus were already receiving lower reimbursements. The physicians' view of the legislation prohibiting Medicare balance billing was that their office charges were already less than the Medicare prevailing charge for that locality. Also, some physicians have refused to participate because of the increased paperwork, for which they view themselves as not being paid fairly.

Physicians are also not required to accept Medicaid patients, although in 1985 the Massachusetts Medical Society, in an effort to prevent mandatory assignment, signed an agreement to have 85 percent of the state's physicians take Medicaid patients. Some specialties are particularly reluctant to accept Medicaid patients, particularly obstetricians/gynecologists, because of the low reimbursement levels for a high-risk group of patients.

Low reimbursement levels for physicians from Medicare and Medicaid, coupled with Blue Shield's ban on balance billing, has produced much negative feeling among Massachusetts physicians. One comment from an oncologist is representative of these feelings: "I never could have indulged in the luxury of coming here were it not for the years of practice in Ohio. Reimbursement ratios for Medicare and Blue Cross/Blue Shield were the lowest in the 50 states three years ago. They have now improved, but cuts are threatened. If I were starting off, I would not come to Massachusetts."

Medical malpractice

Premiums for malpractice insurance for Massachusetts physicians are not the highest in the nation, but Massachusetts is the only state to prohibit balance billing, which physicians elsewhere use to pass through the increased cost of malpractice insurance. One unique feature of the malpractice situation in Massachusetts has contributed especially to a high level of physician anger and hostility. In 1983, to delay a 52 percent increase in malpractice premiums, the Joint Underwriters Association (JUA) sued the state Division of Insurance; later in 1983, the Massachusetts Medical Society joined the legal action. During the three-year period (1983–1986) in which the various legal actions took place—suits, countersuits, and appeals—physicians continued to pay the old rates for their malpractice coverage. In 1986, when all the legal issues had been resolved, physicians became responsible not only for their current premiums, but also for the retroactive amounts of the increases for the three years in question. Naturally, for those physicians who have riskier practices, including surgeons and obstetricians, the retroactive amounts were staggering. In fact, in some cases, primarily as a result of the legal actions, the base malpractice premium actually decreased but the retroactive amount covering three years of increases plus interest was far more attention-getting. The responsibility for retroactive premiums was spread over all physicians currently practicing in the state, whether they were in practice or not between 1983 and 1986.

As part of an effort to appease the Massachusetts medical community, a medical malpractice tort reform act (Chapter 351) was passed in 1986. Like so many pieces of legislation passed under a political compromise, this one wound up making almost all of the interest groups unhappy. Lawyers' fees were limited, some out-of-court settlements were streamlined, and, most important to many Massachusetts physicians, the disciplinary powers of the state Board of Registration of Medicine were significantly increased. Caps on financial awards for pain and suffering failed to be included in this piece of legislation.

There was a great deal of public attention drawn to the battle over malpractice in Massachusetts. Between 1983 and 1987, stories in local newspapers about physicians leaving the state of Massachusetts were common. A local television station ran two consecutive editorials criticizing physicians in general and the Massachusetts Medical Society in particular. Many physicians began to talk about the undesirability of Massachusetts as a place in which to practice. A surgeon noted: "Underfunding of Medicaid and reneging on reimbursements to hospitals have put our hospital in jeopardy in spite of its excellent medical staff. The ever-increasing "retroactive premium" for JUA with no serious tort reform and a continued ban on balance billing has made Massachusetts the least attractive state in which to practice." An emergency medical physician made the following comment, which captures the anger of many physicians, as well as the increasingly hostile political environment: "I am actively seeking employment outside Massachusetts, by obtaining licenses in other states. Reasons include soaring and retroactive malpractice insurance costs, a financially dangerous medico-legal climate, the regulatory zeal of the state, paper work, caps on physician and hospital income (without caps on our expenses) and an inept legislature. I am reluctant to leave friends, colleagues, and schools that we value, but the reasons for leaving outnumber the reasons for staying. If we get hit with having to pay even *one* dollar for insurance rate years 1975–1982, or if we ever get retroactively assessed again, I predict that *over half* of the physicians in this state will leave."

The conflict was frequently represented in terms of physicians against legislators, as one internal medicine specialist noted in responding to our survey: "I fear that in the very near future, in lieu of tort reform, my practice and income will be profoundly affected by the malpractice crisis. Tort reform is essential, but I doubt it will ever happen— too many legislators are lawyers and ex-insurance industry people."

Response of the medical community

Into this intensely public and contentious debate, the Massachusetts Medical Society released a 1988 report to the state legislature in which the results of three separate studies all pointed to the same conclusion: the medical practice climate in Massachusetts was unduly restrictive (Massachusetts Medical Society 1988). The first survey involved Massachusetts hospitals, and the major finding was that hospitals were experiencing serious trouble recruiting physicians. A second survey focused on physicians in high-risk specialties, including a variety of surgical specialties and subspecialties. The major finding communicated from this survey was that specialists were increasingly limiting their practice due to increasing malpractice costs. And finally, the Massachusetts Medical Society described the results of their physician opinion poll, in which 72 percent of the responding physicians noted that the "professional liability environment" had become worse within the last year.

At about the same time, three specialty societies—the Massachusetts Chapter of the American College of Surgeons, the Massachusetts Orthopedic Association, and the Massachusetts Chapter of the American College of Obstetricians and Gynecologists—released the results of their membership surveys (Couch and Fisher 1989; Massachusetts Orthopedic Association 1988; Massachusetts Chapter of the American College of Obstetricians and Gynecologists 1988); a separate study on residents and fellows currently in training was also published (Morse 1987). These all reinforced the claims of physician unhappiness with the state's medical practice climate being so extreme that physicians were either leaving Massachusetts or limiting their practices. Because of concerns of physician loss, the public discussion then changed focus somewhat to the question of whether there were enough physicians in Massachusetts to meet the medical needs of consumers. The legislative response was the establishment of a special commission to study the issue of physician supply in 1987–1988. Along with the newspaper articles, which now focused on physicians leaving the state, came more studies and reports, all concentrating on the issue of adequacy of supply. Two reports were distributed; neither were able to draw any conclusions (Massachusetts Health Data Consortium 1988; ABT Associates 1989). Both reports addressed the complicated issue of enumerating physicians, the topic of Chapter 3.

Counterresponses

There is inevitably more than one possible position on most controversial issues, and the situation in Massachusetts is no exception. For example, although many physicians resent what they consider to be Blue Shield's "privileged" position, others have pointed out that Blue Shield is the only insurer that is mandated to provide an open enrollment period, which enables any person to become a subscriber. This policy obviously results in insurance coverage being offered to some small and often high-risk groups. It is the view of Blue Shield—and several active consumer groups in Massachusetts—that the pricing advantages accorded to Blue Shield help offset its increased risk. Blue Shield also argues that it has additional regulations from the state that accompany its price advantage.

The picture of the Massachusetts medical practice climate as painted by the Massachusetts Medical Society is also not without alternative explanations. In fact, the release of the 1988 report on medical practice in Massachusetts stimulated publication of an alternative report by Alan Sager (1988) of the Boston University School of Public Health. The title of his report was "The Sky is Falling: The Massachusetts Medical Society Reports on the 'Physician Shortage'," and it was sponsored by one of the several citizen action committees in Massachusetts, Health Care for All. Sager's report was a careful critique of both the facts and the rhetoric surrounding the several issues involved in what was becoming an increasingly contentious public debate.

One of Sager's conclusions was that a new "social compact" between physicians and society is needed. He enlarges on this opinion by recognizing that physicians need to be paid adequately and simply in light of their skill and the obvious difficulty of their jobs. This notion of a new "social compact" is one that is achieving increased visibility and acceptance as a variety of reforms are suggested for the entire U.S. health care system (Himmelstein et al. 1989; Relman 1989).

As is so often the case, more heat than light was generated by these several studies and reports. It was obvious to many observers in Massachusetts that there were too many facts that were unknown. For example, as Sager (1988) pointed out repeatedly, very little knowledge exists about what physicians in other states think regarding the medical practice climate of their particular state. Furthermore, there is a paucity of information about the different ways in which states choose to regulate medical practices. Because of the emphasis on the national regulatory environment, state level regulation of medical practice has been ignored when, in fact, states can exert a fair amount of control over both the financial and clinical autonomy of physicians. Perhaps the best example of this lies in malpractice, an arena in which a variety of states, including California, Florida, New York, Illinois, Nevada, and Hawaii have participated in major reforms (*Washington Report on Medicine and Health Perspectives* 1985; Williams 1985). Related to the lack of knowledge about different state environments is a lack of understanding of how physicians respond to different regulatory climates. For example, statements made about physicians leaving Massachusetts "because of" the state's regulatory climate revealed a general lack of understanding about physician location changes.

Several things became clarified in the continuing debate in Massachusetts. First, the medical community was not speaking in unison: positions and opinions were generally based on specialty identification. One obvious polarization developed between surgical specialists, medical specialists, and primary care physicians. Second, the various numerical estimates being used to characterize physician supply in Massachusetts were basically incompatible. Many arguments developed over summary numbers that could not be defined, explained, or defended. Third, not enough knowledge was available about physician behavior or physician attitudes to be able to make policy suggestions for Massachusetts. The need for a study that could be objective was recognized and supported by several interest groups. The focus of the study was to be on two major areas: to address physician supply more accurately and to learn more about the perceptions of physicians practicing in Massachusetts. The study was set in the western counties of Massachusetts, including Berkshire, Franklin, Hampden, and Hampshire counties, a substantial representative medical service area (further described in Chapter 3). This region is slightly more rural than the whole state, but the population of 800,000 is clustered around several population centers, including one city.

About This Book

In deciding what from the massive amount of information to include in this book—and what to leave out—we have been guided by basic agreement with Sager's (1988) view of the necessity of a new "social compact" with physicians. To reach this new agreement, the perceptions of physicians must be more clearly understood. Medicine as a profession has changed: being a doctor today is very different from being a doctor twenty or even ten years ago. But the general knowledge base about physicians has not been added to significantly since the 1960s when research on physicians was more common.

The next two chapters of this book are methodological. Chapter 2 provides specific information about this particular study, and Chapter 3 addresses one of the basic themes of this book: the importance of accurate enumeration of the number and types of physicians currently practicing medicine. Arguments about physician supply are intrinsically related to many of the knowledge deficits about physicians. Being able to accurately enumerate physicians is a basic epidemiologic need: without this, additional research is difficult. Chapter 3 is devoted to this topic and includes a recommendation for a new way of enumerating physicians that will be more sensitive to their practice patterns.

The second theme of the book, concerned with increasing the basic knowledge base about physicians, arises from one very important assumption: that it is important to understand the physician's eye view of the health care system and of his or her role within it. Considerable detail is provided to address this theme. Included are the physician's perception of what medical practice is like, as well as the factors that provide satisfaction and those that cause dissatisfaction for practicing physicians. These issues are addressed by looking at the relationship between income, productivity, and satisfaction. Chapter 4 provides background on these important topics, identifying first what is currently known about income and productivity, and about what physicians think about the adequacy of their income. We then use the results of our research to demonstrate what we believe to be serious misunderstandings. Chapter 5 examines these same issues using gender as an important variable. As women increasingly enter the medical profession, gender-based differences become more obvious, especially in income, productivity, and satisfaction. Chapter 5 presents a new conceptual framework that is useful in researching some of these important gender-based differences. Chapter 6 narrows the notion of physician perceptions to that of physician satisfaction and provides a way to measure this.

The final theme of this book is the need not only for more research about physicians, but for research based on different concepts about physicians. The data that arise from the study in western Massachusetts lead to a different understanding of physicians than is commonly represented in the field. The last chapter presents our view of the most important gaps in knowledge about physicians and also suggests several new ways of viewing physicians in order to develop research that reflects the health care system of the 1990s and will therefore be more useful in directing the health policy changes that will extend beyond the 1990s.

References

ABT Associates. *Selected Characteristics of Massachusetts Physicians.* Prepared by ABT Associates for the Massachusetts Medical Society. Cambridge: MA, 1989.

Couch, N. P., and A. H. Fisher. *The Response of Surgeons to the Professional Climate in Massachusetts.* Manchester, MA: Massachusetts Chapter of the American College of Surgeons, 1989.

Friedson, E. *Profession of Medicine.* New York: Dodd, Mead, and Co., 1972.

Fuchs, V. "The Counter-revolution in Health Care Financing." *New England Journal of Medicine* 316 (1987): 1154–56.

Greene, H. L., R. J. Goldburg, H. Beattie, A. R. Russo, R. C. Ellison, and J. E. Dalen. "Physician Attitudes Toward Cost Containment: The Missing Piece of the Puzzle." *Archives of Internal Medicine* 149 (Sept. 1989): 1966–68.

Haddad, A. "Billing Restrictions Galling to Doctors." *Daily Hampshire Gazette,* April 27, 1988.

Hafferty, F. W. "Physician Oversupply as a Socially Constructed Reality." *Journal of Health and Social Behavior* 27 (1986): 358–69.

Harvey, L. K., and S. C. Shubat. *Physician and Public Attitudes on Health Care Issues.* Chicago, IL: American Medical Association, 1989.

Himmelstein, D. V., S. Woolhandler, and the Writing Committee of the Working Group on Program Design, Physicians for a National Health Program. "A National Health Program for the United States: A Physicians' Proposal." *New England Journal of Medicine* 320 (January 1989): 102–108.

Knox, R. "What's Ailing Doctors? Examining the National Malaise." *Boston Globe Magazine,* March 18, 1990.

Massachusetts Chapter of the American College of Obstetricians and Gynecologists. Unpublished report. Boston, MA, 1988.

Massachusetts Health Data Consortium. *Physician Supply in Massachusetts.* Special Report Series. Waltham, MA: Massachusetts Health Data Consortium, Inc., 1988.

Massachusetts Medical Society. *Summary History of Massachusetts Blue-Shield Physician Reimbursement Relationships.* February 1987.

Massachusetts Medical Society. *Practicing Medicine in Massachusetts: A Report to the State Legislature.* Waltham, MA: Massachusetts Medical Society, July 1988.

Massachusetts Orthopedic Association. Unpublished Report. Boston, MA, 1988.

Morse, G. "Should I Stay or Should I Go? The 1987 Massachusetts Medicine President-Fellow Survey." *Massachusetts Medicine* (November/December 1987): 29–35.

Reed, R. R., and D. Evans. "The Deprofessionalization of Medicine: Causes, Effects and Responses." *Journal of the American Medical Association* 258 (1987): 3279–82.

Relman, A. S. "Universal Health Insurance: Its Time Has Come." *New England Journal of Medicine* 320, no. 2 (12 January 1989): 117–18.

Sager, A. *The Sky Is Falling: The Massachusetts Medical Society Reports on the "Physician Shortage."* Boston, MA, 1988.

Scott, R. B. "The Doctor in Contemporary Literature." *Lancet* 269 (1955): 341–43. Reprinted in H. M. Vollmer and D. L. Mills, eds. *Professionalization.* Englewood Cliffs, NJ: Prentice-Hall, 1966.

Starr, P. *The Social Transformation of American Medicine,* New York: Basic Books, 1982.

Stevens, R. *American Medicine and the Public Interest*. New Haven, CT: Yale University Press, 1971.

Taylor, H., and A. Paranjpe. *The Equitable Healthcare Survey II: Physicians Attitudes Toward Cost Containment*. Louis Harris Associates for The Equitable Life Assurance Society of the United States. March 1984.

Washington Report on Medicine and Health Perspectives. Washington, DC: McGraw-Hill, 1985.

Williams, S. *Medical Malpractice Resurfacing as Issue for States*. Washington, DC: Alpha Center, 1985.

Chapter 2

Methodological Issues

Every research project has two main methodological problems: the identification of the population or sample from whom information is being gathered, and the development of an appropriate measurement tool. The first two sections of this chapter focus on these activities. The third section provides a description of the survey mechanics with an emphasis on the follow-up procedures utilized. The chapter concludes with a discussion of the response rate.

Development of the Mailing List

On the surface, physicians would not seem to represent a difficult professional group to locate and list, since there are several organizations with either global or specialty listings. However, we discovered that not only are these lists not identical, but, in fact, there is significant variation. We started this process with the three major lists that are generally standard:

1. Folio's Directory (a physician directory that is partially an advertising source)
2. American Medical Association (AMA) Masterfile mailing list, used in a previous study conducted for the Massachusetts Medical Society
3. Massachusetts Board of Registration in Medicine (BRM)

Additional sources included information from 12 specialty organizations, as well as listings from the yellow pages of area telephone books.

Folio's Directory lists 2,014 physicians supposedly practicing in the western part of Massachusetts. Physicians' names are alphabetical by county; other items include license number, date of entry into the data base and last contact, addresses (often two listed for each entry), phone numbers, and specialties for each individual. This list includes those practicing in federal facilities as well as inactive physicians. The book cross-references physicians by town, specialty, and group practice, a feature that was useful in our efforts to create one master list.

The AMA Masterfile mailing list includes 1,029 names for this region, alphabetically entered, and work addresses. It excludes psychiatrists. The version we had was obtained from a consulting company that had used it in a study for the Massachusetts Medical Society and was identified as a list of what the AMA defines as patient care physicians.

The Massachusetts Board of Registration in Medicine list is divided into active and inactive physicians, and within these designations they are further divided by county and then listed alphabetically, with 1,487 included on the active list and 69 on the inactive list for this geographic area. Information includes the physician's name, work address, and primary specialty, and the list was dated April 1988.

Because of the obvious variation in total number of physicians, we did some checking of individual names for each of the three major sources. The variation was too high to accept any one list as being more accurate than another, so we created one comprehensive master list (UMass list). The process began by using Folio's as a basis, since it was the largest and had the most complete set of information. The BRM list (both active and inactive) was checked against the Folio list and corrections were made. The AMA Masterfile list was then checked against this corrected and revised list. Ambiguous entries were checked against the 12 specialty lists and the telephone books.

In all cases, entries were checked for both names and addresses. Addresses were much more difficult to confirm and involved checking all three lists for consistent listings, including the most practice-specific address possible, rather than hospital-based addresses. Calls to specific physician offices were made to check any unclear or uncertain addresses. Out of these three lists, there were dozens of errors related to incomplete addresses, misspelled streets, incorrect zip codes, and duplicate entries due to slight misspellings in names.

Creation of the comprehensive list—the UMass list—from the three separate lists sometimes involved deleting names that were entered twice on one list and those with addresses outside the four-county study area. We also eliminated all duplications between lists, so each name appeared only once. This was a laborious process of checking by hand each of the names on each of the three lists. Each verified name was entered on a simple data sorting mailing list program, which included a number for each entry, the physician's name and title, address of practice, city, state, zip code, phone number, and designation of which of the three lists had originally included the physician's name. This composite list included any physician name included on any one list. For example, if a name were on the BRM list, but not on Folio's, we included it on the UMass list. By doing this, we clearly created a list that was larger than any of the single lists, as was our intention, representing all possible physicians practicing in western Massachusetts, or what might be termed the "potential population."

This mail list program was entered onto a SAS/FSP system, which allows sorting by last name, as well as by several other fields, a feature that enabled us to definitively compare the integrity of each of the three source lists. As questionnaires were returned, the SAS/FSP system provided a profile of the response rates and undelivered questionnaires in relationship to the various lists from which the names were drawn. This data base was also used to keep track of our follow-up efforts, described later in this chapter.

Because of the unexpected differences that were discovered among these three lists, we spent some time analyzing the variation. The results of this analysis, along with some recommendations about comparing the accuracy of the lists and overall limitations of any listing effort for physicians, are included in Appendix A.

Development of the Questionnaire

Questionnaire development is a lengthy process, best accomplished with an appropriate amount of time not only for pretesting, but also for reflecting on the comments of those who have examined the measurement instrument. This process was begun with a series of personal discussions with a variety of physicians in western Massachusetts, including some practicing physicians involved in the leadership of the Massachusetts Medical Society. These personal conversations guided the literature review, which also contributed significantly to the questionnaire design phase. Much of this literature is referred to in the beginnings of Chapters 3, 4, 5, and 6. A first draft of the potential questionnaire was given to eight physicians, all of whom were asked to serve as informants representing their peer group, as well as respondents to the questionnaire draft. In each case, the principal investigator administered the questionnaire, then discussed each item with the respondent. The questionnaire was revised after each such administration. The last of these drafts was reviewed by the consultant biostatistician.

This version was then distributed to a group of 12, all of whom are actively involved in health care research in Massachusetts and who represent several consumer, health, and medical interest groups. After extensive discussions with this group of health professionals, the questionnaire was revised and formatted.

This revised version was then pretested in a more formal manner, by asking a group of physician respondents to complete the questionnaire as a representation of their own personal feelings. Twelve physicians, all known to the principal investigator, completed this pretest. The group included specialists and primary care physicians, physicians who spend a great deal of their time involved in direct patient care services and some who spend relatively little of their time in actual patient care, and physicians who are happy with their practices as well as physicians who are not happy with their practices. These physicians are located in the New England region, and the group included three who are no longer in practice. Appropriate revisions were made at the conclusion of this final pretest.

The final questionnaire as distributed is contained in Appendix B. Information is gathered in four basic areas: demographic characteristics, personal and professional level of satisfaction with medical practice, practice patterns, and information allowing us to calculate the supply of physicians more accurately.

Demographic characteristics

Six demographic variables are identified. Two are specific to the interests of Massachusetts: county in which most of the medical practice is located, and professional society memberships. The other four are of more general interest: years of medical practice experience in Massachusetts, age, gender, and specialty, all of which assisted in the analysis of income and satisfaction.

Personal and professional level of satisfaction

The perception that Massachusetts has a large number of physicians who are unhappy with the medical practice climate of the state is based primarily on anecdotal evidence, much of which can be found in news media coverage. Two sets of items were designed to collect information systematically about the level of professional satisfaction, and responses to these were used to develop a scale to measure physician satisfaction. Several additional questions provide more detail on physicians' perceptions of the medical practice climate of the state.

Two questions also address the knowledge base physicians have about what medical practice is like in other states, and one question addresses whether a respondent is practicing at what he or she defines as full professional capacity. Although these latter items do not directly measure occupational satisfaction, they do provide an important context for interpreting physician perceptions. And, as we will see further on, whether a physician perceives himself or herself to be practicing at full professional capacity is an interesting variable.

Physician respondents are also allowed three opportunities to provide open-ended responses, indicating what they like least and most about medical practice in Massachusetts. The last page provides space to add any additional comments that are appropriate. Responses to these items are included throughout this book to add context to the numerical analysis.

Practice patterns

Several items gather information about practice patterns, including description of practice types, financial arrangements, malpractice, and hours worked in a typical week. Physicians were also asked to indicate whether these practice characteristics have changed over the past five years.

Physician supply

Accurately estimating physician supply in a particular geographic area is one of the major reasons for this study. Several data sources were used, the most obvious being some list of physicians practicing within the region. As discussed previously, however, the available lists are not accurate enough to designate the supply. Therefore, the questionnaire itself also contributes to estimating physician supply, primarily by providing information used to characterize a physician as either being in practice, and thus part of the available supply, or not practicing, and thus not part of the supply estimate. This subject is fully described in Chapter 3. Three specific items (Q-1, Q-9, and Q-18 in Appendix B) are used to provide this information.

Using information from the questionnaire to help determine physician supply produces a potential bias since complete information is produced only for those who respond to the mailed-out questionnaire. This potential bias necessitates careful attention to survey mechanics, particularly the follow-up phase, to ensure as high a response rate as possible.

Survey Mechanics and Follow-up Procedures

Each physician on the UMass list received a survey packet, including the questionnaire (formatted as a booklet), a cover letter personally signed by the principal investigator, and a postage-paid return envelope. The design of the survey packet, as well as the overall follow-up procedure, was guided by Dillman's (1978) concept of the total design method of mailed surveys.

Each questionnaire was numbered so that returned questionnaires could be so noted on the data base. All who did not return a questionnaire within two weeks were sent a reminder postcard. The initial responses along with postcard-induced responses combined to produce a 59 percent response rate.

The telephone follow-up phase began three weeks after the surveys were initially sent out; all practices that had not returned surveys were contacted over a period of three to four weeks. This telephone phase actually served two distinct purposes. The first, of course, was to encourage responses from those who had not responded. However, the second purpose was even more important. The telephone phase definitively identified those physicians included on the UMass list who were not actually in active practice in Massachusetts. It was this information that permitted the development of an accurate population estimate, and made it possible to differentiate between nonrespondents and physicians who were not part of the population.

At the conclusion of the telephone phase, we sent out one more postcard to the remaining nonrespondents, allowing one month for all questionnaires to be returned. Data collection was closed on Friday, September 15, 1989, with 70 percent of the population of practicing physicians responding.

Response Rate

The first requirement for calculating a response rate is to determine the population, which may or may not be identical to the number of questionnaires distributed. Questionnaires were mailed to all 1,811 names included on the UMass list, which was viewed as a description of the potential population. The combination of information from the questionnaire itself and calls to all nonrespondents in the follow-up phase enabled us to determine the actual population of practicing physicians available to this geographic region.

Table 2.1 shows the determination of the actual population. Each of the 1,811 questionnaires was placed into one of the five response groups shown in Table 2.1 based on specific information obtained from the physician or from some other reliable contact. Group 1 (908) are the final respondents in the study because they returned a questionnaire. Group 2 (394) are the nonrespondents: these are physicians verified to be in practice in western Massachusetts who did not return a questionnaire.

Each of these physicians' offices was contacted in the telephone follow-up phase.

A total of 509 physicians (28 percent of the potential population of 1,811) are ineligible for inclusion in the definition of the population. This total includes three groups: physicians known to have practices outside the western Massachusetts area (Group 3), physicians who were not practicing for some known reason (Group 4), and physicians who could not be located (Group 5).

Group 3 includes physicians who have left western Massachusetts and their current location is known, which required at least the designation of a state and preferably a specific address. Out of the 110 who fall into this group, specific out-of-state addresses were obtained for 80; for the remainder, a state or geographic region was indicated by their previous practice or a close family member.

Group 4 includes 183 physicians who have stopped practicing for any one of several reasons noted in Table 2.1. This group provides examples of individuals that formal lists with voluntary updating procedures have the most trouble identifying and keeping current.

The most troublesome category, of course, is Group 5. This group of 216 was subjected to vigorous follow-up efforts. Some names were expected to fall here, since some of the 1,811 on our UMass list were marginal entries, meaning that their name was present on only one of the three original lists, and could not be verified by any other list. Almost 90

Table 2.1   Definition of Population of Physicians Actually in Practice in Western Massachusetts

Group 1	Completed and returned questionnaires	908
Group 2	Physicians who received a questionnaire but never responded, or who refused to answer (all known to be practicing physicians in western Massachusetts)	394
Group 3	Physicians who have left western Massachusetts and whose current location we know	110
Group 4	Physicians who had stopped practicing for one or more of the following reasons: retired; died; closed their practice; involved in a residency program; removed from practice for 12 months due to chronic illness; loss of license, or otherwise have indicated to us that they are inactive	183
Group 5	Physicians we were unable to locate despite all aggressive measures	216

percent of Group 5 represent this type of marginal entry. The remainder we expected to find practicing in western Massachusetts but could not locate despite rigorous efforts, including calling medical practices located near their last known addresses, as well as consulting several telephone books, directory assistance, and specialty lists.

Although it is theoretically possible that, because of a series of errors, some of these might be practicing in western Massachusetts, it is very unlikely. We did ultimately manage to locate two people who were originally placed in this group whose addresses were wrong on the list. However, our best guess is that the rest of Group 5 are physicians who are not practicing in western Massachusetts.

As a result of the aggressive follow-up phase, we can clearly identify the population of physicians located in the four western counties of Massachusetts to be 1,302, including 908 who responded to our survey, giving us a 70 percent response rate. We could have attempted to characterize the 394 nonrespondents in some way, such as specialty, gender, or years of experience, in order to further analyze any possible response bias. However, our confidence in the various lists was understandably low and time pressures prevented another telephone follow-up phase to ascertain this information.

Although we do now know the number of physicians who actually have a medical practice in western Massachusetts, we do not know the extent to which they see patients. In other words, we would like now to further refine the notion of "physician known to be in practice" to something more specific, which we will term "patient care physician." In order to address this question, we need to present some results from selected items on the questionnaire. Chapter 3 provides a further description of these patient care physicians. We will also apply this concept to the larger problem of enumerating physicians in a given geographic area.

Reference

Dillman, D. A. *Mail and Telephone Surveys: The Total Design Method*. New York: John Wiley and Sons, 1978.

How Many Physicians Are Really Practicing in Western Massachusetts?

A Case Study Presenting a New Model to Estimate Physician Supply

For the past 30 years, much of the health policy in the United States has been directed by physician supply. Massachusetts health policy is no exception. As noted in the first chapter, a major objective for this particular research is an ongoing discussion about how many physicians are practicing in Massachusetts. What began as an effort to increase objectivity in an acrimonious political atmosphere in one state ends with the insight that the same problems permeate national health policy.

This chapter presents the results of the analysis of physician supply in Massachusetts, but it must begin with a discussion of some of the more important conceptual issues. Physician supply is a complicated topic, and it is also a topic about which much has been written. However, this literature does not lead to an integrated body of knowledge; rather, there is a startling lack of common conceptualization about physician supply that contributes to such diversity that a concise summary of the literature is impossible. The two beginning sections of this chapter extract some of the more important considerations of this field. We must begin with a brief history of research and policy efforts in the area of physician supply. Of necessity, attention must be devoted to the work of the Graduate Medical Education National Advisory Committee (GMENAC), although many of their results lie outside the scope of our interest. The second section is an analysis of the diversity that exists about the very concept of physician supply. The following two sections provide the results of what is essentially a case study: the data base from western Massachusetts is utilized to suggesta modification for enumerating physicians. This modification incorporates practice patterns into the actual estimates of physician supply, analogous to an adjusted or standardized rate. Important to this case study is a discussion of some of the assumptions and limitations of this approach.

The results of this case study lead to a reconsideration of the whole question of physician supply, and the following section presents some of the ongoing discussions and disputes. It is our belief that many of these still-unsettled issues could be resolved by the use of the standardized estimate of physician supply presented in this chapter.

The chapter concludes with some specific recommendations that attempt to smooth out many of the inconsistencies encountered in research on physician supply in western Massachusetts. These recommendations bring some badly needed standardization to this field of inquiry.

Appendix C contains an important addendum to this chapter. It concerns the often ignored, overarching methodological problem in physician supply: the nomenclature related to defining specialty categories. This is particularly problematic in determining primary care specialties. As demonstrated in Appendix C, the major issue is whether to include internal medicine in the category of primary care or in the category generally termed "medical specialties." Two different categorization methods are used with our western Massachusetts data base to demonstrate the effect of these two approaches.

The length of this chapter reflects the enduring debate on this issue, as well as the variety of methods employed in human resources research. Past inattention to some fundamental definitional problems has resulted in a proliferation of research without a shared conceptual structure. There is no doubt that concern about adequacy of physician supply continues to be a major driving force behind much of the research and policy in the 1990s. We hope this chapter will be a significant contribution to conceptualizing physician supply.

A Brief History

One of the earliest assessments of the number of physicians needed for the nation was made in the Flexner report (1910), when the author asserted that 31 medical schools with an annual total number of 3,500 physicians would be sufficient for "two generations." The policymakers at the time implemented only about half of Flexner's recommended controls, reflecting an intuitive feeling (even at this early date) that too many doctors are preferable to too few. This response also demonstrated something that has been repeated many times: policymakers rely on and respond to human resources research in such a way that the actual numbers of physicians are directly affected. Consequently, it is incumbent upon investigators in this field to be fully aware of the practical ramifications of their work.

In 1932, the Commission on Medical Education compared the physician/population ratios in the United States to those of several major European countries and concluded that the United States had too many physicians. It is difficult to determine whether it was the commission's report or the general economic climate that caused the AMA in 1934 to suggest decreasing the number of medical schools by 50 percent (Ginzberg 1989). During this time, utilization of medical services also decreased since people could not afford medical care, and as a result physician incomes also decreased. Between 1934 and 1940, the number of physicians produced decreased significantly—the first drop since the Flexner report in 1910 and the last drop before the 1980s. In 1940, the number of physicians per 100,000 population was 140 (Hafferty 1986). After World War II, the preoccupation with reduced numbers of physicians turned strongly to a fear of not having enough. The number of medical schools increased dramatically and the number of graduating physicians almost doubled. By 1958, the number of physicians per 100,000 population was estimated to be 148 (Hafferty 1986).

During the 1960s, concern about the number of physicians as well as geographic and specialty distribution became part of several social justice agendas, with an important philosophical conviction growing out of the civil rights movement that not only was equal education a right, but so also was equal access to health care. Discussions of a national objective related to ensuring equal access to health care created several significant programs, including Medicare and Medicaid, as well as the Neighborhood Health Centers program and the National Health Service Corps.

Despite many political barriers to these social programs, most groups shared the perception that an inadequate physician supply existed for meeting the health needs of populations with limited access to health care. Although the perception was defined as a shortage, it was also viewed as an effect of maldistribution, both of too many specialists in relation to generalists and as an unequal distribution of all physicians in low-income urban and rural areas.

A total of nine major reports were published by either private foundations or medical associations; all concluded there was a shortage of physicians (Iglehart 1986; McConnell and Tobias 1986; Tarlov 1983, 1988). This enormous activity contributed to the naming of this time period as the "era of debate and funding for health manpower" (GMENAC 1980a). Policymakers paid attention to the results of these reports and enacted many pieces of legislation aimed at increasing the supply not only of physicians, but also of all other health care professionals. Some of the more important legislation included the Health Manpower Act of 1968 (PL 90-490), which gave construction funds for medical schools to increase their enrollments; the Comprehensive Health Manpower Training Act of 1971 (PL 92-157), which gave capitation grants to increase medical school enrollments, especially in family practice departments; and the Health Professions Educational Assistance Act of 1976 (PL 94-484), which was specifically geared to increasing the number of primary care physicians (GMENAC 1980a).

The effect of the legislative activity was direct and dramatic. Medical schools increased in number from 87 in 1963 to 126 in 1980, and average enrollment also increased (Harris 1986). The number of physicians increased also, although the estimates vary depending on the years being covered. For example, Harris (1986) uses the years 1967–1980, during which he estimates that the ratio of actively practicing doctors/population rose by over 50 percent. Iglehart (1986) indicates that 152 nonfederal physicians/100,000 were practicing in 1970, and that this increased substantially to 199/100,000 by 1981. Ginzberg (1989) notes that, as a result of the many federal and state initiatives between 1960 and 1975, the number of physicians went from 140 to 180/100,000. In 1984, Ginzberg and Ostow (1984) estimated that there were 200/100,000, a figure 30 percent higher than in 1970 and 40 percent higher than in 1960. The American Medical Association (1986) estimated that a 54 percent increase occurred in numbers of physicians between 1970 and 1983, from 156 to 208/100,000, while the general population increased only by 15 percent. Other AMA reports indicated 199 physicians/100,000 (Iglehart 1986). Although no consensus existed on the exact number of physicians, all estimates pointed to a substantial increase over a 20-year time span.

By the late 1970s, the pendulum had begun to swing back, and reports and articles started to appear that mentioned a possible surplus of physicians beginning to develop. In 1976, the Graduate Medical Education National Advisory Committee (GMENAC) was charged with determining not only how many physicians were in practice, but also how many would be required so that the nation could move to balancing what exists (supply) and what would be required or needed. GMENAC's conclusions were completed in 1980 and have become perhaps the most widely quoted and argued reports ever produced (GMENAC 1980a–d).

The theoretical basis of GMENAC actually comes from a very early effort by Lee and Jones (1933) to try to determine need for medical services. In 1933, Lee and Jones devised criteria for need for medical services based on expert opinions concerning amount of care required for what was at the time an exhaustive list of diseases. And, in fact, a major activity of GMENAC was defining norms for physician services based on expert opinions, which were then adjusted by a committee to take account of "economic, social, behavioral constraints" (GMENAC 1980b, 18). The overall methodology of GMENAC is therefore considered to be an "adjusted needs–based" one. An example of the factors taken into account by the adjusting or modeling committee illustrates some of the complications. The panel of experts indicated that gallbladder surgery should take three hours: the modeling technical group modified it to two hours. The modeling panel agreed with their experts about otitis media (that all cases should be seen by a doctor), but disagreed with the same experts about a variety of eye problems (including refractive errors) and decided that a high percentage of these problems could be dealt with by an optometrist rather than an ophthalmologist (Harris 1986).

In order to move from estimating current supply to predicting future supply based on projected requirements, GMENAC developed and used three separate models. The first was a supply model that was used to project the future supply of a variety of specialists. Policymakers could choose from several sets of assumptions that they felt were most likely, and the supply model would reveal what the physician supply would be if those assumptions were true. Some of the assumptions involved trends in medical school enrollment, physician specialty choice, productivity, immigration, retirement, and mortality rates. The second model (requirements) made adjustments for physician demand by projecting future requirements for physicians based on trends in disease incidence, consumer income, health insurance coverage, physician fees, and population demographics. This epidemiologic approach also had a variety of assumptions identified. The third model—far beyond our scope of interest here—was the graduate medical education model, which identified systematically for the first time all the different pathways to various specialty designations.

GMENAC was obviously a massive effort: the reports contained a total of 107 recommendations with over 800 pages of analysis and supportive material. Over 300 consultant experts assisted in the work, and a full-time staff of over 20 people was employed. Five technical panels addressed nonphysician health care providers, geographic distribution, educational environment, and financing medical education as well as the more well-known work on modeling physician supply requirements (GMENAC 1980a–d). Its total budget was somewhere between $4 million and $5 million.

The GMENAC reports are now over ten years old and the overall effect of this work on the field of human resources planning should not be underestimated. GMENAC has created its own literature, and many of these published articles were written simply to describe GMENAC and outline their recommendations (for example, McNutt 1981 and Bowman

1985). Criticisms of GMENAC are legion, many of them based on philo-sophical disagreements. And, of course, the first projections made in 1980 can now be compared with the real world of 1990. However, this does not mean that GMENAC has provided the final word on physician supply. In fact, as we will soon see, one of the major contributions of GMENAC has been almost completely overlooked.

One contribution of GMENAC about which there is consensus is the framing of the discussion around the concept of physician surplus rather than shortage, although there is not total agreement on whether such a surplus is a positive or a negative thing. Between 1979 and 1983, four separate academic—as opposed to all the previous professional—studies suggested that an oversupply of physicians was either present or impending (Aiken et al. 1979; Schwartz et al. 1980; Newhouse et al. 1982; Williams et al. 1983). Not all investigators viewed this over-supply negatively: for example, Newhouse et al. (1982) argued that the oversupply of physicians would be beneficial because it would cause physicians to move to rural areas in response to increased competition among physicians in crowded urban areas. This "diffusion theory," based on a market model of physician supply, has generated many articles, some of which use physician supply data to support the diffusion theory while others use exactly the same data to disprove the diffusion theory.

In general, there seems to be a gradual acceptance of the idea of a physician surplus. A national study sponsored by the American College of Hospital Administrators in 1983–1984 discovered that 63 percent of the physicians surveyed believed there was—or shortly would be—a physician surplus in urban areas; 71 percent believed this to be true in suburban areas, and 42 percent in rural areas. A vast majority of these respondents (81 percent) also predicted a decline in quality of health care due to an increasing competition between physicians (Anderson 1984). The AMA also reported on this phenomenon: 33 percent of physicians surveyed in 1981 thought there were too many physicians currently practicing in their communities. By 1982, this had risen to 41 percent and by 1984 it was 43 percent (Freshnock 1984).

It is outside the scope of our interest to enter this debate, but it is important to acknowledge the complexity involved in any potential resolution. GMENAC is invariably given the credit for causing this con-ceptual shift to considerations of a physician surplus. Hafferty (1986) challenges this conclusion by observing that GMENAC was established just as the first graduates emerged from a medical education pipeline expanded to correct a perceived physician shortage in the 1960s and early 1970s. Because of the long delay between entrance to medical school and active practice (especially considering the increasing trend toward specialization), these graduates would have had only a very small effect on actual physician supply by 1976, when GMENAC was first established. Additionally, the so-called GMENAC era was also a time during which significant changes, many of them economic, took place in the social environment of medical practice. The national health policy turned from expansion to a preoccupation with costs and cost-containment programs; physicians began to be viewed as important gate-keepers of resources to be allocated, rather than as sources of services to be provided. A link began to be established between physician supply and health expenditures.

At the same time, a fundamental change occurred in medical practice; during the 1970s patient visits dropped, and physician incomes began to lag behind inflation. By 1979, a majority of office-based practitioners did not believe they were operating at full capacity (Owens 1979). The reason seemed to be the perception that there were now too many physicians, which was causing physician incomes to decline. Peers, previously regarded as colleagues, increasingly came to be viewed as competitors.

Hafferty's basic premise is that this perception of a surplus has arisen primarily because of the identification of the physician as part of the link in health care expenditures, and secondarily because of the shift in medical practice patterns from a general orientation to a more specialized practice pattern—a shift that has caused a decrease in patient visits and a leveling off of physician incomes. Physicians are more likely than patients to believe that there are too many physicians. For example, in 1984, only 12 percent of the general public believed there was a physician surplus, but almost 60 percent of physicians believed there were too many physicians (Ginzberg 1982). The physician perception sometimes conflicts with reality; in Minnesota, 55 percent of physicians in one metropolitan area thought there were too many physicians when, in reality, this particular county had the second-lowest physician/population ratio in the whole state (Hafferty 1986).

Hafferty concludes by reminding researchers of the importance of the social construct, noting that shared perception becomes reality. The reality of a physician surplus is not located in physician/population ratios or in any other statistic but in social action or behavior, especially by physicians who implement changes in their practice patterns based on a belief of a surplus.

For us, the arguments and counterarguments summarized in this section indicate that there is, in fact, a lack of shared social construct right now in terms of physician supply. This lack is not so much in terms of the argument about numbers of physicians, but rather in how physician supply is conceptualized. In reading the five technical reports of GMENAC, we find that three conclusions are important for our work, and two of these contribute to this conceptualization issue. The first conclusion of GMENAC has been consistently the most visible recommendation, and it focuses on the numbers argument. GMENAC predicted that the physician/population ratio in the year 2000 will be 247/100,000 unless some controls are instituted. GMENAC went further by indicating this to be too many physicians; their recommendation of a more appropriate ratio was 191 physicians for a 100,000 population base.

Two other conclusions are repeatedly stated in every one of the technical reports. These two have been almost totally ignored, but they are among the most important of the observations arising from GMENAC. Both are phrased as problems that limit not only GMENAC's work, but also the work of others in this area. The first problem is theoretical: there is no agreement about the definition of a physician who is to be counted as part of the U.S. supply and thus included in the numerator of the physician/population ratios. The second problem is related to this theoretical concern but is more practical and concerns the actual recording in the data bases of physicians being counted. Each of the five technical panels noted both the theoretical problem and the resulting inaccuracies that significantly limited their work. These two problems make it hard to accept either GMENAC's projection of 247/100,000 in 2000 or their suggestion that 191/100,000 is the "ideal" ratio of physicians/population.

This lack of a standardized nomenclature symbolizes a lack of a shared social reality. We do not have agreement on exactly what defines physician supply. Despite this lack of understanding, even more sophisticated numerical models continue to be developed based on GMENAC's work (Weiner 1989). In our view, one of the strongest suggestions made by the GMENAC project has been largely overlooked: a basic understanding and shared definition of the very concept of physician supply needs to be developed before the process of constructing more complicated and quantitatively sophisticated models of health human resources needs is continued. It is within this area that our work in estimating physician supply is located.

What Is Physician Supply?

Several definitions of physician supply have been formulated by health planners and subsequently buried in the archives of now-closed regional planning offices. For example, one particularly well-accepted report, prepared for the federal government in 1976, gives a careful discussion of supply, both from a conceptual view and from a methodological perspective (Kriesberg et al. 1976). Supply was described as being one of several estimates: it may be the number of persons in a specific area qualified to practice an occupation, whether actively practicing or not; the number actually practicing the occupation at any given time; or the number of entrants, including newly qualified practitioners entering the market as well as previously qualified practitioners reentering the market after a period of nonavailability. These estimates imply that there is a distinction between active supply (those currently employed and those actively seeking work) and potential supply (those active workers plus any inactive workers who might be brought back into the labor force if either working conditions or personal circumstances were different). Ginzberg (1982) terms this concept of active supply an "effective" supply, that is, the number of physicians who are actually available to serve consumers.

The American Medical Association is one of the major sources of estimates of physician supply; over the course of the last 30 years, the definition of who should be included in the AMA data bases has ranged from all-inclusive efforts that count all licensed physicians to the more precise recent differentiations, which include categories of federal and nonfederal; active and inactive; and the important designation of patient care physician, defined as a physician involved with patients at least 20 hours per week (Blumberg 1971; Roback, Mead, and Pasko 1984).

When reading the literature on physician supply carefully to determine who is being counted, one is struck by the tremendous variation in definition. It is common to use data from the AMA Physician Masterfile (Roback, Mead, and Pasko 1984), and to limit the count to the category of nonfederal physicians since they make up 94 percent of the nation's physicians (Fruen and Cantwell 1982). Not infrequently, this definition is modified, as when Kindig and Movassaghi (1989) used both federal and nonfederal physicians from the AMA Masterfile and also used osteopaths from their association's masterfile, but eliminated interns and residents.

An increasingly common approach today is to enumerate only board-certified physicians since an overwhelming percentage of graduates now obtain board certification (Schwartz et al. 1980; Moore and Priebe 1991). The study by Moore and Priebe (1991) is an example of this approach. They used data from five national agencies, including the Association of American Medical Colleges, Educational Council for Foreign Medical Graduates, American Board of Medical Specialties, National Resident Matching Program, the Division of Survey and Data Resources of AMA, as well as the AMA Physician Masterfile. Their enumeration involved several specific corrections, including holding certificates in two separate subspecialties—very valuable for demonstrating trends in specialization as well as for measuring the output of the medical education system. For example, they were able to show how many women are being trained in various specialties and subspecialties. Unfortunately, they also make conclusions about the total physician work force based on the board-certified enumeration, suggesting that the work force did not increase as rapidly in the 1980s as in the 1970s. Board-certified physicians are clearly only a part of the physician work force and national supply estimates should not be based on this subset.

An additional variation in the literature on enumerating physicians is how to count physicians involved in the medical education process, including academic physicians as well as interns and residents. In some studies, residents are explicitly excluded, in others they are included but counted separately, and in still others they are counted as less than one physician (McConnell and Tobias 1986; GMENAC 1980c; Kindig and Movassaghi 1989; Garg et al. 1991). In fact, GMENAC (1980c) estimates themselves counted residents as only 0.35 FTE. The effort to include estimates of those involved in residency programs is a reminder of the uncomfortable lack of a standardized definition of the concept of physician supply. Much of the variation centers on the practice patterns of physicians. There seems to be an implicit understanding that knowledge about practice patterns of physicians should be taken into account in defining physician supply, but there is little explicit effort to do so.

Practice patterns of physicians do seem to have changed over time. One of the first studies of practice patterns found that only 9 percent of physicians in 1966 were doing something other than patient care (Blumberg 1971). In 1986, the AMA Masterfile data base showed that the actual number of physicians providing patient care had increased by 63 percent since 1966, but the number of physicians who indicate a preponderance of professional activities other than patient care has increased 139 percent and the number of doctors who designate research as their primary activity has increased 330 percent (Ginzberg 1986).

One impetus for analyzing practice patterns of physicians more carefully was GMENAC. In refuting GMENAC's conclusions, Schwartz, Sloan, and Mendelson (1988) removed from their numerator 16 percent of all possible physicians, based on their calculations of decreased productivity of female physicians and on the elimination from the estimates of those physicians who primarily are involved in administration, medical teaching, or research. Various investigators have all argued that the estimates from GMENAC are erroneous because there are an increasing number of physicians involved in HMOs and they have different practice patterns, most of which involve using supervised nonphysician providers to decrease physician supply estimates (Weiner et al. 1987; Tarlov 1986; Steinwachs et al. 1986).

These studies have something important in common: they are all based on an assumption that the appropriate definition of a "physician" for the purposes of coming up with an estimate of physician supply should be based somehow on the actual practice patterns of the physicians, or a concept of effective supply. GMENAC did attempt to link practice patterns with the enumeration of physicians. They focused on the decreased productivity of female physicians—estimated to be 78 percent of males—and they counted interns and residents as 0.35 FTE of a regular full-time physician (GMENAC 1980c). Both of these are found in the requirements models, but they are not part of the supply models.

We wondered what would happen if practice patterns of physicians were incorporated into the actual estimates of physician supply, by weighting the numeric estimate depending on the average time spent in direct care each week for the physicians being counted—not unlike common practice in the health field when a rate or ratio is adjusted or standardized, as for example, an age-adjusted death rate. This adjustment, of course, requires exact knowledge of the population itself, as well as information about practice patterns of physicians that can be used to modify the estimates of supply. The technique is not new, but actually using it to modify the estimates of physician supply is.

Of course, this technique does require a slightly different methodology for enumerating physicians, one based on primary survey data collected directly from physicians. Surveys of physicians to gather information about practice patterns have been done, but the link between practice patterns and physician supply has never been established. Some of the earliest surveys directly observed physician-patient encounters to gain information about quality of care (Peterson 1956; Clute 1963), while others recruited physicians to report directly on care (Marsland, Wood, and Mayo 1976). These studies tended to be small, mainly limited to certain geographic areas and involving a small sample of physicians. These reports were used as the basis for the later studies of the 1970s and early 1980s on physician productivity (Aiken et al. 1979; Marsland, Wood, and Mayo 1976; Noren et al. 1980). More recent studies of medical practice are based on larger samples of physicians, usually drawn from national registrars to whom physicians self-report about their practice patterns. Greenwald and Hart (1986) summarized some differences in studies on medical practice based on data gathered by the National Center for Health Statistics National Ambulatory Care Survey (NACS), University of Southern California (USC) Medical Activities and Manpower Projects Physician Surveys, and Medical Economics Continuing Survey (MEDECON). They noted that although there were clear and important differences in both wording and response rates, these primary surveys contributed important and valuable information not available from other sources.

The AMA has an extensive network of primary survey information as well as secondary data base information collected on a variety of samples of physicians. The oldest and best known secondary data base is the Physician Masterfile, established in 1906; it is contributed to by numerous organizations, including medical schools, hospitals, medical societies, national boards, and state licensing agencies. Each physician is entered into the data base upon entry into medical school. The historical part of the data base includes birth date; medical school information including year of graduation, internship, and residency training; state licensure data; and any relevant board certification information. Other information includes geographic location of practice, type of practice, degree of patient care responsibilities, specialties, and employment (AMA Center for Health Policy Research 1986; Roback, Mead, and Pasko 1984). Physicians are responsible for updating their entries on the list; some of the problems related to that are discussed in Chapter 2 and Appendix A.

In addition to this extensive secondary data base, information is also collected directly from physicians through two separate surveys conducted by the AMA. Every four years, a sample of physicians receive mailed questionnaires that ask for information on professional activities, including the proportion of time in direct patient care activities (Roback, Mead, and Pasko 1984). Since 1981, the AMA has also conducted periodic surveys of samples of physicians under the Socioeconomic Monitoring System (SMS), which focuses on several characteristics of medical practice, including physician earnings, productivity estimates, practice expenses, fees, and various health policy issues. The sample is limited to nonfederal physicians and also to patient care physicians or those "who spend the greatest proportion of their time in patient care activities" (Noren et al. 1980; Greenwald and Hart 1986; Reynolds and Ohsfeldt 1984; Gonzalez and Emmons 1989). In order to be counted as a patient care physician, a physician must spend at least 20 hours a week in direct patient care activities. Also excluded are residents and all those who cannot be located by mail or telephone after exhaustive tracking efforts are made or who have no current address available. Other exclusions include doctors of osteopathy, and foreign medical graduates who are only temporarily licensed to practice in the United States (Reynolds and Ohsfeldt 1984).

Although both of these primary surveys collect valuable information about physicians and medical practice patterns in the United States, these data are not integrated into the Masterfile, which is the primary source for estimating available physician supply. We propose that even more precise definitions of practice patterns, with a particular emphasis on productivity, can be made available through a primary survey of physicians, and that this information can then be used to modify the numeric estimates of physician supply.

Using Practice Patterns to Modify Estimates of Physician Supply: A Case Study

Three initial steps were required to classify a physician as being primarily involved in patient care; this information was then applied to the estimate of physician supply. The first step created an eligible pool of physicians thought to be practicing in western Massachusetts. This was achieved by the compilation of the UMass list, as described in Chapter 2. As noted, we viewed this as the potential supply of physicians.

The second step verified that these physicians had some type of medical practice in western Massachusetts. This was achieved by enumerating those who responded to the questionnaire and considering them with nonrespondents, all of whom were contacted by phone to ensure they actually had a practice of some sort in western Massachusetts. These two groups total 1,302 physicians, 908 of whom responded to the survey, as shown in Table 2.1. This verification procedure is necessary for accuracy and is also a necessary step in order to identify the whole population. The third step designated what we have termed a "patient care physician," or one who spends at least 10 percent of his or her time involved in direct patient care activities. From responses on the questionnaire, we know that about 88 percent identify themselves within our "patient care physician" category.

Table 3.1 presents several estimates of physician supply for western Massachusetts. The first two estimates are the "official" ones; the first is from the AMA Masterfile and the second from the Massachusetts Board of Registration. Estimate 3 comes from counting returned questionnaires and then verifying whether nonrespondents have any kind of medical practice in western Massachusetts. This estimate is much more accurate since we at least know that this group of physicians (1,302) actually has some kind of medical practice in western Massachusetts, rather than depending on the accuracy of either the AMA or state Board of Registration list. This table will also be used to develop several other estimates of the physician supply available in western Massachusetts.

After the accomplishment of these three initial steps, further refinements of the supply estimate are made based on analysis of practice patterns from the information gathered by the questionnaire. These adjustments are made assuming that the major resource of interest is that of availability of physician time for actual patient care, or the effective supply. The first refinement, of course, is to identify those respondents who have characterized themselves as meeting our definition of patient care physician; this is 88 percent, and assuming that the nonrespondents are no different from the respondents, then 88 percent of the 1,302 physicians originally defined as being involved in some kind of medical practice in

Table 3.1   Comparison of Estimates of Physician Supply for Western
Massachusetts

	Total Number of Physicians	*Physicians per 100,000 Population*
1. Patient care, nonfederal physician supply (Roback, Mead, and Pasko 1984)	1,481	185
2. Massachusetts Board of Registration	1,464	183
3. University of Massachusetts total estimate	1,302	163
4. Physicians who see patients at least 10 percent of the time (patient care physicians)	1,145	143
5. Direct care–equivalent physicians (contact hours based on individual ratio analysis)	961	120
6. Full-time-equivalent physicians (based on 40 hours per week)	1,259	157
7. Full-time-equivalent physicians (based on 58 hours per week)	1,145	143

western Massachusetts are actually in active practice. Thus, there are actually 1,145 patient care physicians available for consumers in western Massachusetts, for a physician/population ratio of 143/100,000, which is substantially lower than other estimates.

To continue this line of thought one step further requires additional information on practice patterns. Exhibit 3.1 shows the relevant question from our survey that was originally included on the AMA Socioeconomic Characteristics Survey. Using the data from this question we can continue to refine the notion of enumerating physicians based on additional information on how they spend their time each week.

Table 3.2 shows the results from the 784 respondents who are our patient care physicians. For this table we have collapsed the nine categories of professional activities into two: direct care activities and other professional activities. For general/family practice and medical specialties, direct care activities include office visits, any contact with patients in other settings (including hospitals, nursing homes, etc.), and other contacts with patients (including telephone conversations). For surgeons this direct care category includes surgery, and for obstetricians it also

Exhibit 3.1 Item from Questionnaire Used to Gather Information about Practice Patterns

One of the most important parts of this study is our effort to determine how many practicing physicians are generally available to consumers in western Massachusetts. To do this, we need an approximate distribution of your time. We are using the same categories as the AMA Socioeconomic Characteristics of Medical Practice Survey.

Please answer all of the following based on a typical week of practice during the last 12 months. Give us your best estimate to the nearest hour.

Q-18 During a typical week of practice within the last 12 months, about how many hours a week do you spend with:

a. Office-based patients including all offices if your practice involves multiple sites .... About ____hrs.

b. Surgery patients—time in surgery, labor or delivery .... About ____hrs.

c. Hospitalized patients, including all hospital rounds .... About ____hrs.

d. Hospital emergency room patients .... About ____hrs.

e. Hospital outpatient clinics .... About ____hrs.

f. Patients in nursing or convalescent homes, or some other extended care facility .... About ____hrs.

g. Telephone conversations with patients or their families, consulting with other physicians, providing other services to patients such as interpreting lab tests and x-rays. (Please do not include any other time reported in other activities) .... About ____hrs.

h. All other activities related to your professional responsibilities, including administrative, teaching, supervising medical residents, medical staff functions, and professional reading, writing, and research .... About ____hrs.

i. Any other professional activities we have left out ... About ____hrs.

j. Total number of hours you work in activities related to medicine per week... About ____hrs.

involves labor and delivery. This category captures all direct patient contact as well as other more removed but still patient-oriented activities such as telephone conversations with patients and their families, as well as providing supportive medical services to patients such as interpreting laboratory tests and x-rays. All other aspects of a physician's

Table 3.2   Hours Worked per Week for Western Massachusetts Patient Care Physicians, by Specialty Groupings

Specialty Grouping	N	Distribution in Sample (%)	Hours per Week in Direct Care Activities (mean)	Hours per Week in Other Professional Activities (mean)	Total Hours per Week (mean)	Proportion of Time Spent in Direct Patient Care Activities (%)
1. General/family practice	83	10.6	48	11	59	81.3
2. Medical specialties	242	30.9	50	8	58	86.2
3. Surgical specialties	219	27.9	52	10	62	83.8
4. Other specialties	240	30.6	42	14	56	75.0
Total	784	100.0	48	11	58	81.3

time, including administrative activities, teaching, and professional reading, writing, and research, are captured together as "other professional activities." Table 3.2 gives the results for the respondents by four general specialty groupings, following a similar system used by the AMA, which places internal medicine into the medical specialty category. (See Appendix C for a discussion on an alternative categorization, using the somewhat more functional categorization of internal medicine as one of the primary care specialties.) The category "other specialties" on Table 3.2 includes anesthesiology, psychiatry, pathology, and radiology, among others.

As Table 3.2 demonstrates, physicians in western Massachusetts work an average of 58 hours per week and spend an average of 49 hours per week in direct patient care activities. These figures are similar to the national averages reported in the AMA's 1988 Socioeconomic Monitoring Study: 58 total hours a week with about 48 hours a week spent in direct patient care activities. The respondents in the AMA study spent about 84 percent of their time in activities that could be categorized as involving direct patient care, which was about the same proportion of time that western Massachusetts physicians spent in direct patient care activities. There is some variation among the four specialty groupings, but the similarity of these practice patterns between the western Massachusetts study area and the national profile, based on AMA data, suggests that our target area was not significantly different from the nation as a whole.

Now the final step is incorporating this information about practice patterns into estimates of physician supply. The final three estimates shown on Table 3.1 are the result of this application. These are simple methods for standardizing or adjusting numbers to represent the physician work force more accurately. As we noted previously, such adjustment is actually a very common activity; as a matter of fact, it is rare to use an unadjusted rate or ratio in the health field. An age-adjusted death rate is perhaps the most widespread example of controlling for the effect of an obviously important confounding variable. Private industry also frequently adjusts or standardizes work force estimates to provide greater comparability. There are two primary ways to provide an adjustment to a work force estimate. The first is to make an adjustment based on some type of functional activities, commonly termed "contact hours." Estimate 5 is the result, and we are suggesting the term "direct care equivalent (DCE) physician" to represent this. The DCE physician estimate is calculated by applying the proportion of time spent in direct patient care activities (84 percent) to the number of patient care physicians. This results in a physician/population ratio of 120 DCE physicians for 100,000 people.

Estimate 6 is the result of the second common approach to standardization: the use of a full-time-equivalent method based on hours worked per week. For this, 40 hours per week is used to define one full-time equivalent (FTE) employee: someone who works 60 hours a week would be considered to be a 1.5 FTE employee while someone who works 30 hours a week would be considered a 0.75 FTE. Estimate 6 (Table 3.1) is derived by dividing the average number of hours worked per week for each of the patient care physicians by 40 and adding the resulting individual ratios for one summary figure. This results in 1,259 full-time equivalent physicians or 157 FTE physicians per 100,000 population. This is a higher number than the others in Table 3.1 because physicians work more than 40 hours per week. Through the survey, we discovered that the western Massachusetts physicians work the national average for physicians, 58 hours per week. The last estimate on Table 3.1 shows that when using 58 hours per week as full time, there are 143 FTE physicians per 100,000 population. This is the same as Estimate 4 derived from our definition of patient care physicians because this sample works the average number of hours used as a basis for the definition of a full-time equivalent, that is, 58 hours/week.

Which number to use?

Table 3.1 presents six possible numbers representing physician supply for this geographic area. The resulting physician/population ratios vary from 120/100,000 to 185/100,000, a variation that is too large for us to accept all these estimates as being equal.

The first two estimates are "official" approaches, based on the best that the current lists can provide. Estimate 3 provides a verification of office address in the study area in question: this estimate includes both re-spondents and nonrespondents to the study. As such, this is a substantial improvement in accuracy since each of these 1,302 physicians is known to be currently involved in a medical practice within the target area. In a sense, this estimate provides a correction of the currently available lists, an obviously significant improvement. However, this number does not provide enough information about the extent of patient care involvement of this group of physicians. Estimate 4 is a still more accurate count of physicians who are verified to be in the geographic area and who also fit our liberal criterion of patient care physician (one who spends at least 10 percent of his or her time in patient care activities). This method produces an estimate of physician supply that is 22 percent less than the official estimates.

The last three estimates take this line of reasoning a step further by using the concept of standardizing or adjusting a ratio in order to have a comparable estimate over many different settings. Estimate 5 depends on a functional activities analysis or a contact hours approach, while

Estimates 6 and 7 use a full-time equivalent approach based on hours worked per week. Of these two approaches, the functional activities analysis (contact hours) is the most viable. First of all, utilizing the FTE approach immediately raises the very difficult question of assessing the number of hours that physicians work per week. Using the standard 40-hour workweek is clearly not appropriate since, as demonstrated in Table 3.2, physicians obviously work more than 40 hours per week. Using the average hours per week (58) as the denominator shows no improvement over the simple verification efforts demonstrated in Estimate 4.

The functional activities analysis is an explicit recognition of exactly what is being counted: the physician supply actually available to patients, or Ginzberg's "effective" supply. To distinguish this from other estimates of physician supply, we suggest the term "direct care equivalent (DCE) physician estimate."

Before expanding this discussion to include the implications of using the DCE physician estimate, we would like to make clear some of the assumptions upon which this work is based, and to address their implications.

Assumptions, Definitions, and Limitations

First, we define a patient care physician as one who spends 10 percent of his or her professional time seeing patients. This is obviously a minimum time and is, in fact, more liberal than the definition of patient care physician used by the American Medical Association, which sets an expectation of 20 hours per week (Reynolds and Ohsfeldt 1984). Based on an average workweek for most physicians (60 hours), 20 hours is about 33 percent. We set this more liberal estimate intentionally so that we would capture the largest possible number of physicians, and 88 percent of the total respondents in fact fit into this initial designation. Of course, consequent inclusion in the DCE physician estimate depends on the physician's direct patient care activities. The AMA itself has acknowledged the importance of actual physician availability to consumers by distinguishing between total physician supply, nonfederal physicians, and patient care physicians. Additionally, as we have shown, many researchers today argue that practice patterns of physicians must be more seriously considered in estimating physician supply. Although direct patient care activities are not independent of a physician's other activities (such as reading, teaching, and research), they can be counted separately. The assumption here is not necessarily that direct patient care time is inherently more valuable, but that specificity is important. Since direct patient care time is a valuable resource, it is only logical that the ability to measure it be developed, and using the direct care equivalent measure would allow us to do so.

We are suggesting that a refinement or adjustment based on functional activities (direct care equivalent physician) be used rather than one based on hours worked per week (full-time equivalent). Using an adjustment based on functional activities avoids the very problematic area of deciding the number of hours a week physicians work. (Among our respondents, only 10 percent worked fewer than 40 hours a week, and 62 percent worked between 40 and 67 hours a week.) A problem that is not so easy to deal with is the type of professional activity left out. As many respondents observed, at least one major activity was not included: hours "on call." This category of hours is especially difficult to evaluate, since not all on-call hours are spent in direct patient care, but neither are they truly "off" hours.

The survey item from which our data are derived is not perfect: the question directs physicians to indicate activities during a "typical" week of practice, a fuzzy concept at best. There is a fair amount of variation in actual hours reported for each of the nine categories shown in Exhibit 3.1, although not as much variation in the overall proportion of time spent in direct patient care activities or in total hours worked. This question obviously depends on recall and requires detailed information that respondents generally do not like to give. However, the estimates that arise using this approach are better than any other option, including the assumption that physicians spend all their time seeing patients, which is clearly not true.

A second limitation in defining the total population is our specific exclusion of those involved in medical education. They were excluded because in western Massachusetts they do not make up a source of physician supply large enough to justify the time and effort it would take to fit them proportionately (intern, resident, fellow, or academic physician) into the equivalent time of a direct care physician. This delineation can and should be made, however, so that the total physician supply of a particular geographical area is captured. In order for the direct care equivalent physician concept to be maximally useful, activities of medical interns, residents, and fellows, as well as their clinical faculty must be appropriately allocated. This will be difficult, since education, research, and patient care are so obviously interwoven at academic medical centers and teaching hospitals. However difficult, the issue of academic medicine has been mentioned in the literature. For example, GMENAC (1980b) suggests that an intern or resident should be counted as 0.35 FTE. The issue of those physicians who are involved in teaching medical students has also been explored (Garg et al. 1991; Gavett and Mushlin 1986), particularly in light of the problem of decreased revenues from academic physicians, which in Garg's study was 30–40 percent. Garg et al. concluded that academic physicians should be counted as 0.70 FTE.

What about the lists?

This methodology clearly depends on collecting primary data directly from physicians, a time-consuming and expensive task, but not an impossible one. The high response rate to our survey demonstrates that physicians will respond to carefully defined and administered surveys specifically of interest to them.

The DCE physician estimate produces a number that is about 35 percent less than the official estimates for our western Massachusetts counties. This difference should not necessarily be viewed as a statement about the validity of the lists, but rather as a consequence of utilizing a more careful and limited definition of who should be counted in estimating physician supply.

It is well recognized that the official lists available to researchers, regardless of whether they come from the AMA or a state board of registration, are subject to errors. Appendix A identifies the various errors in the different categories of physicians and also discusses two distinct sources of error for any type of list. One source of error (Type I) leads to an underestimate of the population by not including all those who should be included—almost always the result of the passage of time and the problem of keeping the list current. The second possible error involves those who are on the list but should not be, which results in an overestimate. This overestimate often occurs because of definitions; for example, physicians generally hold licenses in several states. If so, they are counted as part of each state's supply, even though they may practice in only one of those states. Analysis of our three source lists showed, not surprisingly, that each of the three lists has both types of error. In general each of the lists produced an overestimate of what we later discovered to be the true population. Whether this is appropriate depends on the nature of the research and the definition of supply that is being used. In this research project, we wished to determine the actual availability of physicians to serve consumers' health needs in this four-county area.

We are not the first ones to document such discrepancies in lists: Pearse (1988) did a study of one specialty (obstetrics/gynecology) and found a discrepancy of 17 percent between the specialty list maintained by the AMA and the list maintained by the American College of Obstetricians and Gynecologists (ACOG). Unfortunately, in that study no way was available to determine which of the lists was more accurate, while this part of our research had that as a major objective.

A final caveat should be noted here: this study does not address the *adequacy* of physician supply in western Massachusetts. This issue is important enough to merit some explanation, along with a more general discussion of why it is important to be careful about both the conceptual understanding of physician supply and the practical way in which physicians are actually counted.

Supply: Why Does It Matter?

The numeric estimate that is used to represent the number of physicians available is important—first in an inherent sense, since summary numbers should be valid in and of themselves. Second, the number used to represent physician supply has an additional importance, since it is used to represent the numerator in the ubiquitous physician/population ratios, which in turn are clearly linked to significant changes in health policy, legislation, and even social expectations (as the beginning of this chapter pointed out). In this case, therefore, much can be lost when inaccurate estimates are allowed to influence health policy. Physician/population ratios are widely used because they are the primary empirical tool used by both academic researchers and policymakers. These summary numbers are so frequently used that the many assumptions upon which they are based are usually ignored, as well as the several limitations that are produced by the reliance on these assumptions.

The denominator represents the population, which implies that need for medical services is distributed evenly over the population irrespective of demographic variables or other variables representing medical need. Obviously, this number is quite dependent on accurate estimates of the population. The denominator is occasionally adjusted, particularly when dealing with specialty-specific data. For example, physician/population ratios for pediatricians are commonly age adjusted, and for gynecologists/obstetricians, the population estimate is frequently adjusted by both age and gender. Adjustments in the denominator could also include socioeconomic factors, including income, education, and insurance coverage. One could adjust the population based on need, using incidence and prevalence estimates, as the GMENAC panel did in trying to determine how many physicians are needed.

It is more common to adjust the numerator, although the action is not frequently recognized as an adjustment. When the AMA differentiates between federal and nonfederal physicians (as well as patient care physicians), this is an adjustment of the numerator. Some of these adjustments are actually based on information about practice patterns, including specialty and case mix, as well as physician productivity, including the utilization of nonphysician providers. Studies frequently depend on the AMA data base, but investigators usually do not make clear what is being used: only a very close reading can determine whether both federal and nonfederal physicians are being included, or how those involved in medical education are accounted for. For example, Newhouse et al. (1982) adjusted the numerator based on physicians holding multiple specialties; if two specialties were noted they attributed 0.6 FTE to the first and 0.4 FTE to the second. They also modified the numerator by counting physicians involved in medical teaching as 0.5 FTE and excluding all physicians whose major professional activities lie in administration or research. Adjustment of the numerator creates differences in the estimates of numbers of physicians, and as Table 3.1 demonstrates, these differences in estimates of supply create large variations in physician/population ratios.

Actually, physician/population ratios are based on an assumption which in and of itself is not precisely accurate: they are treated as though they are based on a market model, in which it is assumed that all physicians in the numerator provide medical services fairly equally and that those services are provided only to those people represented in the denominator. Also, the population represented in the denominator is assumed not to go outside the defined geographic area for medical care. Yet, the three states with the largest physician/population ratios—New York, Massachusetts, and California—all have patients that extend far beyond the boundaries of the state, primarily due to the presence of large academic medical settings.

This market model assumption is a conceptual limitation, and the nonstandardized manner in which the numerator is adjusted is a numeric limitation. Despite these two important limitations, physician/population ratios are commonly used, primarily because of their ease of understanding. The ratios are now being used in increasingly smaller comparison areas—not just states, but to describe and compare counties, a Health Systems Agency service area, a hospital service area, or even a specific zip code area (GMENAC 1980c). Such utilization in small areas increases the significance of both types of limitations.

One of the primary ways in which physician/population ratios are used is to address issues related to maldistribution of physicians, with the underlying assumption being that the numerator represents physician services that are actually available, and a secondary assumption implying that physician/population ratios across the country ought to be even. However, as perhaps an example of a catch-22, since physician/population ratios are not good measures of physician services, but rather of potential physicians, it is hard to know how to interpret variation among areas in physician/population ratios. Also, Hemenway (1982) provides an interesting counterpoint to the second assumption by suggesting that equity in physician/population ratios between geographical areas is not necessarily a desirable social goal.

It is certainly true that physicians do not locate their practices at random. The literature on location decision is plentiful but very diverse in terms of conceptualization and factors that may affect a physician's decision-making process (GMENAC 1980c; Leonardson, Lapierre, and Hollingsworth 1985; Stamps and Kuriger 1983; Langwell et al. 1986; Langwell, Nelson, and Lenk 1987; Ernst and Yett 1985). This body of literature is only tangentially related to the major point of this chapter, which is to suggest a new way to calculate physician/population ratios. However, the location decision process is obviously important to understand, since maldistribution is an outcome of physicians' decisions on where to locate their practices. Many factors related to the decision-making process have been investigated, including a variety of professional factors (availability of hospital and other health care services; interaction with colleagues); personal factors (educational opportunities for family members, climate, geography, leisure time); and economic factors (income potential, perceived demand for services).

Overlying most of these variables is specialty choice, and much of the research on location decision is increasingly organized around the framework of specialization. One of the technical panels of GMENAC (1980c) dealt with geographic distribution. A primary recommendation was that physician/population ratios are most meaningful when broken down by specialty, based on the observation of different patterns of distribution for general surgeons than for adult medicine (which includes the specialties of general/family practice, internal medicine, cardiovascular disease, gastroenterology, pulmonary disease, and allergy). Other specialties also showed still different patterns of distribution, including obstetrics, pediatrics, psychiatry, orthopedic surgery, urology, and dermatology, among others. Recent research has reinforced this 1980 observation. Both Newhouse et al. (1982) and Schwartz et al. (1980) have suggested the model of oversupply creating a diffusion of physicians into rural areas. Although whether diffusion really occurs is arguable, it does not seem to occur across all specialties, and it particularly does not seem to be true for primary care specialties (U.S. Department of Health and Human Services 1983). A careful case study in Minnesota, in which the analysis was based on physician/population ratios by specialty for counties, demonstrated a diffusion of surgical specialties even into the most rural counties, but no movement of primary care specialties from urban to rural counties (Dennis 1988).

The recent trend in analyzing distribution patterns of physicians is to utilize physician/population ratios on smaller geographic areas (such as counties) and to utilize specialty-specific ratios (see McConnell and Tobias 1986 for an alternative to dependence on physician/population ratios). This trend raises two important issues relevant to the major purpose of this chapter. The first concerns the increased use of specialization as a primary variable to analyze physician supply, including issues related to distribution. Appendix C demonstrates the problem with such dependence on specialty designations without standardizations. Although there is standardization of nomenclature for specialties from the clinical side, the application of these for purposes of supply estimates is not standardized, primarily because of the way in which specific specialties must be combined. Accompanying this is the understanding that what is needed for supply estimates is the actual specialty that the physician practices, which may be different from the clinical designation (Tardiff et al. 1986).

The second issue is related to the use of physician/population ratios to increasingly smaller geographic areas. The geographic distribution technical panel of GMENAC (1980c) cautioned that it was not appropriate to apply national estimates of supply to smaller geographic areas because of increased variation. This panel noted repeatedly the problem of developing accurate estimates of supply because of inadequate data bases, acknowledging several difficulties in monitoring changes in physician supply when inaccurate estimates exist for any one point in time. This panel suggested two remedies, one concerning the geographic area and the other pertaining to the use of physician/population ratios. The first remedy is to develop an alternative unit of analysis to the common geopolitical unit (such as county). Their suggestion is to develop medical service areas that are a functional description of physician services rather than a geographic description. The second remedy the technical panel suggested is the refinement of the numerator of physician/population ratios, based on data about services actually rendered, using claims data from insurers.

Both recommendations have been used in our study: the western Massachusetts area, as defined by the four counties, is a defensible functional medical service area and is generally used that way in a variety of health planning activities. We strongly agree with the need to modify the numerator of physician/population ratios, but this chapter has suggested an alternative to the claims data method by suggesting a system based on primary data collected on several aspects of physician practice patterns. It is our belief that the most standard modification of physician/population ratios is to use as a numerator the direct care equivalent physician estimate and to so designate the physician/population ratio as the DCE physician/population ratio.

Actually, such a modification is not a radically new idea. For example, using estimates derived from AMA secondary data bases, the patient care physician/population ratio for the whole state is 254/100,000, while for western Massachusetts, it is 185/100,000 (Roback, Mead, and Pasko 1984; AMA 1985). This difference is always assumed to be related to the typical maldistribution of physicians between the more rural western portion of the state and the more urban central and eastern portions, in which most of the academic medical centers are located. However, the AMA estimates themselves drop from 331/100,000 to 254/100,000 for the state as a whole when only patient care physicians are counted. This 24 percent drop suggests that there must be many physicians in Massachusetts whose major professional role is something other than direct patient care. Thus, there may be reasons for maldistribution in the state quite apart from the traditional urban/rural differentiation.

Use of the DCE physician/population estimate for both western Massachusetts and the state as a whole (or the eastern part) would help correct—or at least provide a weighting for—differential practice patterns that may exist between urban and rural areas. For example, in this study we know that physicians in western Massachusetts spend about 81 percent of their time in direct patient care, and surgeons spend about 85 percent of their time in direct patient care. There may be more physicians per population in the more urban areas of Massachusetts, but they may spend significantly less time in direct patient care activities, perhaps because of their academic work. There may be significant differences in the practice patterns of physicians in the western and eastern part of the state that may have little to do with the traditional urban/rural distinction. Without incorporating such information about practice patterns into the estimates themselves, it is unwise to conclude anything about the variation of physician supply between these geographic areas of the state.

Adequacy

This methodological discussion skirts around the conceptual issue, commonly termed "adequacy," but which may be translated as asking whether a particular geographic area has enough physicians. Determination of adequacy—or how many physicians are needed in any particular geographic area—was of course part of the GMENAC report, and they concluded that an ideal number of physicians for the nation as a whole is 191/100,000 (GMENAC 1980a, 1980c; Schloss 1988). It is difficult to know how to relate to that suggestion, given the variation in how physicians are counted.

We are not commenting on whether an oversupply exists in this geographic region, or whether it is good or bad to have an oversupply in any area. The published literature can be used to support practically any position. There are those who agree with Newhouse et al. (1982) that an oversupply of physicians is positive because it would help reduce geographic maldistribution by a form of a market model where physicians would be forced to locate in less desirable (that is, rural) areas. Others argue that an oversupply of physicians increases competition and thus quality (Schwartz, Sloan, and Mendelson 1988). Opposing this view are those who cite the many disadvantages from too many physicians, including complications from unnecessary care, increased costs, and physician dissatisfaction due to lowered incomes (Harris 1986; Schroeder 1984; Menken and Sheps 1985).

When one examines physician/population ratios from an international perspective, one is even harder pressed to identify the ultimate answer to how much is enough (Schroeder 1984; Menken and Sheps 1985). For example, in 1969, there were 155 active physicians/100,000 population in the United States, which put the United States ahead of most countries at that time. Countries with more at that time included Italy (175), Denmark (175), Australia (167), Austria (159), and West Germany (159). Countries with fewer physicians included Switzerland (147), Norway (127), Canada (120), New Zealand (120), Netherlands (116), Great Britain (115), and Sweden (114) (Blumberg 1971). By 1980, the United States had relatively fewer physicians per capita (191/100,000) than several countries, including Belgium (240/100,000) and West Germany (229/100,000). The United States was comparable to the Netherlands (190/100,000) but more than Great Britain (162/100,000). Projections for 1990 at that time were as follows: Belgium, 340/100,000; West Germany, 316/100,000; United States, 247/100,000; and Great Britain, 171/100,000 (Schroeder 1984).

The United States does have a much higher ratio of specialists to generalists, and both the United States and Great Britain have a much higher proportion of foreign-trained physicians than other countries. In comparison with physician concentrations in many European countries, the concentration in the United States is not that much greater, but the mix of physicians is such that there is a much higher concentration of specialists, which makes the United States more vulnerable to physician-associated increases in cost of medical care services (Schroeder 1984). The troublesome issue of being able to address the important variable of specialty is raised again here, reinforcing our view that standardized nomenclature needs to be developed that can be applied to estimates of physician supply.

We are not the first to notice this. The one consistent finding of the five GMENAC technical panels is that data bases for physician supply are inaccurate because the theoretical definition of whom to count is unclear. And, as Appendix C demonstrates, this definitional ambiguity is particularly true for specialty designations. Although, as mentioned earlier, much research indicates that distribution patterns differ among primary care specialties and between primary care specialties and other specialties, the variation in definition of primary care specialties makes it very hard to generalize. This lack of accepted, standardized operational definitions significantly weakens the results of research into areas that are of great importance to the health field. This chapter concludes with a few recommendations to help the process of coming to some shared conceptualizations.

Recommendations: Let's Take a Step Backward

This part of our research into physician practice patterns demonstrates the need to reconsider the basic method currently in use for enumerating physician supply. This chapter has shown that too many different assumptions are used to define who should be counted. Practice patterns of physicians seem to have changed significantly over time, with the major result being a diversification of the professional activities of a physician. If all physicians used to do only patient care, that seems not to be so true today, which means that supply estimates based on that assumption will be likely to produce an overestimate. We are not arguing that physician/population ratios should be abandoned: rather, there should be a more standardized and explicit approach to the problem of enumerating physicians, and this definition should be used to adjust the numerator in the physician/population ratios. We recognize that the use of physician/population ratios is arguable since they are an imperfect measure of physician availability. However, these ratios remain the primary level of analysis of physician supply, and given the continuation of their utilization, it is important that they be standardized.

In this chapter, we have tried to demonstrate that it is necessary to take the proverbial step backward in order to reexamine a seemingly simple activity: that of enumerating physicians to produce estimates of the availability of this specific health care resource for consumers of a particular geographic area. In some ways, what we are demonstrating here is simple and straightforward. First, the methodology of the study allowed the collection of information directly from physicians, and the follow-up phase was targeted and aggressive. Consequently, we were able to produce a more accurate estimate of the complete or potential population of physicians available to provide services to this geographic area. Second, by utilizing some simple information on practice patterns, we are able to identify those physicians who spend 10 percent or more of their professional time seeing patients and who might be called "accessible" physicians. Third, by calculating direct care equivalents, we are able to produce a more specific enumeration of what Ginzberg has termed "effective" physician supply. By using this methodology we have been able to show that there are about one-third fewer physicians available to consumers in western Massachusetts than originally thought. However, this conclusion will obviously take on more meaning when comparable estimates are available from other states and regions of the country. Although the results regarding physician supply are of specific interest to Massachusetts, the larger issues raised are of general interest and have been unresolved for the more than ten years that have passed since GMENAC completed its work. The following five recommendations are offered to help create more standardized research, which should then improve subsequent policy decisions arising from research into physician supply:

1. *The concept of supply should be redefined so that two separate estimates are included.* The first estimate should be the potential population of physicians, including all active, licensed physicians, both federal and nonfederal. The second estimate should be a more precise enumeration adjusted by information about practice patterns.

2. *Direct care equivalents should be the standard primary comparison unit for the second supply estimate.* The most appropriate adjustment or standardization is to use a functional analysis that we have termed the "direct care equivalent (DCE) physician." This estimate should be utilized in the various personnel models, including comparisons of states and regions such as urban/rural analysis.

3. *More research needs to be done to perfect this direct care equivalent estimate.* The most important refinement that needs to be made is to include an estimate of the medical education system. Interns, residents, and fellows should be counted as 0.35 FTE, as GMENAC does, and academic faculty be calculated at 0.70 FTE, as suggested by the research of Garg et al. (1991). Although the use of physician extenders is important, we suggest that the direct care equivalent concept should apply only to physicians. That GMENAC included nonphysician extenders in their requirements model simply adds to the already unacceptable variation.

4. *A correction factor based on replication of the refined direct care equivalent estimate should be developed and applied to the existing data bases.* We do not think that the massive data bases maintained by the American Medical Association should be replaced. In fact, the AMA periodically collects primary survey data from samples of physicians. The lack is not in the data collection, but in the application of the information to the data base itself. We suggest that the AMA—as well as other researchers—develop a correction factor to be applied to the current estimates of physician supply and that these corrected estimates be utilized as the direct care equivalent estimate for physician supply, adjusted for the medical education system as noted above. This adjusted number would become the numerator in the physician/population ratios.

5. *Standard nomenclature and standard combinations for specialty designations should be developed and utilized.* The variation in specialty designation and the variation in numeric estimation of physicians compound the errors, since specialty designation is such an important part of physician supply. At present, comparison of studies is almost impossible because of differences in specialty designation. All studies should follow the AMA specialty designations, which provide detail by separating out subspecialties (such as gynecology and obstetrics). In combining specialty designations for larger categories, however, a more functional combination is appropriate, one that uses a primary care categorization including general and family practice, internal medicine, pediatrics, and gynecology/obstetrics. The importance of this standardization cannot be overstated. There is sufficient preliminary evidence that distribution patterns of primary care physicians are substantially different from those of other physicians, with some indication that primary physicians are even more underrepresented in rural areas than other specialties and subspecialties. In order to develop an appropriate health human resources policy directed at primary care physicians, it is imperative that studies categorize primary care specialties in the same way. Appendix C gives a clear example of the difficulties involved when using different combinations of specialty categories for primary care specialties.

A Final Word

Utilization of the direct care equivalent physician estimate will not solve all of the problems raised in this chapter, but it will at least make enumeration of physicians more standard and also more precise. This approach will make health policy and analysis that flows from research in physician supply more meaningful, and it will also help to avoid contentious political arguments such as have been seen in the state of Massachusetts. Throughout our work on this particular aspect of physician practice patterns in western Massachusetts, we have been amazed at the inaccuracies that result from ambiguous nomenclature, in clear contrast to the precision in the many other areas of health research. For example, in the area of health status indicators, there is a wide variety of precisely defined and uniformly used standardized or adjusted rates and ratios. This attention to precision is in contrast to research in the general area of physician supply, including analyses of physician distribution. For example, in two very recent studies, definitions of full-time equivalent physicians were used, but in neither study was this concept defined (Gonzalez and Emmons 1989; Mulhausen and Gree 1989). In fact, in one of the studies, which was calculating physician need for HMO populations, they even noted that there "was no standardized definition of 'full-time-equivalent' other than that used by the individual plans" (Mulhausen and Gree 1989, 1932). It is only appropriate that we develop well-respected standardized measures to address physician supply, which has such a direct bearing on important pieces of health policy and legislation. The data are now available to do so, and when applied to the estimates of physician supply in western Massachusetts, the differences were very large (Table 3.1).

We are not necessarily arguing against the obvious increasing emphasis on forecasting and modeling. Weiner et al. (1987) have noted: "Physician supply forecasting will always be shrouded by statistical, economic and clinical minutiae; yet, at its heart, it is not a purely technical enterprise. Its purpose is to provide policymakers and managers with information and perspectives that allow them to select more rationally among alternative decision options" (p. 436).

Although this is clearly true, it is crucial to make assumptions more clear in the models that are used. The "minutiae" need to be clearly defined and used in a standard way. This can best be done by refining the definition of the numerator to be more narrow, based on practice patterns of physicians.

References

Aiken, L. H., C. E. Lewis, J. Craig, R. C. Mendenhall, R. J. Blendon, and D. E. Rogers. "The Contribution of Specialists to the Delivery of Primary Care: A New Perspective." *New England Journal of Medicine* 300 (1979): 1363–70.

AMA Center for Health Policy Research. *Physician Supply and Utilization by Specialty: Trends and Projections*. Chicago, IL: AMA, 1986.

American Medical Association. Characteristics of Physicians: Massachusetts: AMA, 1985, Table 17.

Anderson, A. *Health Care in the 1990's: Trends and Strategies*. Chicago: American College of Hospital Administrators, 1984.

Blumberg, M. S. *Trends and Projections of Physicians in the United States 1967–2002*. Berkeley, CA: Carnegie Commission on Higher Education, July 1971.

Bowman, M. A. "GMENAC Revisited: Medical Manpower in the Late '80's." *Journal of Medical Practice Management* 1 (1985): 66–72.

Clute, K. F. *The General Practitioner: A Study of Medical Education and Practice in Ontario and Nova Scotia*. Toronto: University of Toronto Press, 1963.

Dennis, T. "Changes in the Distribution of Physicians in Rural Areas of Minnesota, 1965–85." *American Journal of Public Health* 78 (Dec. 1988): 1577–79.

Ernst, R. L., and D. E. Yett. *Physician Location and Specialty Choice*. Ann Arbor, MI: Health Administration Press, 1985.

Flexner, A. *Medical Education in the United States and Canada: A Report to the Carnegie Foundation for the Advancement of Teaching*. New York: The Carnegie Foundation, 1910.

Freshnock, L. G. *Physicians and Public Attitudes on Health Issues*. Chicago: American Medical Association, 1984.

Fruen, M. A., and J. R. Cantwell. "Geographic Distribution of Physicians: Past Trends and Future Influences." *Inquiry* (Spring 1982): 44–50.

Garg M. L., J. F. Boero, R. G. Christiansen, and C. G. Booher. "Primary Care Teaching Physicians' Losses of Productivity and Revenue at Three Ambulatory-Care Centers." *Academic Medicine* 66 (June 1991): 345–53.

Gavett, J. W., and A. I. Mushlin. "Calculating the Costs of Training in Primary Care." *Medical Care* 24 (1986): 301–12.

Ginzberg, E. "The Future Supply of Physicians: From Pluralism to Policy." *Health Affairs* 1 (1982): 6–19.

Ginzberg, E. *From Physician Shortage to Patient Shortage: The Uncertain Frontier of Medical Practice*. Boulder, CO: Westview Press, 1986.

Ginzberg, E. "Physician Supply in the Year 2000." *Health Affairs* (Summer 1989): 84–90.

Ginzberg, J. E, and M. Ostow. *The Coming Physician Surplus: In Search of a Policy*. Landmark Studies, Rowman and Allanheld: San Francisco, 1984.

Gonzalez, M., and D. Emmons. *Socioeconomic Characteristics of Medical Practice 1989*. Chicago: Center for Health Policy Research, AMA, 1989.

Graduate Medical Education National Advisory Committee. *Vol. 1: Summary*. Washington, DC: Department Health and Human Services, Publication No. (HRA 81-651), 1980a.

Graduate Medical Education National Advisory Committee. *Vol. 2: Modeling Research and Data Technical Panel*. Washington, DC: Department Health and Human Services, Publication No. (HRA 81-652), 1980b.

Graduate Medical Education National Advisory Committee. *Vol. 3: Geographic Distribution Technical Panel.* Washington, DC: Department of Health and Human Services, Publication No. (HRA 81-653), 1980c.

Graduate Medical Education National Advisory Committee. *Vol. 4: Technical Panel on Educational Environment.* Washington, DC: Department of Health and Human Services, Publication No. (HRA 81-654), 1980d.

Greenwald, H. P., and L. G. Hart. "Issues in Survey Data on Medical Practice: Some Empirical Comparisons." *Public Health Reports* 101 (Sept–Oct. 1986): 540–46.

Hafferty, F. W. "Physician Oversupply as a Socially Constructed Reality." *Journal of Health and Social Behavior* 27 (1986): 358–69.

Harris, J. E. "How Many Doctors Are Enough?" *Health Affairs* 5 (1986): 73–83.

Hemenway, D. "The Optimal Location of Doctors." *New England Journal of Medicine* 36 (Feb. 1982): 1342–48.

Iglehart, J. K. "The Future Supply of Physicians." *New England Journal of Medicine,* 314 (March 27, 1986): 860–64.

Kindig, D. A., and H. Movassaghi. "The Adequacy of Physician Supply in Small Rural Counties." *Health Affairs* (Summer 1989): 64–76.

Kriesberg, H. M., J. Wa, E. D. Hollander, and J. Bow. *Methodological Approaches for Determining Health Manpower Supply and Requirements: Analytic Perspective.* Aspen: DHFW, Publication HRA 76-14511, 1976.

Langwell, K., J. L. Czajka, S. L. Nelson, E. Lenk, and K. Berman. *Survey of Factors Influencing the Location Decision and Practice Patterns.* Washington, DC: U.S. Department of Health and Human Services: ODAM Report 4-86, 1986.

Langwell, K, S. Nelson, and E. Lenk. "Effects of Community Characteristics on Young Physicians Regarding Rural Practice." *Public Health Reports* 102 (1987): 317–28.

Lee, R. I., and L. W. Jones. *The Fundamentals of Good Medical Care.* Chicago: University of Chicago Press, 1933.

Leonardson, G., R. Lapierre, and D. Hollingsworth. "Factors Predictive of Physician Location." *Journal of Medical Education* 60 (Jan. 1985): 37–42.

Marsland, D. W., M. Wood, and F. Mayo. "A Data Base for Patient Care, Curriculum and Research in Family Practice; 526,196 Patient Problems." *Journal of Family Practice* 3: (1976) 25–28.

McConnell, C. E., and L. A. Tobias. "Distributional Change in Physician Manpower, U.S. 1963–1980." *American Journal of Public Health* 76 (June 1986): 638–42.

McNutt, D. R. "GMENAC: Its Manpower Forecasting Framework." *American Journal of Public Health* 71 (Oct. 1981): 1116–24.

Menken, M., and C. G. Sheps. "Consequences of an Oversupply of Specialists: The Case of Neurology." *Journal of the American Medical Association* 253 (April 5, 1985): 1926–28.

Moore, F. D., and C. Priebe. "Board-Certified Physicians in the United States 1971–1986." *New England Journal of Medicine* 324 (Feb. 21, 1991): 536–43.

Mulhausen, R., and M. J. Gree. "Physician Need: An Alternative Projection from a Study of Large, Prepaid Group Practices." *Journal of the American Medical Association* 261 (1989): 1930–34.

Newhouse, J. P., A. P. Williams, B. W. Bennett, and W. B. Schwartz. "Where Have All the Doctors Gone?" *Journal of the American Medical Association* 247 (1982): 2392–96.

Noren, J., T. Frazier, I. Altman, and J. Delozier. "Ambulatory Medical Care: A Comparison of Internists and Family-General Practitioners." *New England Journal of Medicine* 302 (Jan. 3, 1980): 11–16.

Owens, A. "Working at Full Capacity? A Lot of Your Colleagues Aren't." *Medical Economics* 56 (1979): 63–71.

Pearse, W. H. *Manpower Planning in Obstetrics and Gynecology.* American College of Obstetricians and Gynecologists Report, Feb. 1988.

Peterson, O. L. *An Analytical Study of North Carolina General Practice 1953–54.* Evanston, IL: Association of American Medical Colleges, 1956.

Reynolds, R., and R. Ohsfeldt. *Socioeconomic Characteristics of Medical Practice 1984.* Chicago: Center for Health Policy Research, AMA, 1984.

Roback, R. L., D. Mead, and T. Pasko. *Physician Characteristics and Distribution in the U.S.* 1989 Edition. Chicago: Survey and Data Resources, AMA, 1989.

Schloss, E. "Beyond GMENAC—Another Physician Shortage from 2010 to 2030?" *New England Journal of Medicine* 318 (April 7, 1988): 920–22.

Schroeder, S. "Western European Responses to Physician Oversupply." *Journal of the American Medical Association* 252 (July 20, 1984): 373–84.

Schwartz, W. B., J. P. Newhouse, B. W. Bennett, and A. P. Williams. "The Changing Geographic Distribution of Board-Certified Physicians." *New England Journal of Medicine* 303 (1980): 1032–38.

Schwartz, W. B., F. A. Sloan, and D. N. Mendelson. "Why There Will Be Little or No Physician Surplus Between Now and the Year 2000." *New England Journal of Medicine* 318 (April 7, 1988): 892–97.

Stamps, P. L., and F. H. Kuriger. "Location Decisions of National Health Service Corps Physicians." *American Journal of Public Health* 73 (Aug 1983): 906–8.

Steinwachs, D. M., J. P. Weiner, S. Shapiro, P. Batalden, K. Coltin, and F. Wasserman. "A Comparison of the Requirements for Primary Care Physicians in HMO's with Projections Made by GMENAC." *New England Journal of Medicine* 314 (1986): 217–22.

Tardiff, K., D. Cella, C. Seiferth, and S. Perry. "Selection and Change of Specialties by Medical School Graduates." *Journal of Medical Education* 61 (Oct. 1986): 790–95.

Tarlov, A. "The Increasing Supply of Physicians, the Changing Structure of the Health Services System and the Future Practice of Medicine." *New England Journal of Medicine* 308 (1983): 1235–44.

Tarlov, A. R. "HMO Enrollment Growth and Physicians: The Third Compartment." *Health Affairs* 5 (1986): 23–35.

Tarlov, A. "The Rising Supply of Physicians and the Pursuit of Better Health." *Journal of Medical Education* 63 (1988): 94–107.

U.S. Department of Health and Human Services, Health Resources and Services Administration, Bureau of Health Professions, Office of Data Analysis and Management. *Diffusion and the Changing Geographic Distribution of Primary Care Physicians.* Washington DC: DHHS, ODAM Report 4-83, June 1983.

Weiner, J. P. "Forecasting Physician Supply: Recent Developments." *Health Affairs* (Winter 1989): 173–79.

Weiner, J. P., D. M. Steinwachs, S. Shapiro, K. L. Catlin, D. Ershoff, and J. P. O'Connor. "Assessing a Methodology for Physician Requirement Forecast: Replication of GMENAC's Need-based model for the Pediatric Specialty." *Medical Care* 25 (1987): 426–36.

Williams, A. P., W. B. Schwartz, J. P. Newhouse, and B. W. Bennett. "How Many Miles to the Doctor?" *New England Journal of Medicine* 309 (1983): 958–63.

Chapter 4

Physician Income: How Much, Why, and What Do Physicians Think about It?

Interest in physician incomes elicits a spectrum of responses, depending on the audience. The general public is often derisive of the high incomes that many physicians enjoy, policymakers generally focus on how physician incomes can be limited, and physicians themselves are frequently defensive. A fair question to ask is why we should bother considering determinants of physician income as one of the major topics of this book. Although empirical information about physician incomes exists, it is mostly descriptive, and as we shall see in this chapter, the nature of income calculations and comparisons for physicians has been subject to considerable misunderstanding.

For some, income of physicians is reduced to being a function of reimbursement patterns, which, although true, is far too simplistic. There is an amazing variety in the ways in which physicians may be paid in the United States today, and increasingly physicians are paid by some combination. Some of the more corporate reimbursement systems may include profit-sharing, which is the basis for Relman's (1980) famous concern about for-profit medicine and possible conflicts of interest for physicians. That some of these organized reimbursement systems also frequently contain arrangements for physicians to share financial losses is much less well known, but common (Hillman, Pauly, and Kerstein 1989; Hillman 1987; Hemenway 1990). Of course, individual organizational reimbursement systems are subject to the health insurance industry, both "private" and "public." Many of these reimbursement schedules have historical roots in a model of physician behavior that is based on the assumption that physicians are primarily sensitive to economic incentives.

A variety of cost-containment legislation has arisen from these same assumptions, and, as noted in Chapter 1, the result of these regulatory attempts is mixed at best.

One of the clearly negative consequences of the reimbursement system is the large income differential, largely dependent on specialty, that exists among physicians. Typical of the American health care system is the response to these differences—the Physician Payment Reform Commission's suggestion of a different way to reimburse physicians, based on time rather than procedures (Hsiao et al. 1988; Hsiao, Braun, and Dunn 1988; Roper 1988). Although many applaud this proposed solution, it will probably create other, still unanticipated negative consequences, which in turn may be used to suggest further reforms.

What is more appropriate is to reevaluate what is known about physician incomes—not only how much money they make, but also what determines that amount, and what physicians think about their incomes. We began this whole research project thinking that we understood physicians and medicine as a profession. However, as we continued with our investigation—including an extensive survey of the literature, discussions with the medical leadership in Massachusetts as well as with practicing physicians, and analysis of the respondents in western Massachusetts—we realized that much of the understanding of the field of medicine is based on descriptive or anecdotal data. Although this source of information is obviously important, it is not sufficient to provide an adequate understanding of physician behavior and attitudes, particularly for examining income, which is used as a human resources supply issue by some, and as a cost-containment issue by others. Descriptive data on income of physicians, such as those collected by the AMA, do not provide the insight necessary for an understanding of what influences income, whether physicians are motivated by income to make practice changes, and how income affects physician satisfaction.

This chapter provides an opportunity to reexamine physician income with the hope of increasing the level of understanding of this important part of medical practice. We begin with a brief background, primarily into how other researchers have addressed income, although this section will also provide a rudimentary statement on the nature of reimbursement patterns today. Also included here is a description of the type of information maintained by the AMA. The next section focuses on methodological issues that arise in any study of income and concludes with a description of the most important limitations specific to our own study. The empirical results of the survey done in western Massachusetts are presented after that, beginning with a description and comparison of these findings with the several national profiles gathered and maintained by the AMA. We then examine some variables important in the determination of income. This section concludes with an analysis of what physicians in our study think about their incomes.

The chapter concludes with some thoughts about physician income, as well as some suggestions for further research that we propose are necessary before further financial reform can occur.

Background

The literature concerning money is fairly extensive, but it is largely focused on arguments about the incentive value of different ways to reimburse physicians, or various administrative problems involved in physician reimbursement. Although these two factors are obviously critical to any policy decisions regarding fiscal reform, our emphasis is more fundamental, that is, we concentrate on the determinants of physician income and what physicians feel about their income levels.

There are three major categories of literature concerning physician income, excluding the descriptive work of the American Medical Association, primarily represented in the Socioeconomic Monitoring System, which produces annual reports (Gonzalez 1991). The first general category of literature uses income to bolster research on physician supply. This impressive group of studies uses changes in average income of physicians over time to support the argument that there are (or will be) either too many or too few physicians (Luft and Arno 1986; Tarlov 1988; Ginzberg et al. 1981; Schwartz and Mendelson 1990; Sloan and Schwartz 1983). As one might suspect after reading Chapter 3, we are troubled by these articles mainly because of the nonsystematic way in which the concept of supply is used.

The remaining two categories of literature regarding physician income are more specific. One focuses on the relationship of financial incentives to choice of specialty. The intent of most of these studies is to understand the barriers to recruiting medical students into primary care, since this group of specialties is relatively underpaid (Kassler, Wartman, and Sillman 1991; Hough 1988; McCarty 1987). After a careful review of this group of studies, Langwell and Werner (1980) concluded that income expectations do not have a significant effect upon specialty choice. The remaining category of studies concerning income focuses on the relationship between physician behavior and reimbursement method and is the largest single category of articles concerning physician income. Perhaps the first to undertake a systematic study of this was David Mechanic (1975), who noted that fee-for-service physicians have different practice patterns than prepaid physicians. He used the term "assembly line practice" to describe prepaid care, and he suggested that fee-for-service physicians work longer hours and spend more time in direct patient care activities. This initial supposition has led to a long line of research into how organizational arrangements affect physician behavior. Some articles question whether financial arrangements affect clinical judgments (Hillman, Pauly, and Kerstein 1989), while others focus on physician response to financial incentives, including the differential utilization of a variety of services by patients as dictated by physicians (Hillman 1987; Hemenway et al. 1990; Hickson, Altemeier, and Perrin 1987).

In the health field, there is frequently a close association between research and policy enactment; this association is evident in the area of physician income, as it is in health human resources, as observed in Chapter 3. Many of the articles just noted end with some sort of policy directive about the optimal way to reimburse physicians. The study that produced the relative value scale is a good example of such translation of research into policy (Hsiao et al. 1988; Hsiao, Braun, and Dunn 1988; Roper 1988). This resource-based reimbursement system was phased in to replace Medicare's customary payment method beginning in January 1992. Whether this will decrease income differentials or simply reorder them remains to be seen.

Most of the research depends on data collected and reported by the AMA, which is careful to define "income" as net income (after expenses but before taxes). But they also report income trends; for this analysis, inflation-adjusted income, also known as "real income," is utilized. Real net income expresses physician earnings in terms of the purchasing power of a dollar in 1981, which includes an inflation adjustment. Unadjusted net income is referred to as "nominal income" (Gonzalez 1991; Gonzalez and Emmons 1989). Whenever one is reporting trends or growth in income, it is obviously important to consider inflation. Despite the precision of AMA data, in many articles it is sometimes difficult to determine which income figure is being used. One example is found in the effort to determine whether physician incomes have increased or decreased over the last ten years. Physician incomes are at the high end of the national distribution; in fact, they are about five times that of the average American worker (Crozier and Iglehart 1986). In 1989, according to AMA data, the average physician income increased 7.7 percent, which is above the 4.6 percent increase for inflation (Gonzalez (1991). This same 7–8 percent annual rate of increase for physician income is also reported by others, although not consistently. For example, Schwartz (1986) noted that physician incomes in 1984 represented only a 2 percent increase over 1983, which followed a 6.8 percent growth rate of 1982–1983. He noted that physicians' incomes increased less than the rate of inflation in 1984. Some researchers look at a longer time span and examine both real and nominal income. This usually produces a slightly different conclusion: either no increases occur in real income from 1970 to 1985, although nominal physician incomes rose dramatically during this time period (Sammons 1982); or (when the decade 1975–1985 is used) a 5 percent decline shows up in the real median incomes of physicians (when inflation is taken into account) (Clare et al. 1987).

This example demonstrates two problems, the first of which is a measurement problem. Income is a complicated variable and needs to be reported precisely with the appropriate comparative figure. Second, physician incomes are as much a political statement as anything else. Income levels are used on both sides of the supply argument. Sloan and Schwartz (1983) are particularly well known for their argument about physician incomes: they feel that real income of physicians has remained virtually constant over the 1980s. They also compare the increase in physicians' incomes (1.7 percent over 1970–1974) to the increase of lawyers, accountants, and engineers (from −4.2 to +2.3 percent) in the same period. Their major point is that these highly trained professional groups are all well below the nearly 20 percent increase in the real per capita income of the population as a whole during this period.

Because of the controversy over physician incomes, we were initially reluctant to gather information about this variable. However, concerns about physician incomes are magnified in Massachusetts, since there are several income-restricting pieces of legislation that are unique to the state. For example, Massachusetts physicians (unlike those of any other state) are prohibited from billing patients for the difference between their customary charge and what Blue Shield is willing to pay. Another example concerns malpractice premiums, with a unique retroactive billing method that was explained in Chapter 1. These two factors are significant contributors to physician dissatisfaction in Massachusetts.

Physicians in the New England area have always had lower incomes than physicians in the rest of the country; net income for New England physicians was $128,300 in 1989, compared to $155,800 for all physicians. This is the lowest average income of any region, with the next closest being $142,600 in the Mountain region, and the highest average incomes ($170,300) coming from the West South Central region (Gonzalez 1991).

These lower incomes and the general negative response of physicians to regulations and restrictions on their medical practice has made the issue of income part of the generally contentious public atmosphere that is the backdrop of this whole study. As a result, we wanted to collect income data in a way that would enable us to address some of the larger issues that were being raised, rather than simply to redescribe income levels.

Methodological Issues and Limitations

In general, income is recognized as a variable for which it is difficult to gather good information. First of all, respondents are usually sensitive about revealing income. Second, the accuracy of any self-report is questionable since both honesty and recall may be problematic. Gathering income data on physicians is viewed as being even more difficult than for the general population, and, in fact, income is a complicated variable for the physicians. Many physicians are self-employed, and so the definition of what to count as income usually involves elaboration of a variety of practice expenses, as well as precision about net or gross income, and before or after taxes. Also, physician incomes are in the high end of the overall income distribution in the United States, so their incomes are frequently discussed in the media, often negatively. Since many researchers do not appreciate the complexity and since physicians' incomes are often used as a political statement, physicians often are reluctant to report income. For these reasons, few investigators ask physicians to report on income directly, and use data from the periodical reports of the AMA's Socioeconomic Monitoring System.

We decided to include income on our questionnaire and to word the question the same way as in the 1989 AMA Socioeconomic Characteristics Monitoring Survey (Gonzalez 1991). This question asks for an estimate of income for the past 12 months, after all expenses but before taxes. The specific wording is the following (Q-14, Appendix B):

> What is your net annual revenue from your medical practice activities for this past 12 months? (To make this comparable to the AMA Socioeconomic Characteristics Study, please estimate this after all expenses but BEFORE taxes. Be sure to include the value of all fringe benefits that may be paid on your behalf, i.e., Keogh Plan.)

The AMA asks physician respondents to indicate actual net (unadjusted) income to the nearest thousand. We altered the response mode by providing respondents with a choice of eight income categories starting at "less than $40,000" up to the top category of "over $160,000." The question was worded in this fashion to decrease the sensitive nature of the information and increase the likelihood of physicians responding.

Using this response mode created two complications that produced some limitations in our ability to analyze the income data. The first is that the upper income category has no maximum and, thus, no clear range. Seventeen percent of all western Massachusetts respondents fall into this category. If many of these 130 physicians have incomes above $180,000, based on the $19,000 range of the other categories, it would result in calculations for mean incomes that are too low. Second, for analysis purposes, we frequently calculated exact income from the categories. This is commonly done and is an easy calculation. For example, a group's mean income of 4.87 is equivalent to $97,530: Category 4 is $81,000–100,000; 0.87 × $19,000 (range of category) = $16,530, which is added to the beginning point of the category ($81,000) to obtain $97,530.

It would have been more accurate to utilize the response mode of the AMA, which would have produced exact income for each individual. In fact, only 50 out of the 791 patient care physicians responding to our survey withheld this information. This 8 percent nonresponse rate was higher than the 1–2 percent nonresponse rate for the other demographic questions, but clearly it was acceptable given the sensitive nature of this question. In retrospect, physicians were not as reluctant to report income as we had feared.

Two additional specific limitations emerge from the utilization of just this one question to determine income. The question is worded to elicit income generated from "medical practice activities." We should have included two additional, specific types of income-generating activities. The first oversight is not asking respondents about income from other investments, especially medically related. These sources would include rental/ownership of equipment, medical space, and other service sites such as nursing homes. This oversight may be significant, because some respondents may have included this income while others may not have. Second, on-call hours were not specified in the estimate of income. Once again, some respondents may have included it while others did not; for those physicians who are reimbursed specifically for on-call hours, this may affect income. The AMA does not collect this type of detail either, although it does address deferred payments, requesting that these be included in the physician's net income.

The analysis of incomes presents a whole different range of problems, two of which should be mentioned here. The first problem is choosing the most appropriate summary measure of central tendency. For most variables, the commonly used measure of central tendency is the mean or average value. When means and medians for physician income are examined, it is typical to observe that the median income is lower than the mean, indicating that the distribution around the mean has been skewed by the presence of higher incomes. This skew is reflected in the AMA's national profile: in 1989, the mean income for all physicians was $155,800, but the median income was $125,000 (Gonzalez 1991), which means that half of all physicians earned below $125,000. In our study, there is a similar direction of difference between the mean and median income, but the difference is not as pronounced, probably because of the open range allowed for the highest income category of over $160,000. The AMA and most economists suggest that median income is a more accurate measure of central tendency. However, mean incomes are frequently reported, so we will utilize both measures of central tendency, as appropriate.

The second general problem in analyzing incomes is that the distribution of incomes is often as important—and in some cases, more important than—the median or mean value. Throughout the presentation and discussion of results, which is the topic of the next section, we will do comparisons of distributions as well as comparisons of median and mean values. To accomplish this, we will follow the analytic model used by many economists, which is to use the income distribution of the whole group of respondents as the "expected" distribution. The "observed" distribution will then be the income distribution as affected by the particular variable being examined, such as specialty, age, or practice setting.

Results

In this section, we would like to present some of the most interesting and relevant results that arise from this survey. This section is organized so that descriptive results will be presented first and compared to the national information, using the AMA data. Included here will be a discussion of the effect of specialty on incomes, since this is such an important determinant. Following this will be three additional types of variables that help determine income: demographic variables, practice characteristics, and productivity. This section will conclude with additional results that focus on what physicians think about their incomes, including their level of satisfaction and their perception of how productive their medical practices are.

Descriptive and comparative results

The mean income for all patient care physicians responding to the survey is $97,500, while the median income is $94,400, suggesting some skewing of the sample toward upper income levels, but not as pronounced as the national data. In the Socioeconomic Characteristics Monitoring Survey covering the years 1984–1989 and published in 1989, the mean net income for all physicians nationwide was $144,700 and the median net income was $120,000 (Gonzalez and Emmons 1989). These income data were collected by the AMA in 1988. Our data were collected in June and July of 1989 and referred also to 1989; therefore we will use the 1989 AMA data (Gonzalez 1991) for comparison purposes. It is also important to note that we are using for comparison purposes the values reported by the AMA for net unadjusted (or nominal) incomes. This is the appropriate comparison since we do not have data over time, but rather cross-sectional data. The results presented here (and elsewhere in this volume) refer only to the 791 patient care respondents.

As we noted previously, distribution of income is usually just as important as measures of central tendency; Figure 4.1 shows the distribution of incomes of our respondents. About one quarter of the patient care physicians in western Massachusetts make over $141,000, with 17 percent falling into the highest-income category. Twenty-eight percent make below $80,000, while close to half of all respondents fall between $81,000 and $140,000.

Specialty. There is a relatively unusual aspect of this income distribution that is included in Table 4.1 showing income by specialty. For surgeons, radiologists, OB/GYNs, and pathologists in western Massachusetts, the median income is higher than the mean income, which indicates a distribution that is particularly skewed to the lower end.

In order to put these figures in context, it is necessary to compare them to regional and national figures by specialty groups. Table 4.1 and Figures 4.2 and 4.3 show these comparisons, using the specialty categories that are utilized by the AMA in their data summaries. (See Chapter 3 and Appendix C for our discussion of specialty categories.) From these, it can be seen that the mean and median income values for each of the nine specialty groups in western Massachusetts are substantially lower than either the national (Figures 4.2 and 4.3) or regional (Table 4.1) figures. New England as a region has had lower median incomes than the nationwide estimates for some time (Gonzalez and Emmons 1989). Western Massachusetts physicians have even lower incomes than the New England region as a whole. The regional comparisons drawn from the AMA are frustrating since there were fewer than 20 respondents from New England in seven of the nine specialties. These low counts reflect a weakness of the AMA Socioeconomic Monitoring Survey, since the sample size is not large enough for very many specific regional comparisons. In our study of western Massachusetts we had 74 pediatricians, 48 obstetricians, 41 radiologists, 33 anesthesiologists, and 15 pathologists among our respondents, demonstrating the usefulness of intensive, targeted follow-up efforts to increase the response rate.

Table 4.2 shows the rankings from highest median income to lowest median income using the national AMA data and our western Massachusetts data for the same nine specialties. Although there are some differences in dollar figures, the ranking of the specialties for the western Massachusetts population is the same as for the AMA national sample. Figures 4.2 and 4.3 show this schematically and also demonstrate the large discrepancies between the median incomes of the specialty groups.

Figure 4.1 Income Distribution of Western Massachusetts Physicians

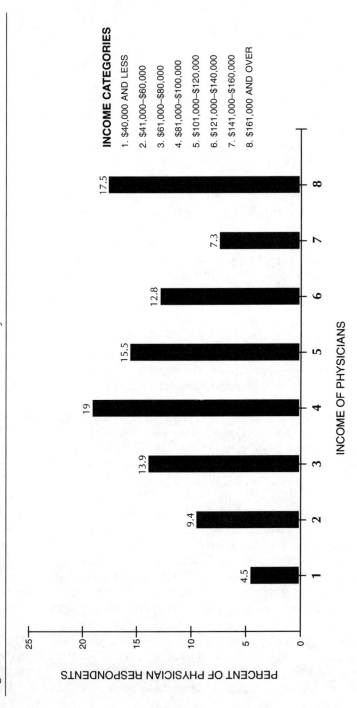

Table 4.1   Comparison of National Mean and Median Income by
Specialty with Massachusetts Data

	National		New England		Western Mass.	
	*Mean Income**	*Median Income**	*Mean Income**	*Median Income**	*Mean Income*	*Median Income*
All Patient Care Physicians	155.8	125.0	128.3	117.0	97.5	94.4
Specialties						
General/Family Practice	95.9	90.0	—†	—	64.8	62.1
Internal Medicine	146.5	120.0	123.1	105.0	76.2	76.2
Pediatrics	104.7	93.0	—	—	72.4	68.6
OB/GYN	194.3	164.0	—	—	121.0	124.8
Surgical	220.5	180.0	169.4	158.0	124.8	136.2
Radiology	210.5	180.0	—	—	141.0	150.5
Anesthesiology	185.8	180.0	—	—	121.0	121.0
Pathology	154.5	148.0	—	—	108.6	112.4
Psychiatry	111.7	100.0	—	—	78.1	76.2

Source: National and regional data from AMA Socioeconomic Monitoring System 1990
core surveys, published 1991.
*Income is after expenses and before taxes; reported here in thousands of dollars.
†Data are not reported where there are fewer than 20 observations in the core study.

For example, the difference between the national median income of the
highest three specialties (anesthesiology, surgery, and radiology) and
the lowest-income specialty (general/family practice) is $90,000. In fact,
the median income for the highest three specialties is twice the lowest
specialty nationally. In our western Massachusetts study, the highest-
income specialty is radiology; the lowest, general/family practice (Tables
4.1 and 4.2). There is an income differential between the medians of these
two specialties of $88,400, although both western Massachusetts medians
are lower than the national figures.

The fact that physician incomes in western Massachusetts are significantly lower than the national averages is obviously of particular
relevance in Massachusetts. There are several possible explanations. One
that is often suggested is that low incomes are prima facie evidence
that there are too many physicians practicing in Massachusetts. As we
have demonstrated in Chapter 3, this does not seem to be true, at least
in the western part of the state that served as the study area. Others
argue that it is those regulations unique to Massachusetts that primarily

Figure 4.2   Median Physician Net Income: Western Massachusetts
Physicians Compared to National Figures

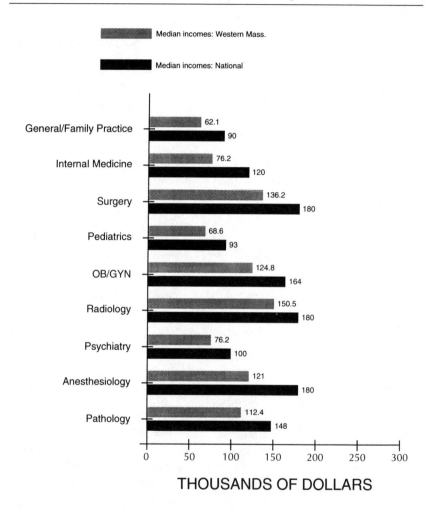

□ Median incomes: Western Mass.

■ Median incomes: National

General/Family Practice — 62.1 / 90
Internal Medicine — 76.2 / 120
Surgery — 136.2 / 180
Pediatrics — 68.6 / 93
OB/GYN — 124.8 / 164
Radiology — 150.5 / 180
Psychiatry — 76.2 / 100
Anesthesiology — 121 / 180
Pathology — 112.4 / 148

0   50   100   150   200   250   300

THOUSANDS OF DOLLARS

Source of national figures: American Medical Association Socioeconomic Monitoring
System 1990 Core Survey.

restrict physician incomes. This argument is somewhat mediated by the
fact that physician incomes in the New England region have historically
been low; in fact, other income measures have also been low, especially
manufacturing wages (U.S. Bureau of the Census 1972, 1982, 1990). Of

Figure 4.3   Mean Physician Net Income: Western Massachusetts
Physicians Compared to National Figures

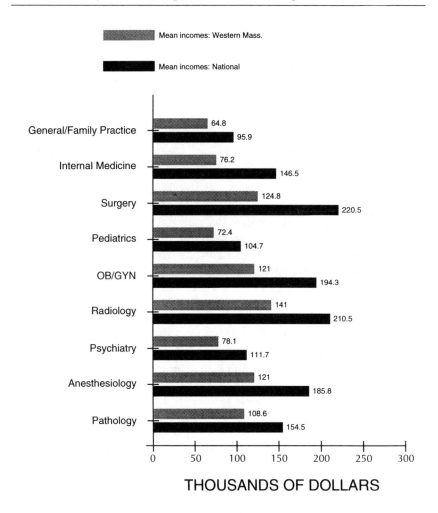

Source of national figures: American Medical Association Socioeconomic Monitoring
System 1990 Core Survey.

course, it is also true that the western Massachusetts area does not
include a major metropolitan area. The national median income for what
the AMA characterizes as a nonmetropolitan physician is $107,000, which
is much closer to the western Massachusetts median.

Table 4.2 Ranking of Specialties by Median Income

National Data, Based on Gonzalez (1991)	*Western Massachusetts Study*
1. Surgical ($180,000)	1. Radiology ($150,500)
2. Radiology ($180,000)	2. Surgical ($136,200)
3. Anesthesiology ($180,000)	3. OB/GYN ($124,800)
4. OB/GYN ($164,000)	4. Anesthesiology ($121,000)
5. Pathology ($148,000)	5. Pathology ($112,400)
6. Internal Medicine ($120,000)	6. Internal Medicine ($76,200)
7. Psychiatry ($100,000)	7. Psychiatry ($76,200)
8. Pediatrics ($93,000)	8. Pediatrics ($68,600)
9. General/Family Practice ($90,000)	9. General/Family Practice ($62,100)

About 36 percent of western Massachusetts patient care physicians are in one of the primary care specialties (general/family practice, internal medicine, pediatrics, or obstetrics/gynecology), which tend to have lower incomes. However, this proportion is not significantly higher than the national figure, which is estimated to be about 33 percent (Crozier and Iglehart 1986; Roback, Randolph, and Seidman 1990).

Making an observation about whether a physician's income is too high or too low is obviously a value judgment, although the median income of general and family practitioners in western Massachusetts ($62,000) would probably be judged low by any observer. The income differentials of $90,000 nationally ($88,400 in western Massachusetts) between the highest- and lowest-income specialties is remarkable and encourages reflection on reimbursement patterns, as representing what is more highly valued in the American medical care system. These income differences have been noted by other investigators, and the variation seems to be constant over time (Crozier and Iglehart 1986; Schwartz 1986). The observation of these income differences has caused a lot of research concerning the relative importance of income in specialty choice, with some arguing that medical students select specialties for reasons other than income (Kassler, Wartman, and Sillman 1991), while others note that income is more important to those who select procedure-intensive specialties (Hough 1988). Regardless of whether these income differences affect choice of specialty, they do affect the professional identity of physicians. These income differentials encourage physicians to be more closely identified with their own specialty than with their profession—a trend, which although not new, is accelerating as income discrepancies among specialists continue to increase.

Demographic variables. We examined the relationship of income and three demographic variables: age, years of experience, and gender.

Age and years of experience are obviously closely related, although many researchers (including those in the AMA) suggest that years of experience is more sensitive. A correlation of age and years of experience in Massachusetts (which is what we specified in the questionnaire) provides a Pearson correlation coefficient of 0.82, indicating a close alignment of these two variables. Table 4.3 shows the age distribution of the respondents, along with mean and median incomes. This age distribution is quite close to the national profile, as provided by the "Physician Characteristics and Distribution" publication from the AMA (Roback, Randolph, and Seidman 1990). The primary difference is that there are fewer physicians over the age of 65 practicing in western Massachusetts than nationally.

Table 4.4 shows the relationship between years of experience and income (both of which are postresidency), for the western Massachusetts respondents in comparison to the national data using information from one of the SMS interim reports (AMA 1989). Tables 4.3 and 4.4 show that income seems to peak somewhere between 45 and 54, which in western Massachusetts coincides with between 11 and 15 years of experience. As Table 4.4 shows, this pattern is true for physicians nationwide, as well as in western Massachusetts. Others have shown a very similar income pattern with respect to age and years of experience (Langwell and Werner 1980). This pattern of income is not unique to physicians as Figure 4.4 demonstrates, showing income levels for the general male population for five levels of education. For each of the educational levels, income peaks between 45 and 54. The higher the educational level, the more pronounced is the peak. It is very striking that the shape of the curve for the highest educational level is very similar to the curve for physicians that would be drawn from Table 4.4.

Table 4.3 Age and Income (Mean and Median) for Western Massachusetts

Age Category*	n	Percent	Mean Income	Median Income
30–44	409	55.3	93,540	88,600
45–54	183	24.7	113,768	112,400
55–64	103	13.9	101,000	98,100
65 and over	45	6.1	66,489	58,100
Total	740	100.0		

*For one-way ANOVA, the effect of age on income is significant at $p = .001$.

Table 4.4   Mean Income by Years of Experience for National Data and Western Massachusetts Physicians

Years of Experience	National Data		Years of Experience in Massachusetts	Western Massachusetts	
	Males	*Females*		*Males*	*Females*
1–4	110,600	74,000	1–3	97,150	64,232
5–9	145,200	84,900	4–10	101,570	68,790
10–14	158,200	99,400	11–15	107,460	71,260
15 or more	127,200	72,800	16 or more	91,830	61,000

Source: National data from American Medical Association (1989). Income data from 1988.

Table 4.4 raises the important issue of gender as a possible determinant of income, since it shows that women earn less than men for every level of experience, both nationwide and in our particular study area. In our western Massachusetts study, female physicians have a mean income of $67,210 as compared to male physicians' mean income of $103,260. Because of the interest in women in medicine and because there are many complex issues surrounding income differentials due to gender, we will devote Chapter 5 to an examination of women in medicine, with a further analysis of the incomes of male and female physicians, as well as several other variables of interest.

Practice characteristics. There is a relationship between the type of practice arrangement in which physicians work and their level of income. The linkages are not straightforward, due to factors such as specialty and the variety of organizational and financial arrangements used by physicians. Mechanic (1975) set the framework for most research in this area: his survey results indicated that fee-for-service physicians spend more time in direct patient care activities than those in prepaid practice and that fee-for-service physicians work longer hours. This article, which was published during a time in which group practice in general and prepaid arrangements in particular were viewed with distrust, concluded with suggestions related to "improving the responsiveness of prepaid practice."

Despite the historic mistrust of organized group settings, the number of group practices has increased in the United States, as has the number of prepaid practices. The number of groups increased by almost 70 percent from 1969 to 1980, and the number of physicians with some type of group affiliation more than doubled in that period of time. The growth

Figure 4.4 Income Levels for Men by Years of Education

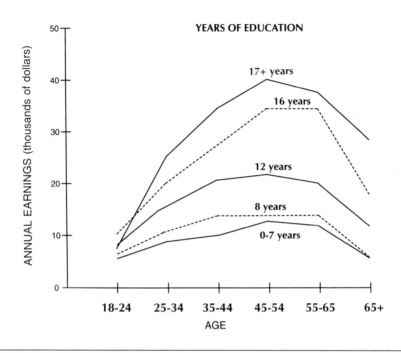

Source: U.S. Bureau of Census data are for males, 1982. Table originally appeared in C. R. McConnell. *Economics: Principles, Problems and Policies,* 10th ed. New York: McGraw-Hill, 1987, p. 665. Copyright 1987 by McGraw-Hill. Material is reproduced by permission of McGraw-Hill, Inc.

of group practice physicians as a percentage of total active physicians rose from 16 percent in 1969 to just over 25 percent in 1980 (Sammons 1982). This increase continued in the early part of the 1980s: between 1980 and 1984, there was an increase of 58 percent in physician positions in group practices. The 1980s also saw an increase in the number of large groups—groups with 100 or more physicians (Crozier and Iglehart 1986). Growth in organized group practices has been dramatic, but not exclusive, since 38 percent of patient care physicians remain in solo practice, although only 20 percent of the youngest physicians (under age 36) are in solo practice (Marder et al. 1988).

Of course, the payment mechanism is also important to consider here, since group practices may be a traditional fee-for-service or they may be prepaid, with physicians receiving income via a fee-for-service model or a salary or capitation model, or some combination. Much of the literature has focused on the effect of these alternative reimbursement patterns on physician behavior. Surveys of physician behavior have been specific to an HMO setting (Hillman, Pauly, and Kerstein 1989), a resident training program (Hickson, Altemeier, and Perrin 1987), and a for-profit ambulatory care center (Hemenway et al. 1990). In all three cases, method of reimbursement seemed to be related to physician behavior, with fee-for-service–reimbursed physicians spending more time in direct patient care. However, the organizations that may employ physicians and their alternative methods for reimbursing physicians are multiple and complex, seldom falling into the neat categories suggested by some of this research. Even HMOs, which have expanded enough to be called the "third compartment," have very diverse organizational structures and several ways of reimbursing physicians, some of which include an agreement that the physicians share revenue losses (Hillman 1990; Tarlov 1986). One can no longer use organizational structure as a proxy for financial arrangement; the two should be accounted for separately.

An additional complication is that physicians represent a more dynamic work force than most research is able to acknowledge. Physicians not only change their practice location, but also their practice specialty. For example, in 1982 the AMA found that 18 percent of physicians in the sample changed their medical specialty in the study period from 1974 to 1978, and 24 percent changed their practice setting (Sammons 1982). Increasingly, it is appropriate to directly survey physicians rather than be dependent on data bases that may be two years old.

Several items were included on our questionnaire to attempt to gather information about several aspects of practice characteristics. Some were more successful than others in terms of quality of data. Perhaps the most successful was the item where physicians were asked to indicate which one of twelve possible practice arrangements was most indicative of their practice (Q-11, Appendix B). For analysis purposes, the four most common categories were identified: solo practice, group practice of three or more, an HMO (in this geographic area, this is a staff model), or a hospital-based practice. Most of the other arrangements had frequencies that were too small to provide meaningful analysis. Although these four categories represent discrete and different practice types, the categories cannot be considered to be immutable. For example, one respondent noted as an aside to this seemingly straightforward question: "Although I describe my practice as a group practice, I am responsible for my solo practice and am accountable for my overhead and my benefits."

Table 4.5 shows the mean and median incomes of these four practice arrangements, the distribution of income within each of the four practice arrangements, and the proportion of respondent group within each practice arrangement. Most of the respondents are involved in either solo practice (30 percent) or in a private group of three or more (35 percent). About 15 percent practice in a hospital setting, and about 10 percent are involved in an HMO-based medical practice.

When comparing the distribution of incomes to what might be expected in the whole sample (reading down this table), those in solo practice have a greater proportion (23 percent) than would be expected (14 percent) in the lowest-income category and smaller proportions (22 percent and 21 percent) than would be expected in both of the two upper-income categories (28 percent and 25 percent). Just the opposite is true for those who practice in a group, since they have a higher proportion than would be expected in the two upper-income categories (32 percent and 39 percent, compared to the expected 28 percent and 25 percent) and a much lower proportion in the lowest-income category (7 percent as compared to 14 percent). In the middle range, there are greater concentrations of HMO physicians and hospital-based physicians. About half of the HMO physicians (49 percent) fall into the middle-income range ($61,000–$100,000), although only 33 percent are expected to be in this category. Hospital-based physicians are also concentrated in the two middle-income categories, between $61,000 and $140,000.

These observations are reinforced by looking at Table 4.5 in another way (reading across): of those who are in the highest-income category, half are involved in group practice. Of those who are in the lowest-income category, half are involved in solo practice. Those in the middle ranges are primarily HMO and hospital-based physicians.

The summary figures for income shown at the bottom of Table 4.5 further support these distributional observations: mean income is highest for those involved in a group practice of three or more ($114,300), followed by hospital-based practices ($96,200), solo practice ($82,900), and HMO physicians ($81,000). These differences are statistically significant, as shown by an analysis of variance test. The difference in median income between the highest and the lowest groups based on practice arrangements is smaller than the $88,400 high-low difference based on specialty designation, but it is still a substantial gap at $33,300.

Considering the types of practice arrangements most often chosen by certain specialty groups, the differences in income are largely (but not completely) explained. Table D.1 (in Appendix D) shows this. The most interesting part of this table comes from reading the table across. For example, the vast majority (78 percent) of the highest-income group (radiologists) are likely to choose to practice in groups of three or more, which is the most lucrative practice arrangement. Anesthesiologists are also very likely to be practicing in a group of three or more. This arrangement does not hold as strongly for surgeons since 58 percent of

Table 4.5 Income Profile of Patient Care Physicians by Practice Arrangement

Income Categories	Distribution in Sample		Practice Arrangement								Totals of Four Practice Groups	
			Group 3 or More		Hospital		Solo Practice		HMO			
	N	%	n	%	n	%	n	%	n	%	n	%
$60,000 or less	103	13.9	18	7.4 (17.5)*	8	7.7 (7.8)	50	23.3 (48.5)	10	14.3 (9.7)	86	13.6
$61,000–$100,000	244	32.9	52	21.5 (21.4)	41	39.4 (16.9)	71	33.0 (29.2)	34	48.6 (14.0)	198	31.4
$101,000–$140,000	210	28.4	77	31.9 (36.7)	38	36.5 (18.1)	48	22.3 (22.9)	22	31.4 (10.5)	185	29.3
$141,000 or more	184	24.8	95	39.2 (51.6)	17	16.4 (9.2)	46	21.4 (25.0)	4	5.7 (2.2)	162	25.7
Total	741	100	242	100 (35%)	104	100 (15%)	215	100 (30%)	70	100 (10%)	631	100.0
Mean		97.5		114.3		96.2		88.6		81.0		
Median		94.4		116.2		92.4		82.9		81.0		

*Numbers in parentheses are calculated across rows; these represent the percentage in that particular arrangement, at that income level. The row percentages do not equal 100% because seven less-common practice arrangements are not reported for each income level.
For a one-way ANOVA, the effect of these four practice arrangements on mean income is statistically significant at $p = .0001$.

general surgeons and 43.5 percent of surgical specialists are practicing in the lower-income solo practice arrangement.

In the lower-income primary care specialties, there is more diversity of practice and also a lower proportion involved in groups of three or more. For example, 54 percent of general and family practitioners shown on this table are involved in solo practice and only 19 percent are in a group of three or more; internists are slightly more balanced, with 27 percent in solo practice and 46.5 percent in a group; pediatricians show the greatest balance, with 27 percent in solo practice, 27 percent in a group practice, and 29 percent in an HMO. For these three primary care specialties, a substantial number (from 18 percent to 29 percent) are in the lowest-income practice arrangement, the HMO model.

In the middle-income range are OB/GYNs and pathologists. Interestingly enough, OB/GYNs have a practice pattern arrangement closer to that of the primary care specialties, with 38 percent involved in a solo practice and 36 percent involved in a group practice, but their incomes are significantly higher than the primary care specialists. Pathology, with an income very similar to OB/GYN, has a more diversified practice pattern, with 64 percent involved in a group practice and only 9 percent in solo settings. Far more pathologists and psychiatrists are found in the second-highest income practice arrangement, the hospital.

Although there is clearly a trend toward locating the higher-income specialties in the higher-income practice arrangements, the relationship is not definitive. For example, 21 percent of those involved in a group practice are internal medicine, while 14 percent of those involved in a group practice are radiologists. As was noted previously, radiologists make almost double what internists make.

It has been a common perception that solo practice is the most lucrative, with HMO-based or hospital-based physicians having the lowest incomes. In our study, solo practice is not as lucrative as either group practice or a hospital-based practice; in fact, it is only more lucrative than an HMO-based practice, which is the lowest-income practice arrangement. Although the AMA data are not as specific as ours, the finding that solo practice is less lucrative than other practice arrangements is also demonstrated in the national data. In the 1990 Socioeconomic Monitoring Survey, the issue of practice patterns is not addressed, but in the 1984 Socioeconomic Monitoring Survey, the AMA noted that physicians in solo practice had a mean income of $100,000, while those in nonsolo practice had a mean income of $111,300 (based on 1983 incomes) (Reynolds and Ohsfeldt 1984). When we divided our practice arrangements in the same way, western Massachusetts physicians who had a solo practice had a mean income of $88,600, and those in a nonsolo practice had a mean income of $102,200. (Nonsolo practices in our study were identified as one of eleven primary practice arrangements, including dual practices, groups of three or more, closed panel/staff model HMOs, hospitals, clinics, nursing homes, federal facilities, etc.) The income differential between solo and nonsolo practice of $13,600 is very similar to the 1984 AMA study.

Another practice arrangement that could affect income is the location of work. In the 1984 AMA study, there was a substantial difference between nonmetropolitan and metropolitan (but still less than 1 million in population) practices, with mean incomes of $87,200 and $111,000, respectively (Reynolds and Ohsfeldt 1984). There are no major metropolitan areas in our study area, but there are more-rural and less-rural medical practices as well as practices located near or in one major urban area. One item in the survey asked physicians to agree or disagree with the statement "I view my practice as being essentially rural." A comparison of responses to this question shows that those who view their practices as primarily rural have a mean income of $91,000, while those viewing their practice as not primarily rural have a mean of $101,000. Once again, the $10,000 differential is very similar in direction to the national figures. As noted earlier, the lack of a large metropolitan area in western Massachusetts may also partially account for the lower average incomes found for our respondents in comparison to the AMA averages for New England and the nation.

Financial arrangements. Although this is an important group of variables to take into consideration in analyzing physician incomes, we had mixed success in being able to collect meaningful information. First, we did not attempt to gather detailed information about practice expenses, choosing instead to use net income as a way to eliminate the need to account for practice expenses, which in 1989 were 44.9 percent of gross revenues for all self-employed physicians (Gonzalez 1991).

We attempted to gather information about various methods of reimbursement, with limited success. For example, respondents were asked to indicate their primary payment method: salary, capitation, or fee-for-service. Since increasingly physicians are paid by a combination of these methods, we asked for an indication of how frequently they receive reimbursement in that way—always, partially, or never. Table D.2 shows that roughly equal proportions of respondents reported salary or fee-for-service as the method of payment they always use. (About 10 percent of our respondents note they have some other arrangements, and these are not shown on this table.) Fee-for-service generates the highest median income; this payment method includes both solo practice, which as we have seen is not very lucrative, and also group practice, which was the highest-income practice arrangement. Table D.3 also suggests this trend: as fee-for-service is used more, income increases, and as salary is used more, income decreases. Of course, it is impossible to determine the exact role of reimbursement method versus practice arrangement in this analysis.

We also gathered information on two other variables related to financial arrangements, but with less success. These will be briefly described here in an effort to share our mistakes so others may benefit and be able to gather more meaningful data. The first of these two variables was the proportion of income that originates from third party payers and the type of third-party reimbursement. We asked physicians to indicate which of several payer categories represented at least 25 percent of their patients, including cash, Medicare, Medicaid, Blue Shield, other commercial carriers, capitated patients, and workers' compensation. Table D.4 compares the "expected" distribution for the whole sample to the distribution by payer, using four income categories. For example, most (65 percent, or 486) patient care physicians have at least 25 percent of their patients paid for by Medicare, and the income distribution for this group is the closest to the expected distribution as found in the total sample. About the same proportion (63 percent) indicated that at least 25 percent of their patients are paid for by Blue Shield, and the distribution across the income groups is also quite similar to what exists in the total sample. Medicaid, which 40 percent (about 299 physicians) indicate represents at least one quarter of their patients, has slightly fewer than expected in the highest-income group and slightly more in the lowest-income group. Only 8.5 percent indicate that at least one-quarter of their patients are paid for by workers' compensation. This payer category is responsible for the greatest divergence from the overall distribution of incomes, with more than expected in the highest-income group.

Although these differences in distribution of incomes are suggestive, there are no conclusions that can be made because of the limitation of the wording of the question. A respondent who says "yes" to Medicare, for example, is indicating that at least 25 percent of his or her patients are paid for by Medicare, but the proportion may actually be much higher. This analysis does seem to indicate that a physician who has at least 25 percent of his or her patients paid for by Medicare (or Medicaid) does not necessarily end up in a lower-income bracket. This merits more attention since it is commonly felt by physicians, and often implied in the research literature (Goessel 1990) and popular press, that a high proportion of Medicare and Medicaid patients produces economic hardship for physicians. The low reimbursements to physicians by these two payer sources would certainly seem to result in a lower income, but our results do not demonstrate this effect.

Although we did not collect information on practice expenses, we did attempt to gather information on malpractice premiums. Malpractice premiums are far from the largest practice expense; the largest is nonphysician wages, which in 1989 was 30 percent of practice revenues, in comparison to malpractice premiums, which were about 5 percent of practice revenues (Gonzalez 1991). Even though malpractice expenses are a relatively small proportion of practice expenses, they are the fastest-growing category (Hough 1988; AMA 1989), and they constitute a particularly sensitive topic for physicians. Although the conflict in Massachusetts is similar to other regions of the country, there are also some aspects of the arrangements for malpractice that are unique to Massachusetts, primarily the retroactive arrangement of payment premiums that was described in Chapter 1. Because of this, we did attempt to gather some information about malpractice, but the results were very disappointing in terms of analysis possibilities. Only about one-half of our respondents pay entirely for their own malpractice insurance. Those who do pay for their own have incomes distributed generally like the whole sample, although there is a slight tendency for these self-payers to have incomes skewed toward the lower end. There does not seem to be any clear relationship between income and who pays for malpractice; although 56 percent of the highest-income group pay entirely for malpractice themselves, 65 percent of the lowest-income group also pay entirely for malpractice themselves. The malpractice premium burden is obviously not spread evenly across the specialties, but we did not ask for detailed financial information on the exact amounts that are paid by each specialty.

All of these financial arrangements—including method of reimbursement, type of third party payer, and malpractice expenses—are important variables, affecting income and satisfaction of physicians. In all cases, we needed more detailed information to produce a meaningful analysis.

Hours worked per week. Because of our efforts to standardize or adjust estimates of physician supply as described in Chapter 3, we became interested in how many hours a week physicians work and also what proportion of time they spend in direct patient care activities, since these are more likely to be income generating. There is a fair amount of literature available on hours worked per week as a productivity measure. Historically, physicians have had a pattern of work hours that is closest to the model of the self-employed professional, a group that is well known for working a lot of hours in a week. For example, in 1979 the "wage and salary worker" (a major category used in analyzing labor statistics) worked an average of 38.4 hours/week, while the self-employed person worked 41.9 hours/week; physicians in that same year worked an average of 49.7 hours (Freiman and Marder 1984). Most of the research on hours worked per week is descriptive, often showing trends over time, and is generally drawn from AMA data, although some studies have utilized primary surveys of physicians just for this purpose (Kehrer, Sloan, and Woolridge 1984). Hours worked per week is often used in the supply argument; in that context one may find arguments that are contradictory, such as the contention that physician hours worked per week has increased by 21 percent (Schwartz and Mendelson 1990), while others note that the physician total workweek has remained stable (Hughes 1988). AMA data from the Socioeconomic Characteristics of Practice over the period 1982–1989 indicate a fairly steady level of total professional hours worked per week, as well as number of patient care hours per week and weeks practiced in a year. In 1982, physicians worked an average of 57 hours per week and in 1989 this had risen to 58.8 hours per week (Gonzalez 1991).

Intuition would suggest that working more hours per week would result in higher incomes. Although several articles have addressed the issue of hours worked per week, these have not attempted to relate this measure of productivity to estimates of income. Even Langwell and Werner (1980), who did a very careful economic analysis of the relative importance of income and hours worked on physician location, did not relate productivity to income level. They did conclude that the distribution of physicians by specialty and by urban/rural location indicated that hours worked per week was relatively more important as a decision factor than income. And certainly, the relatively high incomes of physicians are often explained in terms of how many hours per week and weeks per year they practice. Physicians do work a substantial number of hours— our respondents average 58 hours per week (the national average, as shown by the AMA) and, as we showed in Chapter 3, very few work less than 40 hours per week.

It is also important to calculate what physicians do within those working hours, since physicians do a variety of activities, some of which involve direct patient care and some of which represent other professional activities. Even within the category of direct patient care hours, some procedure-intensive activities are more highly reimbursed than are other patient care activities.

As was demonstrated in Chapter 3, data were collected on the various professional activities of physicians in the same format used by the AMA to facilitate comparisons to this national data base. Physicians in western Massachusetts average about 48 hours per week in activities that can be described as patient care activities; the national average from the most recent SMS survey is 53.3 hours per week spent in direct patient care activities (Gonzalez 1991). This varies somewhat by specialty; Figure 4.5 shows our western Massachusetts data and the national data drawn from the AMA. Physicians in western Massachusetts have a remarkably similar pattern of professional activities. The biggest difference is that internists in western Massachusetts spend a lower proportion of their time doing surgery than seems to be true nationally (22 percent compared to 30 percent). For three specialties—internal medicine, surgery, and pediatrics—western Massachusetts physicians are more likely to have a higher proportion of their patient visits categorized as falling into the "other" category.

We are particularly interested in the relationship of these hours worked to income levels, which is not as direct as we had anticipated. Table 4.6 shows the average hours worked per week by four income levels. Physicians who make between $61,000 and $100,000 do work about eight hours per week more than those who make less than $60,000, thus reinforcing the intuitive notion that those who work more hours earn more money. This difference is statistically significant. However, there is essentially no difference in total average hours worked per week between the two upper-income groups, despite the considerable difference in income levels between the two top categories. Those in the lowest-income category clearly spend less time in direct care activities, but there is practically no difference between the upper three income categories in time spent in direct patient care. The ratio of direct care hours to indirect care hours is highest for the $61,000 to $100,000 income range. There is no significant relationship between time spent in indirect care and income.

Since specialty is obviously related to income, particularly through reimbursement patterns, it is important to examine hours worked per week by specialty. Table 4.7 shows this, using the same nine specialty groupings used previously. Three specialty groups average the highest total hours per week (61.6–62.7). These three (anesthesiology, OB/GYN, and surgical specialties) also have three of the highest median incomes. However, the group with one of the lowest total average hours per week, radiologists, commands the very highest median income of the nine groups listed. The incomes of general/family practice, pediatrics, and internal medicine are all significantly lower than for radiology, but the average total hours worked per week is much higher.

Table 4.7 also allows the examination of whether income is related to the proportion of time spent in direct patient care. The top-income group (radiology) spends less hours per week in direct patient care than the other top-income specialties (surgical, anesthesiology, and OB/GYN). Internal medicine specialists spend the same number of hours performing direct patient care, but realize a much lower income. The two lowest-income specialties (general/family practice and pediatrics) spend 84–85 percent of their time in direct care and the two highest-income specialties (radiology and surgery) spend 82–83 percent of their time in direct care.

Figure 4.5 Distribution of Average Patient Care Hours per Week: Western Massachusetts Physicians Compared to National Figures

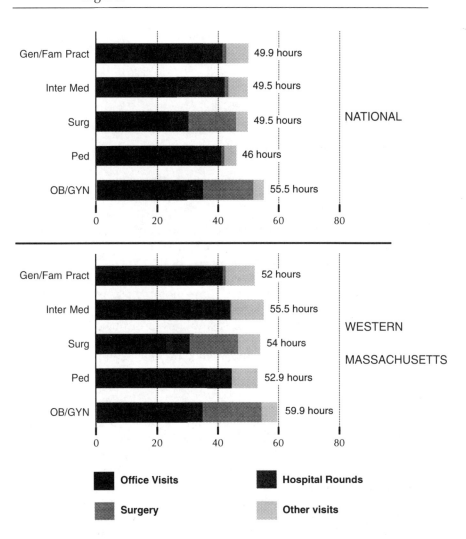

The three "middle income" groups are more variable, spending anywhere from 68 percent to 90 percent of their time in direct care.

There seems to be some relationship between total hours worked per week and income, but not between proportion of time spent in direct patient care and income, and specialty differences may be more

Table 4.6   Average Hours Worked Each Week for Practicing Physicians, by Income Level

Income Categories	Mean Direct Care Hours*	Mean Indirect Care Hours*	Mean Total Hours*	Ratio of Direct Care Hours to Indirect Care Hours
$60,000 or less	39.4	12.0	50.0	3.3:1
$61,000–$100,000	48.5	9.2	56.8	5.3:1
$101,000–$140,000	50.3	12.1	60.7	4.1:1
$141,000 or more	51.5	10.0	60.6	5.1:1

*Figures represent mean hours spent in direct or indirect care and mean total hours, for all active physicians in the indicated income bracket. Indirect and direct hour means do not always equal total hour means, because not every physician reported direct, indirect, and total hours.

important here. The average workweek is about 58 hours per week for all physicians. For those earning under $60,000 per year, this average is less, about 49 hours per week. For those earning $141,000 or more, the average workweek is more, 61 hours. However, the average workweek for those who earn $100,000 is the same as for those who earn more than $141,000, so obviously the differences in hours worked per week do not completely account for the vast ranges of income in the sample. Other factors, such as specialty (reflecting reimbursement patterns), are clearly more important. Also, as we will show in Chapter 5, gender has a significant effect on income.

Summary. All of the preceding tables and discussion provide an array of variables that in some way help to explain the variation in physician income. Of the many factors identified as shaping physician income, questions necessarily arise about which have the greatest influence, especially when the potential interactions of various factors, such as specialty and gender, are considered. For this purpose, a multiple regression analysis was performed to identify which variables created the most explanatory model for predicting physician income in western Massachusetts. The statistical method fit linear regression models by least squares; qualitative variables were transformed to fit a linear analysis (SAS Institute 1988). The following independent variables were used: primary care, solo practice, group practice, hospital practice, HMO, age (rather than experience), gender, hours worked per week, rural location of practice, and fee-for-service. The only reimbursement is fee-for-service (1 = always; 3 = never), since the missing values for the other reimbursement method

Table 4.7 Hours Worked and Income by Modified Specialty Groups of Patient Care Physicians

Specialty Groups†	Average Hours Worked per Week			Income (Thousands of Dollars)	
	Total Hours	Direct Care	Indirect Care	Mean	Median
1. General/Family Practice	57.4	48.0	11.0	66.5	63.8
2. Pediatrics	56.6	48.4	9.3	72.7	69.1
3. Internal Medicine	59.6	52.5	7.7	77.7	76.9
4. Psychiatry	47.6	35.2	13.4	79.0	77.8
5. Pathology	50.1	33.9	30.3	109.6	112.9
6. Obstetrics/Gynecology	64.1	57.4	6.7	121.4	126.2
7. Anesthesiology	61.9	53.5	8.9	122.2	122.7
8. Surgery	61.6	51.4	10.8	125.4	141.0
9. Radiology	50.8	41.6	12.2	141.0	152.1

For a one-way ANOVA, the effect of specialty on the column variable:

$F = 7.94(8df)^*$ $F = 11.64(8df)^*$ $F = 5.59(8df)^*$ $F = 43.74(8df)^*$

$^*Pr > F = .0001$.
†Specialty groups omit "other medical specialty" and all "others." Only half the pathologists record any direct care hours; most (78%) record indirect hours.

questions (capitation, salary, or other financial arrangements) were too high to include in the analysis, and fee-for-service was associated with the highest levels of income.

Table 4.8 shows the standardized B coefficient for each of the independent variables. The range is from +1 to −1, with those values closest to zero having no significance. As can be seen from this table, the best predictors of income are being in a specialty other than primary care, being in a practice arrangement other than solo practice, being a male of a slightly younger age, working more hours per week, and having a less rural location. The adjusted r^2-value reveals that all of these variables taken together account for only about 38 percent of the total variance. This relatively low proportion of variance accounted for may be partly explained by the difficulty in gathering adequate information on an exceptionally complicated aspect of medical practice. As we discovered, collecting accurate information about financial arrangements requires a serious and concentrated effort. Many of the categories offered to respondents do not completely represent reality, which is an indication of the need for more descriptive research. Additionally, not all variables fit a linear model: variations in income due to age, for example, are in a curvilinear pattern, which results in income peaking during middle age.

Despite the relatively small proportion of variance accounted for, the one variable that clearly stands out is that of specialty. As specialty

Table 4.8   Multiple Linear Regression Model for Identifying Predictors of Income

Primary Care	−0.45*
Solo Practice	−0.18*
Group Practice	0.09(n.s.)†
Hospital Practice	−0.04(n.s.)
Health Maintenance Organization	−0.02(n.s.)
Age	−0.09***
Gender	−0.21*
Hours Worked	0.17*
Rural Location	0.08***
Fee-for-Service	−0.05(n.s.)
Experience	—
Adjusted r^2	.3847

*$p < .001$.
**$p < .01$.
***$p < .05$.
****$p < .10$.

†n.s. = nonsignificant.

increasingly predicts income, the disparities between physicians have increased. This suggests that society places different values on the skills and abilities of different types of physicians. The increasing income discrepancy also has consequences for the medical profession itself, primarily by changing the peer group with whom a physician feels most closely identified. Specialty and subspecialty identification has become much more relevant than has the professional identity of "being a physician." The income and job experience of a primary care physician is increasingly removed from the income and job experience of a surgeon. Very little is known about how physicians view their incomes and the incomes of other physicians. We conclude this chapter by presenting some results that reflect the perceptions of physicians about their incomes.

Perceptions of physicians about income

Gathering information about people's perceptions of the adequacy of their income is an interesting process. In this study, we examined this by doing a content analysis of the several personal anecdotes given to us by respondents, by analyzing responses to several questionnaire items that asked for perceptions of income, and by asking physicians about their perceptions of their medical practice and whether they are currently working at full capacity. As might be expected, there is a large variation in these responses, but, in general, the pattern that emerges is one of physicians being motivated by many factors other than just maximizing income.

Personal anecdotes. Specialty identification does not necessarily predict a physician's perception of his or her income, although a radiologist made the comment: "I enjoy my work and feel that I am quite well compensated for it. Probably overcompensated." This physician acknowledged the income differences of primary care physicians by continuing: "I know many primary care physicians who don't feel that they can make an adequate living."

Physicians give a variety of reasons for negative perceptions about their incomes, with many of them directed at the state of Massachusetts. One respondent noted, "Neither the young solo practitioner nor, like myself, the older physician, can afford to practice in Massachusetts because of excessive malpractice premiums that will frequently equal his income, leaving only the independently wealthy available." An emergency room physician targeted the ban on balance billing in his comment: "I work in an extremely busy (62,000 patients/year) intense (30 admissions/day) emergency department. No appointments, turn no one away. We bill for services rendered and have a collection rate of 40 percent. We can't balance bill. We work *hard*, lose money and lose good physicians every year." A gastroenterologist blamed insurance when he noted:

> My hours are increasing, my income falling. The PPOs and BC/BS are squeezing the fees at the same time the malpractice costs are limitless. The press is anti-physician and adds to the depressing environment. If I move into academic medicine I probably would do better financially but I would see less patients and service the community less effectively. The greatest waste in medical costs are insurance forms. My overhead increases every year to fill them out and I get less and less.

For almost all physician respondents, comments about money become comments about their feelings about the medical profession, or sometimes the state legislative environment. One female pediatrician put her current experiences into the context of her expectations by relating the following:

> I did not go into medicine to be rich although I knew I would probably be financially secure in the profession. I used to love to go to work and interact with my patients. Now I can't wait until I can retire; I feel burnt out. I feel like a battered person. I resent the fact that my decisions regarding patient care are preempted by evaluators in a telephone call by people who do not know the patient and make decisions for dollars and cents instead of patient needs.

Many respondents indicated anger; for example, an internist gave us a lengthy comment that details the frustration of primary care physicians with reimbursement:

> I opened my office in 1983—solo practice with the idealistic desire to give "holistic" medical care, with an emphasis on patient education and prevention of disease. In the three years I ran my office, my practice income decreased 5% every year, the hours I worked increased, and I came to feel that my practice was literally killing me. I could not get paid for the actual time I spent with patients.

Several respondents spoke about changes they felt they had been forced to make, primarily as a result of economic pressures. One respondent said, "I retired when my expenses and insurance indicated that I could no longer make a profit in medicine after practicing 35 years.... Following me in retirement soon after were six other physicians on our staff."

Reading over the many comments on the survey and reflecting on the numerous personal conversations that we have had with physicians have caused us to appreciate the complexity of the perceptions that physicians have about their profession. Although these personal anecdotes provide valuable insights, we recognize the difficulty in drawing conclusions based entirely on these comments. The next section presents a more systematic way of evaluating physician perceptions about their incomes.

Responses to questionnaire items. Physicians had two opportunities to respond directly to attitude-type items regarding their incomes. The first item simply asked about how satisfactory the "income of my practice" is. A small minority of respondents noted that their income was either very satisfactory (7 percent) or very unsatisfactory (4 percent). A little over one half view their income as satisfactory, while one quarter view their income as unsatisfactory. A slightly higher percentage of females respond that they are satisfied with their incomes (65 percent), and there are no differences by age. Physicians in HMO practice settings are far more likely to indicate their incomes are "satisfactory"—75 percent of the HMO physicians responded this way. This response is even more impressive in view of the fact that HMO physicians had significantly lower incomes than other practice settings. When responses to this one item are examined by specialty, anesthesiologists have the lowest percentage of a satisfied response (40 percent), while 75 percent of radiologists are satisfied with their incomes.

A second item asked physicians to evaluate their income in terms of "the amount of work I do." Responses to this question produce slightly lower levels of satisfaction, as might be expected. Although still only a minority indicate strong agreement or disagreement, it is interesting to note that this anchor response has shifted to 10 percent strongly disagreeing with this statement. About 40 percent indicate their satisfaction with their income in light of their work load, and close to the same percentage (35 percent) are dissatisfied.

We did examine whether income level predicted the response to these items (Table 4.9). For both items that address perception of income, those in the highest-income category are more likely to agree or strongly agree with these two statements, although a smaller percentage exhibit agreement to the second item, which incorporates perceptions of the work load. Income does not seem to affect overall satisfaction with their medical practice, as the responses to the third item indicate.

Perception of capacity of practice. Many of the comments made by physician respondents focused on the sheer number of hours physicians work—a common emphasis of literature that focuses on physician perception of medical practice, especially when examining the "lifestyle" of physicians. We were interested in trying to identify some additional parameters of this particular perception. Physicians may—and obviously do—work a substantial number of hours, but not all such hours are

Table 4.9 Responses to Three Satisfaction Items from Questionnaire by Income Levels

	Less than $60,000				$61,000–$100,000				$101,000–$140,000				$141,000–$160,000			
	103		13.9		244		32.9		210		28.4		184		24.8	
	Agree/S.A.		Disagree/S.D.		Agree/S.A.		Disagree/S.D.		Agree/S.A.		Disagree/S.D.		Agree/S.A.		Disagree/S.D.	
Distribution in Sample	n	%	n	%	n	%	n	%	n	%	n	%	n	%	n	%
I.	50	54.4	42	45.6	134	61.7	83	38.3	127	65.1	68	34.9	138	78.4	38	21.6
II.	45	46.4	52	53.6	98	45.6	117	54.4	91	47.6	100	52.4	98	61.2	62	38.8
III.	55	66.2	28	33.8	141	68.1	66	31.9	100	59.8	67	40.2	97	65.1	52	34.9

Notes:
I. = Satisfaction with income of my practice (Chi-square is significant at .05 level).
II. = Current income is satisfactory for amount of work I do (Chi-square is significant at .05 level).
III. = All things considered, I am satisfied with my work (not significant).

equally reimbursed. In Massachusetts, some analysts claim that physicians earn less than those in other regions of the country because there are more physicians in Massachusetts competing for limited patients. Of course, this assumes that Massachusetts physicians must be working fewer hours than physicians in other regions of the country. Other arguments about physicians limiting their medical practices are also specific to Massachusetts, including the allegation that some physicians—especially surgeons and obstetricians—were restricting their practices due to increased regulatory pressures, which might result in decreased services for consumers. On a national level, the human resources supply literature increasingly discusses physicians restricting hours of practice for lifestyle choices, and it is commonly alleged that women work fewer hours than male physicians.

All of this—the specific case of Massachusetts and the more general discussion within the published literature—leads us to wonder how physicians define being at whatever they might term "full professional capacity." We used a fairly open question to elicit personal feelings (Q-6, Appendix B): "Are you currently practicing at your full professional capacity? If NO, are you satisfied [or not satisfied] with current level of your practice?" This question allowed participants to define the issue for themselves based on their own expectations and perception.

The overwhelming majority of all patient care physicians (78 percent) indicated to us that they are practicing at what they consider to be full professional capacity, with only 22 percent noting that they are not practicing at their full professional capacity. Interpretation of this particular finding may differ between researchers and policymakers or administrators active in any particular state or region. To a researcher, this is fairly straightforward: 78 percent of the physicians consider themselves to be at their definition of full professional capacity. However, a state planner or an advocate for the medical community would argue that at least one out of five of this region's physicians consider themselves to be underutilized—a significant potential resource.

Table 4.10 provides a profile of the physician respondents' view of whether they are practicing at full capacity, by income and gender. There is some relationship between income and perceived capacity, since a greater proportion of those "not at full capacity" are to be found in the lower income levels, while a greater proportion of those at full capacity are in the upper incomes. It is not clear, however, whether income level determines the perception of capacity or whether professional capacity determines income.

Over all income levels, a greater proportion of men (81 percent) than women (61 percent) perceive themselves as being fully utilized professionally. This distribution is apparently not entirely by individual

Table 4.10 Physicians Practicing at Full Professional Capacity by Gender

| | Totals | | | | Males | | | | Females | | | |
| | At Full Professional Capacity | | Not at Full Capacity | | At Full Capacity | | Not at Full Capacity | | At Full Capacity | | Not at Full Capacity | |
Income Categories	n	%	n	%	n	%	n	%	n	%	n	%
$60,000 or less	51	9.2	51	32.1	36	7.3	28	23.3	15	24.6	22	57.9
$61,000–100,000	184	33.0	50	31.5	155	31.3	38	31.7	29	47.5	12	31.6
$101,000–140,000	174	31.2	32	20.1	161	32.5	30	25.0	13	21.3	2	5.3
Over $141,000	148	26.6	26	16.4	144	29.0	24	20.0	4	6.6	2	5.3
Totals	557	100.0	159	100.0	496	100.0	120	100.0	61	100.0	38	100.0
	$p < .001$		$p < .001$		$p < .001$		$p < .001$		$p < .001$		$p < .001$	

choice, since of those not practicing at full capacity, only 45 percent of the men and 76 percent of the women are satisfied with their current level of practice. Of course, we cannot determine from this whether working at less than full capacity is dictated by personal, professional, or market constraints, but this question will be addressed in more detail in Chapter 5, when we consider the research surrounding women in medicine.

We also examined whether perception of being at full capacity is related to practice arrangements. Solo practice has a lower proportion of physicians who view themselves as being at full capacity, while those in hospitals, group practices, and HMO settings all have higher percentages who view themselves as being fully utilized. These associations are not directly related to income. The higher-income arrangements—group practice and hospitals—seem to have physicians who view themselves as being more fully utilized; of the two lower-income arrangements, solo practice physicians have a low perception of utilization, while HMO physicians are more likely to view themselves as being at full capacity (Table D.5).

Further analysis focused on whether there were any significant differences between specialties in terms of perceiving themselves to be at full professional capacity. Table D.6 shows that there does not seem to be a clear pattern. The lower-income specialties (general/family practice and pediatrics) have roughly the same proportion of physicians who indicate they are at full professional capacity as the higher-income surgical specialties and obstetrics/gynecology. General surgeons (who have a much higher income level) have a significantly lower number indicating that they are at their full professional capacity. Radiology and anesthesiology both have very high rates of physicians indicating that they are at their full professional capacity. Table D.5 shows the perception of full capacity for male and female physicians for the six specialties for which there are enough females for comparison.

The allegation has been made that within Massachusetts surgeons and obstetricians especially have restricted their practices due to the unfriendly medical practice climate. In our study, about one third of general surgeons, 28 percent of surgical specialists, and 22 percent of obstetrics-gynecologists indicate they are not practicing at their full professional capacity. However, 28 percent of general/family practitioners and 20 percent of psychiatrists, internists, and pediatricians also indicate they are not practicing at their full professional capacity.

Being at full professional capacity is something that the physician respondents were allowed to define for themselves. There may be real differences in perceptions and expectations for specialty groups; for example, general surgeons may very well have a different perception of what it means to be "at full professional capacity" than does someone in general and family practice. Likewise, someone in solo practice may have a different perception of being at full capacity than an HMO-based physician, whose schedule is more likely to be controlled by an external organizational schedule. There may also be gender differences in perception of full capacity. Table D.5 seems to support the importance of such expectations. Parts III–V of this table include only those physicians who view themselves as being at full professional capacity. For both practice arrangement and specialty, it seems that there is some variation in average number of hours worked. For example, those who consider themselves to be at full capacity in an HMO setting work 57 hours per week in comparison to the 61 hours per week for those physicians in a group practice setting. The range is larger for specialties: psychiatrists who define themselves as being at full capacity work an average of 49 hours per week while OB/GYN specialists defining themselves as being full capacity work 68 hours per week.

We cannot tell from this limited analysis what personal or environmental factors may contribute to the perception that someone is not practicing at his or her full professional capacity. However, it is important to investigate this further, since understanding the perceptions of physicians in terms of what type of professional work load they expect will help us understand better their perceptions about their income as well as other important aspects of the medical profession.

Summary. The insights gained from examining physicians' perceptions of their incomes in some ways complete the picture resulting from the empirical results and in some ways demonstrate how much more needs to be determined about physician perceptions.

Although physicians—like every other professional group—expect money for their services, physicians in western Massachusetts do not seem motivated entirely by money. A constant theme through the personal comments is that the income-limiting regulations within the state of Massachusetts are often viewed negatively because of inequity or unfairness, not primarily because of income limitations. This is particularly true of the ban on balance billing, which physicians view as providing one company (Blue Cross/Blue Shield) with too much power, and the retroactive malpractice premiums, which physicians view as being unfair. Toward other regulations that are also income restricting, physicians are much more sanguine. For example, 25 percent of respondents found inpatient reimbursements to be at least satisfactory and only 12 percent rated them as very unsatisfactory. Thirty-eight percent find utilization reviews to be at least satisfactory, and 30 percent find professional review organizations to be at least satisfactory. Even a piece of legislation proposing mandatory Medicaid participation was viewed as being satisfactory to 23 percent, although a greater proportion did find this very unsatisfactory. Finally, in response to queries about the reasonableness of the base medical malpractice premiums, 16 percent found these satisfactory; although that is a small percentage, one would not expect any physician to indicate any level of acceptance. Additionally, only 32 percent find malpractice premiums to be very unsatisfying.

The responses of physicians to the more qualitative, perception-based questions presented in this section show that the topic of income is complicated, and level of satisfaction is partly predicted by expectations that seem to be influenced by significant peer groups. Physicians are sensitive to the income inequities in medicine—many respondents acknowledged the vast income differences between primary care physicians and specialists.

Finally, income is more than money to these respondents—income has a very clear symbolic connotation. Almost all the comments regarding money also included thoughts about the professional respect accorded physicians and how they are regarded today. One of the more direct comments was made by an internist who said: "When I started medical school in 1976, I thought I'd make about $60,000/year, in 1976 dollars. That's how much I'm making today in 1989 dollars. I think medicine is a declining profession in terms of power, privilege, and prestige." An emergency room physician noted the following:

> I think that there is a generally negative attitude towards physicians in Massachusetts. It is reflected in increased governmental control of Medicare and the health care industry; increasingly punitive Board of Registration in Medicine; increasingly high priced malpractice insurance; health insurance industry capping amounts that physicians can earn.

A particularly poignant comment comes from an oncologist:

> I feel that we are looked at as "bad, malicious, and malevolent" . . . health care is being rationed—not "unnecessary cost cutting"—and we're the *sole* reason for health cost. We are not! Just look at our salaries. Docs as a whole are just as—if not more—honest and honorable than any other group, and more ethical. We're on your side to help—not hurt.

Summary, Conclusions, and Recommendations

This chapter has focused on physician income including those factors that determine physician incomes, how physicians feel about income, and the various methodological issues involved in examining this important variable. Some of the empirical results from the survey are similar to what others have found. The top income specialties in western Massachusetts mirror the national picture: radiologists, surgical specialists, anesthesiologists, and obstetricians constitute the highest-income categories. The lowest-income specialties are in primary care: general/family practice, internal medicine, pediatrics, and psychiatry. There is a $88,400 differential between the highest-income and lowest-income specialties.

As in the national profile, female physicians in western Massachusetts earn less than male physicians—$36,000 less every year. Because of our interest in this topic, we will devote the next chapter to a further exploration of this gender gap. Also, similar to the national profile, younger physicians earn less. The actual dollar figures for income are substantially lower in all of New England than nationally. The overall median income for respondents in western Massachusetts is $94,400, in comparison to the national median value of $120,000.

Despite our preconceptions, median incomes for solo practice are near the bottom; only HMO physicians make less. Physicians in group practice make substantially more than any other practice arrangement. Another preconception that was not supported by the results of this survey concern productivity, as measured by total hours worked per week and by hours per week spent in direct patient care. Physicians in western Massachusetts—and nationally—work a substantial number of hours per week: 58 is the average, with about 85 percent of these hours spent in direct care activities. Although there is a relationship between hours worked and income, this is only present at the extremes; that is, the very lowest hours worked per week produces less income than the highest hours worked per week. The relationship is not as direct as we had anticipated, since there is very little difference in hours worked per week across income categories that represent a difference of $80,000.

These variables—age, gender, specialty, practice setting, and productivity—are interrelated, although the interactions are not completely clear for all possible combinations. For example, does group practice produce a higher income because higher-income specialties are more likely to be involved in group practices? Although the vast majority of the highest-income group (radiologists) are more likely to practice in groups of three or more, this pattern is not true for surgeons, since 43 percent of this second-highest income group is in solo practice. A multivariate analysis demonstrated that—of all the variables considered—specialty had the highest effect on income, but even considering all four variables, only 38 percent of the variance could be accounted for.

Income is a far more complicated variable for physicians than it is for most researchers. For physicians, it is not only the actual amount of money received for services; it is also a representation of their position within the health care system. Nearly every comment made to us about money was in the context of the professional respect and autonomy that income represents.

Physicians in our study are not unhappy with their incomes, even though these income levels are substantially less than the national comparisons. Interestingly, physicians who demonstrate the highest level of satisfaction with their incomes are those in the lowest-income practice setting, an HMO. Another finding of interest is that the perception of being at "full professional capacity" is not directly related to income: actually, general surgeons have a relatively low proportion of physicians who feel they are at full capacity in comparison to primary care physicians. These findings all suggest the importance of including physician perceptions, and especially expectations, in any study concerning income.

In addition to these results, much of the contribution of this chapter lies in assessing several methodological issues that are critical to being able to successfully analyze physician incomes.

Methodological issues

Most of the information on income currently available to researchers is descriptive, but there is an unfortunate level of inaccuracy due primarily to definitional problems. One example is the general confusion between net and adjusted incomes, especially when the study data are being compared to AMA data. Adjusted incomes should only be used in the context of data over time, since they are incomes adjusted for inflation. Most studies have a cross-sectional design, and the most appropriate comparison (especially when using AMA data) is, therefore, net incomes. Net incomes are also the most appropriate to use for international comparisons, since practice expenses are so different for U.S. physicians.

When gathering information from physicians about income, it is important to recognize the difficulty, since this is a sensitive area. However, we learned that physicians will report actual incomes; it is not necessary to use categories. Using the question worded the same way as the AMA seems acceptable to physicians.

However, it is important to be more clear about all the parameters of physician income. There is a very low level of understanding about the many financial aspects of a physician's practice. For example, on-call hours are often reimbursed separately; these need to be included as a separate category. In our study—as in most of the AMA studies—it is not known whether physicians included these in their net income estimates. Another category that needs to be separately identified is income realized from medical investments, an area that is increasing.

Researchers used to assume that a particular organizational structure implies a certain method of payment. If this once was true, it certainly is no longer so. We learned the hard way in this survey that to collect information on financial arrangements is a daunting task. It is important to consider both method of reimbursement and types of third party payers as well as specifying all sources of income from medicine. In our study, some intriguing trends arose, but, because of the limitations of the data, we are not able to conclude much.

One area that has been almost totally overlooked is that of perceptions of physicians about incomes. Our results indicate this area needs serious investigation. Ignoring physician perceptions, as well as the general misunderstanding of the various complexities about exactly how physicians earn money, has led to physicians being defensive about discussing income—primarily because physicians view income as far more than most researchers: to physicians it is an important symbol of professional respect and trust.

Of course, specialty is a very important determinant of income. Our study showed this, as has every other study. Even this fact reinforces the point made previously, however. It is well known that procedure-intensive specialists make more money than primary care specialists, and certainly the reimbursement system is a large contributor to this difference. However, we feel there are other important differences about which there is inadequate information. Information on financial arrangements, including on-call hours and all practice expenses (including malpractice premiums), needs to be detailed by specialty and by organizational arrangement. This suggestion recalls the nomenclature problem discussed in Chapter 3. It is important to standardize the nomenclature for specialty groups so that accurate income profiles can be developed for each specialty.

Finally, although multivariate analytic techniques are obviously useful here, it is important that the right variables be entered in the analysis. This will only occur after careful univariate and bivariate analysis of this additional information.

Directions for future research

Many of the methodological suggestions noted above are directed at increasing the ability to measure income accurately so that additional avenues of research can be explored. This study, as most others, provides direction for future research primarily by indicating those areas in which a better understanding of physicians needs to be developed. In many cases, the lack of knowledge affects policy development, which will be the subject of the last chapter. The results generated by this study and the several problems we experienced collecting information suggest a general lack of information about what factors influence physician income. There are four specific areas in which more research is particularly important.

The first is in the area of specialty, which, although extensively researched, has also been hampered by the use of nonstandardized nomenclature. What is known is that some specialties make more than others, presumably primarily because of reimbursement. What is not known is what other factors besides reimbursement affect income. Also unknown is the behavioral response physicians make; little is understood about the pattern of practice changes of physicians in response to regulatory pressure. For example, do physicians move from more general to more specialized practices—or move between subspecialties—in order to maximize income?

A second area in which more research is needed relates to practice settings. Physicians are increasingly moving into more organized practice settings, which affects their income and their level of satisfaction, but little is known about what physicians gain and lose by becoming employees. Some physicians choose more organized practice settings, but little is known about factors that encourage them to stay. Physician turnover is a widespread problem among most HMOs, and more knowledge about what physicians expect in organized settings is clearly needed.

Related to both of these areas is the vast morass of what are generally referred to as financial arrangements. It is this area in which we had the most difficulty in collecting relevant and useful data. An instructive example concerns practice costs, a topic that generated many personal anecdotes. One radiologist retired "because malpractice costs are greater than 50 percent of my gross income. When medical license costs, medical education costs, and all other professional costs are added on top of this, my net income was $2000.00." A general surgeon noted that his practice costs were 75 percent of his gross income. These anecdotes are in conflict with the national profile, which generally views practice expenses as being about 45 percent of gross income. Physicians and researchers may be counting different expenses, a difference that needs to be reconciled. Part of this is the problem of measuring productivity. We used a measure of total hours worked per week and number of hours in direct patient care. Not all hours a physician works are equally reimbursable. It is important to standardize this estimate: use of a direct care equivalent standard suggested in Chapter 3 should also be utilized here.

A fourth area in which more research is needed concerns assessing perceptions of physicians—a problem in both perspective and measurement. Researchers, as well as administrators, need to want to better understand physicians and their views without judgment. The physician view of the medical field is understandably their own, but it is a view that needs to be heard and understood. Once it is determined to be valuable to assess physician perceptions, the measurement problem arises. Measuring physician perspectives is admittedly difficult. Personal statements of respondents have been used throughout this book to highlight some of the respondents' feelings, but the limitations of relying exclusively on this type of data are well recognized. Chapter 6 presents a more quantitative measure for physician satisfaction—six separate indexes used to measure physician perceptions about medical practice. Use of these indexes in research will assist in further defining physician perspectives.

References

American Medical Association. *SMS Report: Trends in Physician Compensation.* Vol. 3. Chicago: AMA, November 1989.

Clare, L. F., E. Spratley, P. Schwab, and J. K. Iglehart. "Trends in Health Personnel: Data Watch." *Health Affairs* (Winter 1987): 91–103.

Crozier, D. A., and J. K. Iglehart. "Data Watch: Trends in Health Manpower." *Health Affairs* (Winter 1986): 122–31.

Freiman, M. P., and W. D. Marder. "Changes in the Hours Worked by Physicians, 1970–1980." *American Journal of Public Health* 74 (1984): 1348–52.

Ginzberg, E., E. Brann, D. Hiestand, and M. Ostow. "The Expanding Physician Supply and Health Policy: The Clouded Outlook." *Milbank Memorial Fund Quarterly* 50 (1981): 508–41.

Goessel, E. A. "A Practicing Physician's Experience." *Bulletin of New York Academy of Medicine* 66 (Jan.–Feb. 1990): 64–70.

Gonzalez, M. L. *Socioeconomic Characteristics of Medical Practice 1990/91.* Chicago: AMA Center for Health Policy Research, 1991.

Gonzalez, M. L., and D. W. Emmons. *Socioeconomic Characteristics of Medical Practice 1989.* Chicago: AMA Center for Health Policy Research, 1989.

Hemenway, D., A. Killen, S. B. Cashman, C. L. Parks, and W. J. Bickwell. "Physicians' Responses to Financial Incentives: Evidence from a For-Profit Ambulatory Care Center." *New England Journal of Medicine* 322 (1990): 1059–63.

Hickson, G. B., W. A. Altemeier, and J. M. Perrin. "Physician Reimbursement by Salary or Fee-for-Service: Effect on Physician Practice Behavior in a Randomized Prospective Study." *Pediatrics* 80 (1987): 344–50.

Hillman, A. L. "Financial Incentives for Physicians in HMOs: Is There a Conflict of Interest?" *New England Journal of Medicine* 317 (1987): 1743–48.

Hillman, A. L. "Health Maintenance Organizations, Financial Incentives, and Physicians' Judgments." *Annals of Internal Medicine* 112 (1990): 891–93.

Hillman, A. L., M. V. Pauly, and J. J. Kerstein. "How Do Financial Incentives Affect Physicians' Clinical Decisions and the Financial Performance of Health Maintenance Organizations?" *New England Journal of Medicine* 321 (1989): 86–92.

Hough, D. E. "Indebtedness and Physician Career Choice: or, The Curious Incident of the Dog in the Night-time." *Medical Practice Management* 4 (1988): 62–66.

Hsiao, W. C., P. Braun, D. Yntemo, and E. R. Becker. "Estimating Physicians' Work for a Resource-Based Relative Value Scale." *New England Journal of Medicine* 319 (1988): 835–41.

Hsiao, W. L., P. Braun, and D. Dunn. "Results and Policy Implications of the Resource-Based Relative Value Study." *New England Journal of Medicine* 319 (1988): 881–88.

Hughes, R. G. "A Physician Surplus?" *New England Journal of Medicine* 358 (1988): 954.

Kassler, W. J., S. A. Wartman, and R. A. Sillman. "Why Medical Students Choose Primary Care Careers." *Academic Medicine* 66 (1991): 40–43.

Kehrer, B. H., F. A. Sloan, and J. Woolridge. "Changes in Primary Medical Care Delivery 1975–1979: Findings from the Physician Capacity Utilization Surveys." *Social Science and Medicine* 18 (1984): 653–60.

Langwell, K. M., and J. L. Werner. "Economic Incentives in Health Manpower Policy." *Medical Care* 28 (1980): 1085–96.

Luft, H. S., and P. Arno. "Impact of Increasing Physician Supply: A Scenario for the Future." *Health Affairs* (Winter 1986): 31–46.

Marder, W. D., D. W. Emmons, P. R. Kletke, and R. J. Willkie. "Physician Employment Patterns: Challenging Conventional Wisdom." *Health Affairs* (Winter 1988): 137–45.

McCarty, D. L. "Why Are Today's Medical Students Choosing High-Technology Specialties over Internal Medicine?" *New England Journal of Medicine* 317 (1987): 567–69.

Mechanic, D. "Organization of Medical Practice and Practice Orientations Among Physicians in Prepaid and Nonprepaid Primary Care Settings." *Medical Care* 13 (1975): 189–204.

Relman, A. S. "The New Medical-Industrial Complex." *New England Journal of Medicine* 303 (1980): 903–70.

Reynolds, R. A., and R. L. Ohsfeldt. *Socioeconomic Characteristics of Medical Practice 1984*. Chicago: Center for Health Policy Research, American Medical Association, 1984.

Roback, G., L. Randolph, and B. Seidman. *Physician Characteristics and Distribution in the U.S.* Chicago: Department of Physician Data Services, Division of Survey and Data Resources, American Medical Association, 1990.

Roper, W. L. "Perspectives on Physician-Payment Reform: The Resource-Based Relative Value Scale in Context." *New England Journal of Medicine* 319 (1988): 865–67.

Sammons, J.H. "Health Manpower in the Medical Marketplace." *Health Affairs* (1982): 20–29.

SAS Institute. *SAS/STAT User's Guide*. Release 6.03. Gary, NC: SAS Institute, 1988.

Schwartz, M. R. "Physician Personnel and Physician Practice." In E. Ginzberg, ed. *From Physician Shortage to Patient Shortage: The Uncertain Future of Medical Practice*. Boulder, CO: Westview Press, 1986, pp. 35–74.

Schwartz, W. B., and D. N. Mendelson. "No Evidence of an Emerging Physician Surplus: An Analysis of Change in Physicians' Work Load and Income." *Journal of the American Medical Association* 263 (1990): 557–60.

Sloan, F. A., and W. B. Schwartz. "More Doctors: What Will They Cost? Physician Income as Supply Expands." *Journal of the American Medical Association* 249 (1983): 766–69.

Tarlov, A. R. "HMO Enrollment Growth and Physicians: The Third Compartment." *Health Affairs* (Spring 1986): 23–35.

Tarlov, A. R. "The Rising Supply of Physicians and the Pursuit of Better Health." *Journal of Medical Education* 63 (1988): 94–106.

U.S. Bureau of the Census. *Statistical Abstract of the United States*. Washington, DC, 1972, 1982, 1990.

Chapter 5

Women in Medicine: Have We Really Come a Long Way?

The purpose of this chapter is to examine some of the same variables addressed in the previous chapter, but using gender as the specific analytic focus. As with the previous chapter, we would like to present some of the findings from the western Massachusetts study in the context of other research by comparing some of our results to those of other investigators as well as to national data bases. Doing this raises several analytic problems, which will be described first. This chapter will then present some general background information on women in the medical field before considering whether women practice medicine differently from men. In order to examine whether there are gender-based differences between men and women practicing medicine, we will consider several variables, including specialty, practice characteristics, productivity, and income, as well as some of the relationships among these. This chapter concludes with some thoughts about future research on women in the medical field.

Analysis Problems and Limitations

Considering gender-based differences in the practice of medicine raises two general problems, and our study itself generates two specific areas of concern. The first broad area is one that we have considered previously—whether data gathered from one relatively small geographical area can be generalized to the national scene. With respect to many of the variables included in this study, the respondents from western Massachusetts do not systematically or significantly differ from the national profile. In the case of gender, about 13 percent of the study physician population is female—quite close to the nationwide percentage, between 12 percent and 15 percent of active, practicing physicians (Roback, Randolph, and Seidman 1990). The distribution of female physicians in the four counties is not equal: women physicians account for 21 percent of all physicians in the most urban county, but only 10 percent in the most rural county.

This 13 percent converts to about 100 female respondents, which is the source of the first more specific limitation. This is a small sample, especially when considering specialty differences. However, unlike many other studies that also have small numbers, the respondents are all known to be active, practicing physicians. Also, the information has been gathered directly from the respondents and the nature of the data is more comprehensive than with most studies. Although this small number does limit our ability to make firm conclusions, the data will permit the use of the findings to critique the literature and to suggest directions for further research. Throughout this chapter, we will present a review and synthesis of the literature about women in medicine and then utilize the results from the western Massachusetts respondents to comment further on the literature.

The second general area of concern relates to time and provides a critique of almost all previous research on women physicians. This is an important conceptual limitation appropriate for discussion here. Actually the amount of information on women in medicine is considerable, with the published literature covering almost 40 years. Articles that appeared relatively early in this time period have a sense of examining a very interesting small minority; the overall tone is often one of exploring a curiosity. Later articles frequently retain this same flavor, but empirical data may be used to support a particular ideological position. The larger social changes regarding women in U.S. society have influenced women's role in medicine, but research about women in medicine seems to be oriented toward older, traditional models of the role of women in a profession. Too frequently, women physicians continue to be represented as marginal members of the medical profession, with much research based on continued curiosity.

One of the major sources of information about female physicians is the American Medical Association. As women have increasingly entered the medical field, the AMA has increased its activities related to collecting information specifically about women—as medical students, as medical residents in postgraduate training, and as practicing physicians. In addition to providing data by gender for many variables, the AMA has also sponsored the Women in Medicine Project, which has focused on collecting and presenting data on female physicians (AMA 1987b,

1987c). This project has provided a valuable data base about women in medicine, and most of the published articles incorporate these data in their studies. Articles frequently begin with a summary of the trends of the number of women in medicine. Since the educational "pipeline" is long and complicated, many different numbers are usually included in introductory paragraphs; some focus on women applying to medical schools, others include data on new entrants or recent graduates from medical schools, while more recent articles tend to concentrate on those entering postgraduate medical education—the residency programs. Only a very few focus on women actually practicing medicine. As might be expected, the numbers reported are different depending on which part of the pipeline is being referred to as well as the date of the article itself. All agree that the number of women in medicine is increasing, but at what rate and in which part of medicine generates a fair amount of disagreement, partially due to the lack of consensus about what stages of medicine are most appropriate for analysis. Despite the clear differences between each of these stages, there is considerable variation in the literature with respect to which estimate is being used. Because of this variation, we briefly describe here the stages of the medical profession to illustrate the importance of precision in identifying which time frame is being referred to.

The first step along the medical pipeline encompasses those who apply to medical schools. Having so many more applicants to medical school than actual spots in the schools has, very naturally, always been a source of great pride to the profession. Traditionally, the preferred ratio is about 1.5 applicants to 1 first-year place to ensure well-qualified medical students (Eisenberg 1989). Applications to medical schools continued to increase until 1978, at which time they stabilized for a couple of years; since then, they have steadily fallen. However, when this trend is examined more carefully, it is apparent that the major decline has been among male applicants, while applications from women have increased. By 1989–1990, women made up 40 percent of all applicants to medical school, in contrast to the 26 percent share of the applicant pool they held in 1977 (Bickel 1988; Relman 1989). Eisenberg (1989) makes the point that the number of male applicants had dropped so much that the 1.5 ratio between applicants and first-year places could not be maintained without the addition of female applicants. Indeed, the number of male applicants dropped so much that, by 1988–1989, there were fewer male applicants than available first-year places.

The increased number of female applicants has translated to a similar increase in the proportion of women who are enrolled in medical school: in 1969–1970, women made up 9 percent of new medical students; in 1979–1980, women were 28 percent; and in the 1991 class, 38 percent of the entrants were women (Relman 1989; Allen 1989). This increase is remarkable, representing a tripling of the number of first-year women enrolled in medical schools between 1971 and 1981, a time period that saw only a 14 percent increase in the number of new male medical students (Bowman and Gross 1986). When the time period is extended from 1969 to 1987, male first-year medical students have increased only 16 percent, while the percentage of female medical students has increased 516 percent (Hojat et al. 1990). There has also been a corresponding increase in female medical school graduates: in 1970–1971, only about 9 percent of U.S. medical graduates were women; by 1980–1981, this had increased to 25 percent; by 1985–1986, the percentage of women among medical school graduates had reached 30 percent (Silberger, Marder, and Willkie 1987); and by 1989–1990, women were projected to account for 34 percent of medical graduates (AMA 1987b).

The effect on postgraduate residency programs has also been large: in 1978, women were only 19 percent of medical residents, but by 1988 the proportion had risen to 28 percent (Bickell 1988). However, the first devi-ation from the overall theme of influx of women into medicine is detected here: women are not spreading into all residency training programs in equal numbers. In 1988, women composed 46 percent of all first-year pediatric residents, and an equal percentage were first-year obstetric-gynecology residents (Schaller 1990). These percentages are larger than would be expected based on the overall 28 percent share of female resi-dents. Based on the same analysis, a much smaller percentage of women than would be expected were in a surgical residency program. Increased diffusion of women throughout the various specialties has occurred; for example, in 1981, one-third of specialties had no women in training, but by 1985, only vascular surgery remained as an all-male residency program (Sinal, Weavil, and Canep 1988). This issue of specialty choice is complicated and involves a host of factors, some of which are related to the socialization process within medical school, and some of which are related to larger social factors regarding the role of women in U.S. society. Because specialty choice is critical to most of the analysis of the physician labor pool and to income, as described in Chapter 4, we consider it carefully in this chapter.

Despite the increasing presence of women in the applicant pool, medical school classrooms and postgraduate residency training pro-grams, the effect on the practicing physician pool has been less obvious, partially because of the length of time involved in training physicians. Eisenberg (1989) terms this discrepancy "a legacy of past discrimina-tion (p. 1543)." In the period 1970–1975, only 7 percent of U.S. active physicians were women, a proportion that placed the United States be-low all but four nations in terms of use of female physician power at that time (Jussim and Muller 1975). The percentage had increased to 10 percent by 1979, and even though 10 percent is a small percentage, it represents an increase of almost two-thirds since 1967 (Mitchell 1984). By 1981, women accounted for 12 percent of active physicians (Schloss 1988; Crozier and Iglehart 1986). By 1986, women accounted for 15.2 percent of all active physicians (Moore and Priebe 1991), and this percentage held constant for 1989–1990 (Hojat et al. 1990). Although 15 percent seems—and is—a small percentage, the increase over time is still very large. Between 1979 and 1987 the active female physician population increased by 240 percent, while the active male physician population increased by only 50 percent (Clare et al. 1987; Marder et al. 1988). In the future, this influx of women is expected to occur at an even faster rate. The total number of physicians in the United States is expected to increase about 27 percent between 1981 and 2000; and, at the current rate, the proportion of female physicians will grow by 150 percent. Thus, by the year 2000 at least 20 percent of all practicing physicians will be women (Bowman and Gross 1986). Women currently make up more than one-third of all enrollees in medical colleges, but still are less than one-sixth of all active practitioners, which is one reason for the relative paucity of studies focusing on female practicing physicians. For studies like ours, where the emphasis is on actively practicing physicians, sample sizes are low, especially when trying to analyze specialty differences. The differences in experience for each of these stages—applicants, first-year medical school entrants, graduating medical students, residency places, and practicing physicians—are significant. It is very important when comparing results that the appropriate time frame is selected so the same groups are used.

A related complication is the age distribution of physicians. As would be expected, women make up a larger proportion of young physicians: in 1985, for example, 24 percent of all physicians under age 35 were women (Schloss 1988; Moore and Priebe 1991). Consequently, women in active practice are likely to have fewer years of professional experience (Bobula 1980; Maheux et al. 1990; Kletke, Marder, and Silberger 1990). This pattern is true for our western Massachusetts sample, where 82 percent of the female respondents are under the age of 44, in comparison to 51 percent of male respondents (Appendix Table D.7). About 60 percent of the female physicians have been in practice in Massachusetts for six years or less, in comparison to 24 percent of the male physicians (Figure 5.1). This figure shows that 78 percent of the women respondents have practiced in Massachusetts ten years or less, while only 42 percent of the males have been in practice for ten years or less; 57 percent of the male respondents have been in practice in Massachusetts for eleven or more years, in contrast to only 21 percent of the female physicians.

Figure 5.1   Years of Medical Practice Experience in Massachusetts

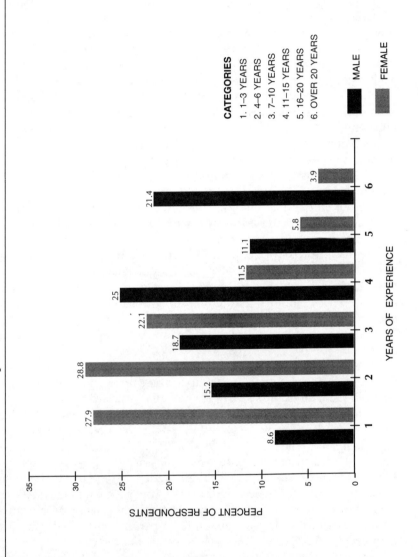

This age and experience profile of the western Massachusetts sample is slightly younger than the national profile. For example, 72 percent of the female physicians in the United States were below age 44 in 1989, in comparison to 81 percent in western Massachusetts. Also, nationally, women physicians make up about 14 percent of physicians over age 55, but only about 6 percent of this age group in western Massachusetts (Roback, Randolph, and Seidman 1990).

As was demonstrated in Chapter 4, age and years of professional experience are important confounding variables, especially when analyzing income and practice arrangements. However, controlling adequately for these variables sometimes creates even smaller sample sizes, especially when the emphasis is on practicing physicians. In this chapter, we will attempt to control for age whenever possible. We will use age rather than years of professional experience in this chapter in order to better facilitate comparisons between our data and other studies. Each of the limitations noted in this section will be further discussed in the context of presentation of our results.

Does Gender Matter in Medical Practice?

It is a common assumption in American society—although often an untested one—that women practice medicine (or any other profession, for that matter) in some way that is substantively different from men. There are three basic answers to the proposition that women practice medicine differently than men. The first is to agree with the assumption, using the many differences that are reported in the literature, including specialty, practice patterns, and productivity, among others, to support the observed assumption. An alternative is to view these same reported differences through a different perspective: yes, there are significant differences in a variety of variables, but these are not due to any inherent differences between male and female physicians. Rather, these observed differences are a result of the many barriers that women face in medicine. If this is true, then it is not useful to continue to describe the differences between male and female physicians: the analytic focus should be on why these differences exist. The third response to the question of gender-based differences in medical practice is, yes, there once were differences, but these do not exist any longer as more women have increasingly entered the medical profession. The tendency for male and female physicians to become more similar is termed the "convergence theory."

We will use our data, as well as evidence presented in other studies, to consider which of these three explanations is the most likely. The variables that will be part of this analysis include specialty, practice characteristics, productivity, and income. The comparison of results from one particular study to the other published literature is a traditional method of research. We want to underscore a particular problem that was discussed in the first section of this chapter: the literature itself. Although much of the literature is descriptive, and thus factual, the choice of data and the interpretation are often based on an ideological view of women. Many current generalizations made about female physicians are actually based on studies done in a period of time in which there were very few women in medicine. Several specific examples of this practice will be included in the later sections of this chapter. They perpetuate a stereotypical view of women in a profession that has been viewed historically as male dominated. It is an inescapable consequence of the demographic trends in medicine that women are becoming more established in the profession. Less obvious, however, is the nature of their influence. Eisenberg reflects an important perspective by choosing as the title of her 1989 article in the *New England Journal of Medicine,* "Medicine is No Longer a Man's Profession or, When The Men's Club Goes Coed, It's Time to Change the Regs."

Professional memberships

Before considering the several practice-related variables, we would like to include one additional measure that may suggest how connected or alienated women physicians feel to the medical establishment: the pattern of joining professional societies or organizations.

Somewhat fewer than half of male physicians join the AMA, a proportion that has remained constant over the last 20 years. Women are less likely to join (about 30 percent), and this percentage has also been constant for 20 years, despite the growth in female physicians (Allen 1989; Bowman and Gross 1986; McDonald 1988). Although professional membership is obviously not a perfect measure of connectedness to a profession, it is one of the few direct measures available. The percentage of both males and females in western Massachusetts joining the AMA is significantly less than the national average—only 32 percent of the male respondents reported being a member, and only 16 percent of female respondents (Table D.8). A higher percentage of both males and females belong to the Massachusetts Medical Society, and the greatest rate of participation is in specialty societies. The pattern of women being more likely to join specialty societies than a state or national professional organization seems to be widespread, although specialty societies do have a substantial variation in terms of proportion of women in the specialty who are members. For example, the American Society of Anesthesiology enrolls the highest percentage of its potential female members, 72 percent (Allen 1989).

Allen (1989) notes several possible explanations for the different rates of involvement of women physicians, particularly in terms of joining the AMA: lack of time, feelings of a lack of opportunity, and an income barrier. Since women make 40 percent less than male physicians nationwide, the organizational dues may actually be a disproportionately high financial burden. Allen's study discovered large differences between the rates at which men and women join all professional organizations, including specialty societies. In our study, rates of membership for specialty societies were similar for men and women, but for all other professional organizations, women were much less likely to be members (Table D.8).

Specialty

In 1953, two-thirds of women were in practice in one of four specialties: pediatrics, psychiatry, obstetrics/gynecology, and pathology. By 1969, specialty choice had changed some: two-thirds of women were in pediatrics, psychiatry, internal medicine, and anesthesiology (Powers, Parmelle, and Weisenfelder 1969). Today, with a larger number of women to consider, it is more common to talk about women being over- or underrepresented in certain specialties. Two specialties that have maintained a clear overrepresentation are pediatrics and psychiatry; other specialties with a relatively high proportion of women include obstetrics/gynecology, pathology, and, some studies suggest, anesthesiology (Bickel 1988; Relman 1989; Hojat et al. 1990; Schaller 1990). It is not an easy matter to determine in exactly what specialties women actually practice medicine: it is easier to count residency places (Silberger, Marder, and Willkie 1987; Schaller 1990), or the percentage of board-certified physicians (Moore and Priebe 1991), both of which answer slightly different questions than functional specialties of currently practicing women physicians. When assessing residency places, women represent 28 percent of all residents, but constitute 52 percent of all pediatric places, 50 percent of obstetrics/gynecology places, 41 percent of all psychiatry places and 38 percent of all pathology places. Closer to the expected distribution are residency training places in family practice (30 percent) and internal medicine (26 percent). Underrepresented are residency programs in all the surgical specialties (Bickel 1988; Schaller 1990).

Specialization—and board certification—is certainly the hallmark of medicine. In 1986, of all male physicians, 58 percent were board certified, but only 40 percent of all females (Moore and Priebe 1991). This difference is probably related to age, since board certification occurs after residency and often after the first few years in a medical practice. There is clearly a relationship between residency training and medical practice, and board certification and medical practice; but it is not always a perfect relationship. For example, medical graduates may do more than one residency program, and their practice may relate to one of those training programs more closely than another. Finding information about practicing physicians is more difficult than finding information about residents or the specialization process, which is an additional reason why there are relatively few studies that focus on the practicing physician.

Two important sources of information do exist about practicing physicians, the first of which is the AMA. According to their figures, 75 percent of women practicing medicine in 1986 were found in the fields of internal medicine, pediatrics, family practice, psychiatry, obstetrics and gynecology, and anesthesia (AMA 1987a). The second information source about practicing physicians is primary surveys of physicians, the most common of which is to question graduates of a particular medical school over time. For example, a recent study of Jefferson Medical College graduates showed the highest proportion of women graduates in internal medicine and family practice (Hojat et al. 1990).

Reviewing the several studies that describe the specialty choice of women physicians produces two conclusions. The first is to categorize women's specialty choices as Bowman and Gross (1986) do: women are more likely to choose anesthesiology and the five "p" specialties— pediatrics, psychiatry, pathology, preventive medicine (public health), and physical medicine. A second conclusion is that women seem to choose all surgical specialties far less frequently than males do, regardless of whether one is counting residency places, board certification, active physicians from the AMA data base, or surveys of practicing physicians.

The specialty distribution of the western Massachusetts respondents is similar to the national profile, with a couple of interesting exceptions. Table C.1 (in Appendix C) shows the frequencies for all 26 specialty choices that were listed in the questionnaire, and Table 5.1 shows the nine specialty groups that we have been using throughout this book for comparison purposes. Table 5.1 also shows the national percentage distribution of male and female physicians for each of these specialty groups. Perhaps the biggest difference between western Massachusetts and what would be expected based on the national specialty distribution is that there are more women practicing in pediatrics (25 percent in comparison to the national 15 percent) and obstetrics/gynecology (13.6 percent in comparison to 8.9 percent nationally). This table shows that there are more female general/family practitioners practicing in western Massachusetts than the national profile, many more pediatricians, more obstetrics/gynecologists, and somewhat more psychiatrists. The one specialty that is particularly different for males, but not so different for females, is the surgical category. Western Massachusetts seems to have a higher proportion of surgical specialists than seems to be true nationwide—29.9 percent in comparison to 14.8 percent. Whether this is due to different categorization or small sample sizes for some specialties, or is a true reflection of the physician distribution in western Massachusetts, cannot be determined without implementing more standardized nomenclature for specialty categories as we discussed in Chapter 3.

Using the expected distribution of male physicians as 85 percent and of female physicians as 15 percent, Table 5.1 demonstrates that there are two specialties that have a higher proportion of women than would be expected—pediatrics and OB/GYN. There are five specialties that have about the proportion that one would expect: anesthesiology, pathology, psychiatry, internal medicine, and general and family practice. In two specialties—radiology and all surgical specialties—there are fewer women than would be expected.

Specialty choice is obviously a complex process and increasingly the literature moves beyond some of the descriptive analysis that we have presented so far to a more analytic focus. The descriptive articles use the differences in practice patterns—in this case, specialty—to answer the question that was posed at the beginning of this section. Yes, male and female physicians do seem to be involved in different specialties. Increasingly, however, research is directed to determine why such differences seem to exist. The first alternative is that differences between men and women regarding specialty choice occur because of the existence of some types of barriers. This body of literature generally focuses on the decision-making process that occurs within the medical school environment. Several investigators have focused on the different ways in which men and women perceive their medical education, with most of these agreeing that women feel they have encountered more barriers than men during their medical school years (Cohen, Woodward, and Femier 1988). One of the most important factors seems to relate to the presence of mentors in medical school, since the mentoring process is viewed as being critical in determining specialty choice, for both males and females. That there are few mentors available for women is noted repeatedly, as is the fact that mentors for women have not been distributed equally across the specialties (Silberger, Marder, and Willkie 1987; Schaller 1990; Cohen, Woodward, and Femier 1988; Levinson, Tolle, and Lewis 1989). Women are present in academic medicine as candidates for mentors for female medical students, but they tend to be concentrated in the lower academic ranks as well as the lower prestige specialties. For example, in pediatrics, 50 percent of all residents are women as are 30 percent of the

Table 5.1   Selected Specialties by Gender

Specialty*	Males n	Males %	Females n	Females %	Total	Males	Females
	Proportion of Sample Found in Specialty					*Gender Proportions within the Specialty (%)*	
General/Family Practice	70	12.6 (11.3)†	13	14.7 (10.9)†	83	84.4	15.6
Pediatrics	52	9.3 (5.8)	22	25.0 (15.1)	74	70.3	29.7
Internal Medicine	104	18.7 (23.3)	20	22.7 (24.1)	124	83.9	16.1
Psychiatry	50	8.9 (3.7)	8	9.1 (5.9)	58	86.2	13.8
Pathology	13	2.3 (1.9)	2	2.3 (2.7)	15	86.7	13.3
OB/GYN	36	6.5 (4.3)	12	13.6 (8.9)	48	75.0	25.0
Anesthesiology	28	5.0 (5.6)	5	5.8 (3.5)	33	84.8	15.1
Surgical	166	29.9 (14.8)	3	3.4 (3.7)	169	98.2	0.8
Radiology	38	6.8 (2.5)	3	3.4 (2.8)	41	92.7	7.3
Total	557	100.0	88	100.0			

*This table deletes the following groups for comparison purposes:
1. All other medical specialties (includes allergy, cardiovascular disease, dermatology, gastroenterology, pediatric specialties, pulmonary disease). There are 42 males and 1 female.
2. All others, including oncology, physical medicine and rehabilitation, critical care medicine, emergency medicine. There are 55 males and 7 females.
†Figures in parentheses are nationwide percentages of nonfederal physicians from Roback, Randolph, and Seidman (1990).

junior faculty. However, 96 percent of the academic chairs who are most responsible for mentoring are male (Schaller 1990).

The specialties that women enter are those that generally involve shorter periods of postgraduate training, carry less prestige, and pay less money, but it is very difficult to determine why (Bowman and Gross

1986; Lorber 1985). Are these specialty fields attractive to women because they are more open to women? Are there more women mentors already available for these specialties? Are women attracted to these specialties because they do not care as much as men do about money, power, or prestige? Or do these specialties involve less prestige primarily because a higher proportion of women are likely to be practicing in them?

These are obviously complicated questions, and the conclusions that the authors draw are varied. Bickel (1988) suggests it is the outcome that matters most: despite few clear-cut differences between men and women while in medical school, women wind up their medical school experience with a strong preference for primary care. Lorber (1987) carries this analysis one step further by noting that there is little actual empirical evidence that women prefer, and thus choose, primary care specialties more than men. She reasons that the weight of the evidence suggests, instead, that women are being tracked (or at least strongly encouraged) to enter the primary care specialties.

The third theory about possible gender-based differences in specialty choices is the idea that although these differences once existed, they no longer exist. Several researchers have suggested support for the so-called convergence theory. Allen (1989) noted that for 1986 graduates, specialty choices for males and females were very similar: 75 percent of both men and women chose internal medicine, pediatrics, family practice, psychiatry, anesthesiology, and obstetrics/gynecology.

Weisman et al. (1980) noted this trend occurring even earlier. Among 1970 graduates, the most frequently selected specialty for men was internal medicine and for women pediatrics; but by 1976 both men and women chose internal medicine most often. In 1980, they reported that distributions across specialties had become even more similar, although some gender differences remained. Women were still overrepresented in pediatrics and pediatric subspecialties, psychiatry, neurology, obstetrics/gynecology, and hospital-based specialties such as pathology. They remained underrepresented in surgery, all surgical specialties, and family medicine. Weisman et al. came to these conclusions by examining seven cohorts of medical school graduates between 1970 and 1976. They also evaluated the switching of specialties and concluded that the specialty areas themselves had become the "salient social contexts in which graduate physicians make career decisions" (p. 823) rather than the medical school environment. Although this may be due to an overall lack of female mentors, Weisman et al. suggest that medicine in the 1970s was in a transition from a profession that was "skewed" (that is, largely male), to one that was "tilted" (having a significant minority of females who were no longer tokens but also who still did not have equal power). They argued that, as women became more of a presence, a continued convergence of male and female behavior patterns would become obvious.

Kletke, Marder, and Silberger (1990) have observed the same trend of underrepresentation of women, particularly in surgical specialties, but they also have noted a weakening of gender-based differences in specialty distribution, as measured by their "index of dissimilarity" (p. 301). This measure decreases even more when the youngest age category of physicians is used, giving more support to the notion that gender-based specialty choice differences are beginning to decrease.

We decided to test this convergence theory by using data from the AMA's 1990 "Physician Characteristics and Distribution" (Roback, Randolph, and Seidman 1990). We used only the youngest physician group (under age 35) to control for the confounding variable of age. Table D.9 shows the 12 most commonly selected specialties, which account for about two-thirds of all physicians. The specialties demonstrating the highest proportion of women physicians are very similar to those that have high proportions of males, with the greatest differences still obvious in the surgical specialties. Perhaps most striking are what the AMA terms "proportionate increases," representing the increase of the under-35 cohort compared to the total. The largest increases are shown on the bottom part of this table: women in the under-35 category are beginning to enter several surgical fields, including general surgery, neurological surgery, orthopedic surgery, and urological surgery. At the same time, males under age 35 are increasingly likely to enter the fields of internal medicine, physical medicine, diagnostic radiology, and family practice.

This table, although suggestive, does not necessarily prove the convergence theory, but it does demonstrate that caution is necessary when attempting to characterize the distribution of women in specialties. One important methodological reminder is appropriate here. The vast majority of these studies use as their time frame the specialty choice process, which focuses particularly on medical school and postgraduate residency experiences. As we have indicated, the actual practice patterns of physicians may be somewhat different, especially when considering a specialty such as internal medicine where there are so many subspecialties available. It is far too early to tell whether the specialty choices of men and women will continue to demonstrate convergence as Weisman et al. (1980) have argued or whether the women entering especially the surgical specialties are the exceptions, defying the tracking phenomenon that Lorber described. In either case, it is very important to try to address this phenomenon from the perspective of actively practicing physicians.

Practice characteristics

In reviewing the current literature regarding female physicians and practice arrangements, we observed a pattern of citations involving literature published in the 1950s and 1960s, used to support research inquiries in the 1980s and even 1990s. The two most commonly cited are by Dykman and Stalnaker (1957), and Powers, Parmelle, and Weisenfelder (1969). Dykman and Stalnaker (1957) were two of the first to report on research into practice patterns of female physicians. The main conclusion of this research was that women were less frequently involved in office-based practice than male physicians. The second commonly cited article, Powers, Parmelle, and Weisenfelder (1969), focused on graduates from 1931 to 1956 and noted that 48 percent of the women were self-employed compared with 75 percent of the men. In this study, they also observed that women physicians (32 percent) were more likely than males (18 percent) to be employed in practice arrangements involving regular hours. These two studies are repeatedly cited in support of similar findings. For example, in a 1971 Detroit study, Heins et al. (1977) noted that although there were equal numbers of male and female physicians involved in solo practice, more women worked in what they termed "non-private" practice. Bowman and Gross (1986) suggest that surveys of medical students continue to demonstrate important differences between men and women: men expect to set up an independent practice—albeit increasingly a group practice—and women are more likely to expect a salaried position. Despite the fact that these surveys were conducted in the 1970s and also utilized medical students—not practicing physicians—as the respondents, Bowman and Gross conclude that "differences in practice setting choices between men and women physicians appear likely to persist" (p. 521). Maheux has done intensive studies of female physicians in Quebec, demonstrating that women are more likely than men to work in the public sector primary care settings and to be paid a salary, although this difference has decreased fairly rapidly. For example, in 1983–1984, for every five female physicians in salaried practice in Quebec, there was one male; but by 1985–1986, this difference had decreased to three female physicians for every one male (Maheux et al. 1990). This observation lends support to the convergence theory, although it is unclear whether female physicians are becoming more like male physicians or males more like females.

There do seem to be some differences based on gender in terms of practice patterns, and we wanted to see if these same practice patterns were true in western Massachusetts. In our study, males are most likely to be practicing in a solo practice (30 percent) or in a group of three or more (35 percent), with a total of 65 percent of the males accounted for by these two practice arrangements. When the hospital setting is included, 80 percent of all men are accounted for. Women physicians seem to have a much more diversified pattern of practice arrangements. The biggest single practice arrangement for women is the HMO setting, representing 22 percent of the women physicians, in comparison to only 7 percent of the men. Another 20 percent of female respondents are in groups of three or more, 18 percent are in a hospital setting, and another 18 percent are in solo practice. These four settings account for 77 percent of the women. Other than the difference in proportion of males and females in an HMO setting, there are also big differences in solo practice, where only 18 percent of women practice in comparison to 30 percent of the men, and in group practices of three or more, where 20 percent of the females and 35 percent of the males practice.

There are two practice arrangements that are primarily male: 91 percent of those in solo practice and 91 percent of those in a group of three or more are males. Using distributional criteria, about 15 percent of each of these practice arrangements would be expected to be women. Dual practice and hospital settings have about the proportion one would expect and the HMO setting has twice as many women as would be expected. Women are relatively overrepresented in HMOs and underrepresented in both solo practice and group practice.

As demonstrated in Chapter 4, there are substantial differences in terms of income of male and female physicians, which we will consider later in this chapter. Men are overrepresented in the most lucrative practice arrangement (group practice), and women are most overrepresented in the lowest-paid practice arrangement (HMOs). However, men are also overrepresented in the second-lowest paid practice arrangement (solo practice). In analyzing other financial variables, it seems that having a larger proportion of a medical practice reimbursed fee-for-service is related to a higher income, and men are more likely to be "always" paid by fee-for-service (47 percent) than women (37 percent). Reimbursement by capitation is related to lower incomes; a similar percentage of males and females (24 percent and 27 percent) indicate that at least 25 percent of their patients are paid for this way. Although the proportion of patients paid for by Medicare did not have an effect on income, it is interesting to observe that in our study 70 percent of the responding male physicians, but only 32 percent of the female physician respondents, indicated that over one-quarter of their patients were paid for through Medicare. Physicians who work for organizations do have less personal responsibility for practice expenses. In our study, about half of male physicians are responsible for their own malpractice expenses, and only about one-third of female physicians have this responsibility.

Attempting to "tease out" the various aspects of practice arrangements, including financial variables, is quite difficult, as was discussed in Chapter 4. When the analysis focuses on possible gender-based differences between actively practicing physicians, sample size problems are exacerbated. This problem is not unique to our regional study. For example, one of the most widely cited articles on gender-based differences in practice arrangements was done by Bobula (1980), who concluded that men were more likely to work in a private solo or group practice while women were more likely to be found in another setting, such as a clinic, student health service, or local government agency. For his study, Bobula used the 1978 AMA Periodic Survey of Physicians, which was a 5 percent national sample. This survey yielded too few female physicians, so he added a second sample of 3,000 female physicians.

The Bobula (1980) article raises another methodological problem: the profound changes in the organization of medical practice between the 1970s and the 1990s. The very terminology that is used in studying practice patterns is significantly different over this 20-year period. For example, currently the term "employed" is used in contrast to "self-employed," with the assumption (sometimes stated but frequently not) that self-employed implies fee-for-service, while employed implies salaried. This concept—self-employed versus employed by others—is a variable that is used to represent a whole set of practice patterns. For example, Silberger, Marder, and Willkie (1987) used data from the AMA's 1986 Socioeconomic Monitoring System telephone survey to find that significantly more male physicians (77 percent) than female physicians (52 percent) are self-employed. However, "self-employed" may not only encompass solo practice, dual practice, and group practice, but also those physicians who subcontract to larger medical organizations. As we learned in Chapter 4, it is no longer appropriate to assume financial mechanisms from practice characteristics.

More recently the terms "incorporated," "ownership," and the old favorite "private practice" have been used with increasing frequency. Some studies use the term "office-based," but this term also may involve several possible financing methods. Gillis and Willkie (1990) offer a description of terminology problems that focus on the use of the term "independent contractor," some of whom may be self-employed and some of whom may be salaried employees. They found it difficult to compare trends over time based on AMA data because of changes made in the AMA's Socioeconomic Monitoring System (SMS) questionnaire in 1987, which decreased the comparability of that data set to the one gathered in 1983–1986.

Across all definitions, women physicians do seem more likely to be working in some type of salaried position, including a variety of institutional arrangements such as hospitals, HMOs, or emergency or home care agencies (Eisenberg 1989; Relman 1989; Maheux et al. 1990). Two studies differentiated between practice arrangements and financial arrangements, and demonstrated similar findings: women seem to be equally likely to be involved in solo practice but seem to be more likely to be in a "nonprivate" practice (Bobula 1980; Heins et al. 1977). Both of these studies are widely quoted, even though one was published in 1980 and used data from the 1978 AMA's Periodic Survey of Physicians, while the other was published in 1977 and represented an earlier survey of practicing physicians in Detroit.

That two relatively old studies still seem to set the standard is an indication that practice pattern is an "interim" variable. It seems important, and there do seem to be differences between males and females, but it is not clear what the differences mean. It is true that specialty choice dictates practice patterns to a certain degree, and therefore practice patterns do not stand alone in their importance.

Gillis and Willke (1990), in an understatement, observed that "overall, trends for physician employees are currently not clear" (p. 38). This lack of clarity is partially due to a lack of consistent terminology. More relevant, however, is that current medical practice patterns are infinitely more complex than at any other time in the past. It is particularly important to separate structural issues of a practice setting from financial issues, since structure does not dictate financing in the 1990s world of medical care. This differentiation, along with more careful descriptions of the variables involved, will assist in developing a better understanding of both structural and financial aspects of medical practice.

Productivity

A recurring theme in this book is methodological problems that consistently limit the generalizability of results from research on physicians. There are basic terminology problems with defining specialty categories, practice patterns, and financial arrangements; the variation makes comparisons very difficult. Difficulties with operational definitions make devising appropriate measurements problematic. The same measurement problems exist in examining physician productivity. There are several approaches to defining productivity, including hours worked per week, weeks worked per year, patients seen, procedures performed, or income generated. We have chosen to use hours worked per week, including total hours and those hours that involve direct patient care activities.

Another limitation is the literature itself, which is another recurring theme in this volume. Traditionally, published literature serves to guide other research efforts. The passage of time may diminish the usefulness of some literature: evolution of concepts, operational definitions, and measurements are frequently observed. When analyzing women in medicine, however, we are amazed by the persistent reliance on conclusions drawn from data collected during a period of time (1950s to 1960s) when women comprised only 5–7 percent of the physician work force. There are also frustrating interpretive problems that stem from the appropriation of research to reify certain philosophical beliefs about women in medicine. Although this phenomenon is present when concentrating on specialty choice and practice arrangements, nowhere is it more clear than in the analysis of possible gender-based differences in productivity. It is not uncommon to find a statement in an article published in the 1980s such as "women physicians work fewer hours than male physicians," supported by a reference to an article published in 1969, based on data collected in 1953.

In this section, as in the others of this chapter, we direct attention to determining whether productivity differences do exist between male and female physicians. The next pages are a summary and critique of previous research, despite the limitations, because this research has created a set of expectations and assumptions about women physicians. We compare our results to the most appropriate current estimates; then we briefly consider possible explanations for observed productivity differences.

The earliest direct study of productivity among female physicians is Powers, Parmelle, and Weisenfelder (1969), and is based on medical school graduates between 1931 and 1956. In this study, women tended to define "full time" as between 40 and 50 hours per week, while men defined "full time" as between 50 and 60 hours; males had an overall yearly total of 2,831 hours of "medically related activity," while women had about 2,000 such hours. Powers, Parmelle, and Weisenfelder calculated that 45 percent of female doctors were working full time in comparison to 95 percent of male physicians. As a result, they concluded that male doctors in 1964 were practicing about 30 percent more hours than women. Despite the definitional problems and obvious time-related limitations, this study is still widely referenced in literature published in the 1980s and 1990s. Another early article (Dykman and Stalnaker 1957), which is also still widely cited, reported that 49 percent of female physicians were in full-time practice, while 89 percent of male physicians were in full-time practice. Several studies published between 1969 and 1971 used "full-time" effort as the productivity measure; all of these studies report that a lower percentage of female physicians work full time than do male physicians (Pennell and Renshaw 1973).

Another approach is to utilize total working time for a female physician over a lifetime as a measure of productivity. Jussim and Miller (1975) calculated that total working time for a female physician over her lifetime of practice was 62 percent of the total working hours of a male physician. This study is also frequently cited; it was published in 1975, but is based on data collected during a period of time in which only about 7 percent of all physicians were women. Continuing the use of this operational definition of productivity, Heins et al. (1977) presented a medical work ratio that calculated full-time months in medical work compared with number of months since medical school graduation, producing the conclusion that men were higher than women, but only by about 10 percent.

This 10 percent discrepancy is in sharp contrast to the earlier suggestion that women work 40 percent fewer hours than male physicians (Jussim and Miller 1975; Powers, Parmelle, and Weisenfelder 1969). It is similar to more recent investigations, especially when hours worked per week is the measure used. Bobula (1980) used 1978 AMA data to determine that male physicians worked 50.9 hours per week versus women's 43.7 and that males practiced about two weeks more every year. This 15 percent differential was consistent across all specialties.

Mitchell (1984) pooled surveys done in 1978–1979 by the National Opinion Research Center to show that male physicians worked about 48 hours per week to females' 45.4 hours per week, a 5 percent difference that added up to 1½ weeks in one year. By the 1980s, the issue of hours worked per week had become politically sensitive, and several studies from the 1980s present conflicting conclusions. Using 1986 AMA data, Silberger, Marder, and Willkie (1987) argued that male physicians spent about 10 percent more hours working per week (58.2 versus female physicians' 52.6), and that male physicians saw about 21 percent more patients per week, but that no difference was found in number of weeks practiced per year. The AMA Women in Medicine Project included results from a study that showed women worked 54 hours per week in comparison to men's 52 hours per week, while their own study showed that women worked only about 7.9 percent fewer hours than men, with some variation by specialty (Lisokie 1986). The most recent estimates of hours worked per week based on AMA data suggest that men work about 59 hours per week and women work about 51 hours per week, a difference of about 14 percent (Hojat et al. 1990; Kletke, Marder, and Silberger 1990).

The productivity measure used in our study is hours worked per week, including differentiating between total hours worked and proportion of time spent in direct patient care activities. It is clearly not a complete measure of work effort but it certainly is an acceptable measure. Data from the western Massachusetts respondents are compared to the most recent research since historical data are of little use here for purposes of comparison. In this analysis of differences in productivity between male and female physicians, we also include specialty, practice arrangement, and years of professional experience, since each may affect productivity.

As Table 5.2 shows, there is a significant difference in total hours worked per week between male and female physicians; in percentage terms, male physicians in our sample work about 10 percent more total hours per week than female physicians, a difference that is statistically significant. The difference in terms of number of hours spent in direct care is not statistically significant. This finding is consistent with recent AMA data. In 1987–1988, male physicians worked 58.7 hours, while female physicians worked 53.8 hours per week, an 8 percent difference (AMA Center for Health Policy Research 1989). Both the percentage difference between male and female physicians, as well as estimated hours per week, seem fairly constant across all recent studies, although Lisokie (1986) indicates a *Medica* survey that shows that women physicians work about 4 percent more hours per week than men physicians. Silberger, Marder, and Willkie (1987) used 1986 AMA SMS data to show that, for self-employed physicians, male physicians work an average of 58.2 hours per week while female physicians work an average of 52.6 hours per week, a difference of about 10 percent, and Kletke, Marder, and Silberger (1990) using 1987 SMS data, came to a similar conclusion, with male physicians working 59 hours per week and females 52.3 hours per week.

Specialty. Table 5.3 examines whether there are any specialty-based differences related to hours worked per week for male and female physicians in western Massachusetts. This table compares males and females in

Table 5.2   Proportion of Time Spent in Direct Patient Care for Patient Care Physicians, by Gender

	Males (n = 683)	Females (n = 104)	t-Test
Average hours per week in direct patient care	48.7	45.7	3.44****
Average hours per week in other activities	11.0	9.0	2.80****
Average total hours worked per week	58.4	53.3	10.58**
Average proportion of time spent in direct patient care activities	83.4	85.7	

*p ≤ .001, using *t*-test of differences.
**p ≤ .01, using *t*-test of differences.
***p ≤ .05, using *t*-test of differences.
****p ≤ .10, using *t*-test of differences.

Table 5.3   Hours Worked per Week for Selected Specialties of Patient Care Physicians, by Gender

Selected Specialties	Frequency		Mean Hours Worked: Direct Patient Care			Mean Total Hours Worked per Week		
	Males	Females	Males	Females	Percentage Difference	Males	Females	Percentage Difference
Pediatrics	51	22	51.2 (85)†	41.9 (86)†	−18.2***	59.8	49.1	−17.9**
Obstetrics/Gynecology	33	11	55.0 (89)	64.7 (92)	+15.0	62.1	70.3	+11.7
Internal Medicine	103	20	54.7 (88)	41.5 (89)	−24.1*	62.0	47.3	−23.7*
General/Family Practice	70	13	49.2 (85)	41.4 (78)	−15.8****	58.2	53.3	−8.4

*$p \le .001$, using t-test of differences.
**$p \le .01$, using t-test of differences.
***$p \le .05$, using t-test of differences.
****$p \le .10$, using t-test of differences.
†Numbers in parentheses represent percentage of total hours spent in direct care.

those specialties where there are at least ten females: pediatrics, obstetrics/gynecology, internal medicine, and general/family practice. First, the overall proportion of time spent by men and women in direct patient care activities is about the same for these four specialty groups, except for general/family practice, where women spend a smaller proportion of their time in direct patient care (78 percent) than men (85 percent). Females in obstetrics/gynecology work more (8.2 hours per week) total hours than males and spend more time in direct patient care activities than males. For the other specialties, women work fewer total hours, with the highest difference in internal medicine, where women work an average of 15 fewer hours a week than men, with most of the difference occurring in the direct patient care category. The results of our study are fairly similar to the current estimates that indicate women physicians work between 10 percent and 15 percent fewer total hours per week, with the clear exception of internal medicine, where the western Massachusetts female respondents work 23 percent fewer hours than male internists, and OB/GYN, where women work 11 percent more hours.

Others have also examined productivity differences by specialty: for example, unlike our results, Bobula (1980) found that the biggest differences occurred in pediatrics, where men worked 21 percent more hours/week than women, and in obstetrics/gynecology, 18 percent more hours/week. Differences were less in internal medicine (13 percent) and general/family practice (16 percent) but still present. Using much more current AMA data (1987 and 1988), Kletke, Marder, and Silberger (1990) concluded that differences in hours worked per week for male and female physicians were much smaller: male physicians in obstetrics/gynecology work 9 percent more hours than female physicians; male pediatricians work 14 percent more than female pediatricians; 18 percent more in internal medicine; and 19 percent more in general/family practice. The percentage differences in internal medicine and general/family practice were the largest observed. The smallest was in radiology, where male physicians worked only 4 percent more than females. In two specialties—pathology and emergency medicine—AMA data for 1987 show that women physicians work 6 percent more hours/week than men. In the study of graduates of Jefferson Medical College, these same types of specialty-specific differences appeared to exist and, in that group, to be primarily related to the increased likelihood of women being employed "part time" (Hojat et al. 1990).

Mitchell (1984) demonstrated a set of results that are slightly different from those others noted here. She used two combined National Opinion Research Center Surveys for 1978–1979. Although she also noted that women physicians worked about 10 percent fewer hours per week, a major exception were female general practitioners who worked about

8 percent more hours per week than male general practitioners. She also found a much smaller differential for internal medicine: male internists only worked 3 percent more hours per week than females.

It is clear from the repeated efforts to analyze differences in productivity between male and female physicians, that this issue is both unresolved and of continuing interest.

Practice arrangement. There is some evidence that an additional important variable affecting productivity is practice arrangement. As we have already seen, it is especially hard to compare studies using this variable because of the nonstandard way in which information is gathered, and because of the changes within the field of medicine that have produced more complex structural and financial arrangements, complicating the analysis of related variables. For example, Silberger, Marder, and Willke (1987) noted several important differences between hours worked per week for males and females in different specialties. For internal medicine, male physicians worked 10 percent more hours each week than females; this magnitude of difference was also true for general/family practice, pediatrics, and psychiatry, but was much smaller for anesthesiologists— only 3 percent. For our study, male internists worked about 23 percent more hours than females. However, the difference between our findings and theirs may be due to Silberger's group calculating the average hours worked per week for physicians who were classified as "self-employed." Eisenberg (1989) suggests that the majority of the 10 percent differential between average hours worked per week for males and females is explained almost totally by the higher ratio of men to women in private practice, which involves working more hours per week.

Table 5.4 shows the difference in hours worked per week for the four major practice arrangements examined in western Massachusetts. Clearly, within the HMO setting, female physicians work significantly fewer hours than male physicians (15.8 percent fewer), and they also spend fewer hours in direct patient care activities. Within the hospital setting, women work about 10 percent fewer hours overall, but they spend slightly more average hours involved with direct patient care than males in that practice setting. In solo practice and within a group of three or more, women work slightly more total hours than male physicians, and they work more hours per week in direct patient care activities than male physicians.

At this point, we are frustrated by a shortage of female physicians which, if alleviated, would enable us to pursue this analysis further within a multivariate model. The one practice arrangement in which women clearly work substantially fewer hours is in the HMO setting, which may explain why women internists work fewer hours than men.

Table 5.4 Hours Worked per Week for Major Practice Arrangements, by Gender

Practice Arrangement	Frequency		Mean Hours Worked: Direct Patient Care			Mean Total Hours Worked per Week		
	Males	Females	Males	Females	Percent Difference	Males	Females	Percent Difference
Solo practice	205	19	49.3	52.0	+5.2	57.9	62.1	+6.8***
Group of three or more	239	21	52.3	54.5	+4.0	60.3	61.1	+1.3
Closed panel/staff model HMO	49	23	48.7	42.7	−12.7	56.2	47.6	−15.8***
Hospital	96	18	38.2	39.6	+3.5	56.3	50.6	−10.1
Other	90	22	48.7	40.5	−17.4***	57.9	47.5	−17.9**

*p ≤ .001, using t-test of differences.
**p ≤ .01, using t-test of differences.
***p ≤ .05, using t-test of differences.
****p ≤ .10, using t-test of differences.

Years of professional experience. Mitchell (1984) has noted that not only is there a relationship between age or professional experience and income, but that there is also a similar relationship between age or experience and hours worked per week, especially for male physicians. In the early stages of their careers, male physicians seem to work more hours per week. According to Mitchell, they reach a peak at about age 44, after which the number of hours worked per week decreases. In her study, female physicians did not demonstrate this same relationship. Kletke, Marder, and Silberger (1990) found that the hours worked per week for patient care physicians peaked at age 37 for male physicians and age 43 for female physicians. They note that the tendency for male physicians to work more hours than female physicians decreases over time. As Table 5.5 shows, the results from our study are very similar to the findings of Kletke's group. The percentage differences in total hours worked per week between male and female physicians is higher in the youngest age category and even then it is only 11 percent, which is not statistically significant. The discrepancy decreases as age increases.

This analysis of possible differences in productivity between male and female physicians leaves us with few firm conclusions, but perhaps encourages a slightly different way of thinking about women in medicine. The first question is whether productivity differs between male and female physicians. Based on current research, it appears that the most likely answer is that if there once were significant differences, the discrepancy is much less in the 1990s. It is interesting to speculate on reasons why some characteristics of male and female physicians—including specialty, practice patterns, and productivity—seem to be converging. Bobula (1980) suggested that this convergence was because women were increasing the number of hours they worked. However, most other investigators attribute the trend to the increasing similarity of men's practice patterns to those of women physicians. Bowman and Gross (1986) and Williams (1978) both found that productivity is converging because men are working fewer hours than they used to. Curry (1983) has also reported this for Canadian male physicians: over time, they are working fewer hours per week and fewer weeks per year.

Of more interest to many investigators is the exploration of the possible explanations for gender-based productivity differences. For example, one common argument is that the specialties that women are more likely to select pay less per hour of activity, and women thus have fewer economic incentives than men (Lisokie 1986). Others acknowledge that it is difficult to determine whether pay per hour reflects a true difference in productivity or a differentiation related to some type of market discrimination (Silberger, Marder, and Willkie 1987). Of course, the most popular explanation is frequently related to special needs of women—

Table 5.5 Average Hours per Week Worked by Males and Females: Two Samples

| | *Kletke, Marder, and Silberger (1990)* | | | | *Stamps and Cruz* | | |
| | *Mean Hours Worked per Week* | | | | *Mean Hours Worked per Week* | | |
Age Categories	*Males*	*Females*	*Percentage Difference*	*Age Categories*	*Males*	*Females*	*Percentage Difference*
30–45	61.5	52.5	15	30–44	58.8	52.3	11.0*
46–55	59.2	54.3	8.2	45–54	60.9	62.2	2.1
55+	52.4	48.8	6.8	55+	54.6	49.3	9.7

*$p \leq .001$, using t-test of differences.
**$p \leq .01$, using t-test of differences.
***$p \leq .05$, using t-test of differences.
****$p \leq .10$, using t-test of differences.

family responsibilities, with a particular emphasis on childbearing and child-rearing.

One of the most common themes in the literature on women in medicine concerns the female physician and family, with particular emphasis on reproduction. Many of these articles focus on how pregnancy affects a medical career—the medical school experience, the residency experience, or the active medical practice (Sinal, Weavil, and Canep 1988; Heins 1983; Potter 1983; Baucom-Copeland, Copeland, and Perry 1983; Sayres et al. 1986; Grunebaum, Minkoff, and Blake 1987).

Issues related to children are also used to explain productivity differentials, although not always in a consistent manner. In 1960, Sloan demonstrated that having children affected hours worked by female physicians, but not male physicians, although in 1970 using the same data set, he could not replicate this result (Sloan 1975). Sinal, Weavil, and Canep (1988) found a relationship between female physicians having children and working fewer hours per week, supporting the earlier finding of Dennis et al. (1990) that female residents who already had children planned on working fewer hours per week than either their male colleagues or their female colleagues without children. However, Kehrer (1976) found that married female physicians worked significantly fewer hours than unmarried women, but that the presence of children had no effect. The AMA (in 1972) suggested that female physicians work fewer hours than male physicians because of overall household responsibilities, and not those specifically related to child-rearing. Both Kehrer (1976) and Mitchell (1984), who showed the same thing later, suggest that married female physicians have fewer economic incentives to work since they are usually married to a high-income professional, often a physician. Bowman and Gross (1986) point out that the lower productivity of female physicians is much more obvious in later years of practice rather than in the prime childbearing ages, when 85 percent of all female physicians have children (Sinal, Weavil, and Canep 1988). This finding is contrary to our results and to those of Kletke, Marder, and Silberger (1990).

There is actually a large body of literature on women in medicine that focuses on the woman as a childbearer or as a part of a domestic household. The primary reason for this literature is to explain productivity differences between male and female physicians. This literature is full of conclusions, statements, and analyses that in the 1990s would be judged to be at the least stereotypical, if not discriminatory. This returns us to the place where we began this section: the difficulty of interpretation when conducting research in an area involving a group considered by many to still be marginal to medical practice.

Perhaps a final question is whether it matters if there are productivity differences between male and female physicians. Certainly one might care about productivity differences in making accurate estimates of physician supply. Some investigators suggest that lower productivity is evidence of higher quality of care delivered by female physicians, since they are spending more time with patients (Eisenberg 1989; Bowman and Gross 1986). Others argue that, from a cost-containment perspective, since women also earn less than men, it would be advantageous to HMOs to recruit more female physicians.

Productivity differences have been widely used to explain the lower incomes that women physicians receive in comparison to men physicians. Certainly, if these productivity differences are declining, one would expect that income differences might also be declining. If the convergence theory holds true for specialty choice, practice characteristics, and productivity, then perhaps it will also hold true for income.

Income

Chapter 4 was devoted to an analysis of income, and one variable of particular interest was found to be gender. In western Massachusetts median income for the female respondents is $61,760; median income for male respondents is $101,000. We are far from the first investigators to find this disparity. Income differentials between male and female physicians have been demonstrated for a long time and are consistent over a variety of income measures. For example, the AMA uses "unadjusted net income" to show that women physicians earn about 60 percent of what men physicians make: $83,000 compared to $137,500 in 1987 (AMA Center for Health Policy Research 1989). Another 1987 report on women physicians noted that the "average net income" for all female physicians was $73,100 as compared to the males' $118,000, or about the same percentage difference. These two estimates establish the range that is generally reported for income differentials between male and female physicians for the 1980s: men physicians earn somewhere between 40 percent and 60 percent more than women physicians. Of course, there are many possible explanations for this impressive differential—that, for example, women are more likely to be in lower-paid specialties or lower-paid practice arrangements, women are younger and have fewer years of experience, and women physicians work less than men physicians. Although some individual studies have addressed one or two of these explanatory variables, none has systematically examined all of these possible explanations with one data set. We perform that examination in this section.

Income is a complicated variable, with many possible measurements. In Chapter 4 we used median income, primarily, since that is generally recognized as the best summary; however, we also examined income distribution and means. Consistent with this approach, median values and income distributions are the primary method of analysis in this chapter; mean income is used when comparing other studies using that summary figure. First, we examine the three variables said to explain the income differences between male and female physicians: specialty, practice arrangements, and age or years of professional experience. Then, we consider productivity. Before presenting the results for these variables, it is appropriate to describe the overall income distribution of the sample.

Table D.10 shows the income distribution of male and female physicians in comparison with the total sample of our patient care respondents. A higher proportion of women than men are in each of the three lower-income categories, about the same percentage of men and women are in the $81,000–100,000 category, and fewer women than men are in each of the four highest-income categories. When the expected distribution of the total sample is compared separately for males and for females, the distribution of males is very similar to the distribution of the total sample, as would be expected given the large proportion of males in the total sample. The income distribution of women, however, is markedly different from that of the total sample: women are underrepresented in the top five income categories and overrepresented in the bottom three categories. Indeed, the actual number of women in the highest income categories is very small. As this table shows, a clear and statistically significant difference exists between the two summary measures—mean and median income—as well as the distribution of male and female physicians' incomes. Figure 5.2 shows the schematic representation of the income distribution of male and female physician respondents.

Specialty. It is obvious that significant income differences exist among specialties. Less clear is whether there are any significant income differences between male and female physicians within the same specialty. Although it has been observed that female physicians seem to make about 38–40 percent less than male physicians within the same specialty (Allen 1989; Bowman and Gross 1986), it is difficult to demonstrate this finding because of the low numbers of women physicians in several specialties, especially the surgical specialties. Table D.11 shows mean and median incomes for twelve specialties, and Table 5.6 shows mean and median incomes for those six specialties for which there are sufficient numbers to compare males and females. Table 5.6 also shows data from Silberger, Marder, and Willkie (1987), who used the 1986 AMA SMS core study data using net income (as we did) and physicians with five through nine years of professional experience.

Figure 5.2 Income Distribution of Physician Respondents by Gender

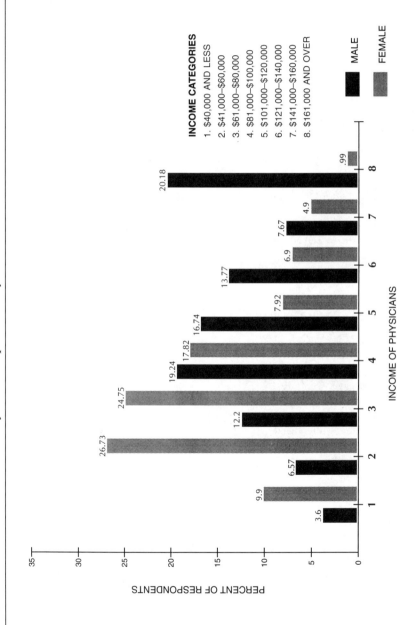

Table 5.6   Comparison of Males and Female, within Specialties

	Stamps and Cruz		Silberger, Marder and Willkie (1987)
	Mean Income, All Physicians	Mean Income, 10 Years or less of Experience	Mean Income, 5–9 Years of Experience
General/Family Practice			
Males (n = 67)	69,507	70,500	76,800
Female (n = 13)	47,769	46,700	66,000
Percentage differential	28%	34%***	14%
Internal Medicine			
Males (n = 102)	83,090	79,050	118,600
Female (n = 20)	55,250	52,590	74,400
Percentage differential	33%	34%	37%
Pediatrics			
Males (n = 47)	83,660	81,760	84,100
Female (n = 21)	48,980	46,130	62,700
Percentage differential	41%	44%*	25%
Psychiatry			
Males (n = 50)	82,520	88,030	93,600
Female (n = 8)	63,280	68,600	61,700
Percentage differential	23%	22%	34%
Anesthesiology			
Males (n = 27)	126,510	126,890	158,700
Female (n = 5)	96,200	101,000	80,500
Percentage differential	24%	20%	49%
Obstetrics/Gynecology			
Males (n = 35)	128,600	123,280	not reported
Female (n = 12)	81,000	94,480	not reported
Percentage differential	37%	20%	

$*p \le .001.$
$**p \le .01.$
$***p \le .05.$
$****p \le .10.$

For all six specialties, women physicians make less than male physicians in that same specialty, according to both our regional data and the national data set. In the national data set, the lowest income difference is in general and family practice, where females make 14 percent less than males. For the other specialties, the income differential ranges from 25 percent less for female pediatricians to 49 percent less for female anesthesiologists. In another AMA report, where income differences between male and female physicians were analyzed, similar results occurred (AMA 1989). Using data from the 1988 SMS core survey, the mean net incomes for four groups of specialties were compared. Within each group, female physicians made less money than males. For general/family practice, females made 33 percent less; for all medical specialties combined, females made 40 percent less; for surgical specialties, women made 34 percent less.

Our data from western Massachusetts are very similar: women make less than men within each of the six specialty groups shown in Table 5.6. The specialty in which women's mean incomes are closest to men's is psychiatry, where the difference is 23 percent. The specialty in western Massachusetts with the biggest income differential is pediatrics, where female physicians make 41 percent less than male physicians.

Silberger, Marder, and Willkie (1987) used mean income for physicians with five–nine years of experience in order to control for the problem that women physicians are generally younger and have less experience than male physicians, which understandably would result in lower incomes. As can be seen in Table 5.6, when we make a similar comparison, using only male and female physicians among our respondents with ten years or less of experience, in almost every specialty the percentage differentials in income cannot be explained by the higher proportion of younger female physicians within each specialty. The "gender gap" in income is still noticeably present, even when controlling for years of professional experience.

It is pretty clear from these comparisons that, on average, women make less money than men practicing in the same specialty, even when controlling for experience. There are exceptions, of course, and our own data set includes some of these exceptions, although the numbers are too low to produce any generalizations. On the whole, our evidence presented here as well as evidence based on AMA data suggest that although it is true that women are more likely to be involved in lower-paying specialties, it is also true that within each specialty, women physicians make between 20 and 40 percent less than male physicians.

Practice arrangements. Women physicians seem more likely to practice in the lower-income practice arrangements, primarily in salaried positions, but documentation is difficult because of the haphazard manner in which practice arrangement has been defined (as we discussed earlier). Specialty and practice arrangements may be related: Silberger, Marder, and Willkie (1987) felt that practice arrangements were the reason for the income differences between male and female specialists within the five specialties they analyzed. We also found differences in incomes based on practice arrangements: the highest incomes were made by those in group practice, followed by hospital-based practice, solo practice, and HMO physicians. There is roughly a 30 percent income differential between the highest-income practice arrangement and the lowest-income practice arrangement (Table 4.5). Just as with specialty, there is a tendency in our sample for women to work in the lower-income practice arrangements. However, just as with specialty, we are curious as to whether income differences between males and females within the same practice arrangement exist.

Table 5.7 shows the mean and median annual incomes for male and female physicians in the four most common practice arrangements for our sample: solo practice, group of three or more, closed panel HMO, and a hospital-based setting. Within each of these practice environments, women physicians make less money, and these differences are statistically significant. The hospital-based setting provides the lowest income differential, but women physicians still make 23 percent less than male physicians practicing in that setting. The largest differential is in group practice, where women make 37 percent less money than males.

Age and years of experience. Income seems to reach its peak somewhere around age 54, often between 11 and 15 years of professional experience, although this may be more true for men than women, since most of these income profiles are drawn from samples that are predominantly male. Women, as we have seen, are more likely to be concentrated in the younger age categories, and therefore are likely to have less professional experience. Table 5.8 shows the relationship between age and mean annual income for our respondents. There are several interesting observations from this table. First, there is an obvious reinforcement of the observation that women physicians as a group are younger. Second, there is the suggestion here of a slightly different profile with respect to age and income for women physicians in contrast to men physicians. Men's incomes drop remarkably once they are over age 55, but incomes improve for the few women in this age category. Within the two age groups for whom we have enough information, the income differential between males and females persist. Gender is the variable that affects income, but age is not statistically significant.

Table 5.9 shows the relationship between years of professional experience in Massachusetts and income for both our data and for data from the AMA 1988 SMS core survey (AMA 1989). There are two technical problems in this table. First, we used different intervals for years of experience than the AMA. Second, our definition of years of professional experience is limited to years in Massachusetts, while the AMA uses a broader definition of total years of professional experience. Despite these two differences, within each category of years of experience, female

Table 5.7 Income by Four Practice Arrangements by Gender

Practice Arrangements	Males			Females			Percentage Difference Between Mean Annual Incomes
	n (%)	Mean Annual Income	Median Annual Income	n (%)	Mean Annual Income	Median Annual Income	
Solo Practice	196 (30.7)	91,469	86,510	19 (19.0)	58,993	47,650	35**
Group of 3 or more	221 (34.6)	118,280	121,380	20 (20.0)	73,350	74,300	37***
Closed Panel HMO	47 (7.3)	90,702	89,930	23 (23.0)	62,653	61,000	31***
Hospital	87 (13.6)	101,218	96,580	17 (17.0)	77,720	73,540	23*
Total	639 (100)			100 (100)			

*p ≤ .001, using *t*-test of differences.
**p ≤ .01, using *t*-test of differences.
***p ≤ .05, using *t*-test of differences.
****p ≤ .10, using *t*-test of differences.

Table 5.8   Income by Age Groups for Male and Female Physicians

Age Groups	Males			Females			Percent Difference
	n	*(%)*	*Mean Annual Income*	*n*	*(%)*	*Mean Annual Income*	
30–44	326	(51)	101,350	83	(82)	65,807	−35*
45–54	170	(27)	116,759	13	(13)	72,692	−38*
55 ≥	143	(22)	90,566	5	(5)	76,200	−16

*p ≤ .001, using *t*-test of differences.
**p ≤ .01, using *t*-test of differences.
***p ≤ .05, using *t*-test of differences.
****p ≤ .10, using *t*-test of differences.

physicians earn substantially less money than do their male counterparts. As the AMA (1989) says, "experience alone does not account for gender differences in earnings" (p. 47). The tendency noted in Table 5.8 for male and female earning power to converge at higher ages (and with more years of professional experience) is not observed here.

Productivity. Our operational definition here is total hours worked per week, and hours per week spent in direct patient care activities. As noted previously, the female respondents work about 7.5 percent fewer hours per week than the male respondents, which averages to about 4.5 fewer hours per week. This productivity differential is important because it is commonly used as one of the explanations for female physicians making less money than male physicians, with others being specialty, practice arrangements, age, and years of experience. As we have seen, although it is true that women are in the lower-paid specialties and practice arrangements and are generally younger, these factors do not fully explain their lower incomes. Women make less money than men within each specialty, within each practice arrangement, and within each age/experience group. That leaves only productivity differences as the primary explanation of the income discrepancy between male and female physicians. Of course, this explanation is based on the assumption that working more hours per week is in fact related to increased income for physicians. Although this relationship between productivity and income is intuitive and may be true for other labor groups, the work described in Chapter 4 demonstrates that hours worked per week are not as directly related to physician income. For example, radiologists as a group have the highest incomes among our respondents and they work almost the fewest hours per week. Table 4.7 shows that those in the two

Table 5.9 Years of Experience and Income for Male and Female Physicians

	Stamps and Cruz		*American Medical Association (1989)*
Years in Medical Practice in Massachusetts	*Mean Annual Income*	*Years in Medical Practice*	*Mean Net Income*
0–3 Years		1–4 Years	
Males (n = 55)	95,440	Males	110,600
Females (n = 27)	64,515	Females	74,000
Percent differential	32%*	Percent differential	33%
4–6 Years		5–9 Years	
Males (n = 97)	98,628	Males	145,200
Females (n = 30)	67,270	Females	84,900
Percent differential	32%*	Percent differential	41%
7–10 Years		10–14 Years	
Males (n = 124)	103,090	Males	158,200
Females (n = 23)	70,880	Females	99,400
Percent differential	31%*	Percent differential	37%
11–15 Years		20+ Years	
Males (n = 159)	107,460	Males	127,200
Females (n = 11)	71,260	Females	72,800
Percent differential	33%**	Percent differential	42%
16+ Years			
Males (n = 204)	103,603		
Females (n = 10)	61,000		
Percent differential	41%**		

*$p \leq .001$, using t-test of differences.
**$p \leq .01$, using t-test of differences.
***$p \leq .05$, using t-test of differences.
****$p \leq .10$, using t-test of differences.

upper-income categories have equivalent average workweeks despite the income differences between the two groups. On average, working more hours does produce more income for those in the four lower-income groups. However, the limited increase in hours do not begin to account for the substantial increase in income.

This same observation is upheld in Table 5.10, which shows the two productivity measures (total hours worked and hours spent in direct care) and income categories for male and female respondents. For men, there is an overall 12-hour differential between the top and bottom income categories: a male physician who makes less than $40,000 works 20 percent less than a male physician who makes over $160,000. For the next four income categories, covering $41,000 to $120,000, however, there is only a 5-hour differential for males. Male physicians seem to hit a productivity "ceiling"; after 61 hours per week, a greater number of hours worked does not contribute to greater income. And for an income range from $121,000 to over $160,000 there is essentially no difference in terms of total hours worked. The same basic pattern holds true for male physicians in terms of number of hours per week spent in direct patient care activities.

For women, a similar profile seems to hold true: there is only a 4.3 hour/week differential for an income capacity that goes from $61,000 to $120,000. There are too few women in the top two income categories to determine if this extends upward.

Men and women physicians in the same income categories exhibit an interesting pattern. In the two lower-income categories, women work fewer hours per week and also spend slightly fewer hours per week in direct patient care. For the three middle-income groups (from $61,000 to $120,000) there is essentially no difference in hours worked per week for male and female physicians. In the highest income category for which there are enough women to analyze ($121,000–140,000) the women work 13 percent more hours than male physicians. Unfortunately, there are not enough women in the top two income categories to continue the comparison.

We also examined specialty and practice arrangements by income for male and female respondents. Table 5.11 shows the mean incomes and hours worked per week for the five specialties in which there are enough women to analyze. Women in this study work fewer hours in each specialty, except obstetrics/gynecology, but the difference in income is far greater than the difference in productivity in most of the specialties. For example for general/family practice and for psychiatry, women work 6–8 percent fewer hours but have incomes that are 23–28 percent lower than the men within these specialties. They work 23 percent fewer hours in internal medicine and their income is 34 percent less; in pediatrics, women work 18 percent less but earn 41 percent less. In obstetrics/gynecology, women work 11 percent more hours than men but earn 24 percent less.

This same pattern is even more pronounced when considering practice arrangements. As noted previously, there are two practice arrangements (HMOs and hospital-based practices) where women respondents seem to work substantially fewer hours than men physicians. However, Table 5.12 shows that the income differential is twice the productivity differential for both practice settings. And in the two practice arrangements in which there is basically no difference in hours worked per week for male and female physicians, the income differential is much larger—38 percent in a group practice setting and 35 percent in a solo practice setting.

Table 5.10 Average Income by Weekly Activities by Gender

Average Hours Spent Each Week	Income Categories							
	Less than 40,000	41,000–60,000	61,000–80,000	81,000–100,000	101,000–120,000	121,000–140,000	141,000–160,000	Over 160,000
Males								
Direct care*	34.0	43.3	48.2	48.9	48.1	51.7	53.1	51.2
Total hours*	48.3	54.0	56.6	57.6	59.5	61.6	61.6	60.4
Females								
Direct care*	30.1	42.0	47.4	49.1	51.6	64.6	44.8†	51.0***
Total hours*	36.4	50.8	54.8	55.9	59.1	70.9	55.6†	62.0***

*$p \leq .001$, using an ANOVA of the effect of hours upon income: $p < .0001$.
**$p \leq .01$, using an ANOVA of the effect of hours upon income: $p < .0001$.
***$p \leq .05$, using an ANOVA of the effect of hours upon income: $p < .0001$.
****$p \leq .10$, using an ANOVA of the effect of hours upon income: $p < .0001$.
†Based on five or fewer cases.

Table 5.11 Gender Differences in Average Income and Hours Worked per Week by Specialty Groups

Specialty Groups	Mean Income		Mean Hours/Week		Income Differential (%)	Hours/Week Differential (%)
	Males	*Females*	*Males*	*Females*		
General/Family Practice (Males = 67; Females = 13)	69,512	49,778	58.2	53.3	−28***	−8
Internal Medicine (Males = 102; Females = 20)	83,242	55,250	62.0	47.3	−34*	−23*
Pediatrics (Males = 47; Females = 21)	83,831	49,151	59.8	49.1	−41*	−18**
OB/GYN (Males = 35; Females = 12)	128,600	98,423	62.1	70.3	−24***	+12
Psychiatry (Males = 50; Females = 8)	82,520	63,375	48.0	45.0	−23	−6

*$p \leq .001$, using t-test of differences.
**$p \leq .01$, using t-test of differences.
***$p \leq .05$, using t-test of differences.
****$p \leq .10$, using t-test of differences.

Table 5.12 Gender Differences in Average Income and Hours Worked per Week by Practice Arrangements

Practice Arrangements	Mean Income		Mean Hours/Week		Income Differential (%)	Hours/Week Differential (%)
	Males	Females	Males	Females		
Solo practice (Males = 205; Females = 19)	91,469	58,993	57.9	62.1	−35**	+7
Group of three or more (Males = 239; Females = 21)	118,280	73,350	60.3	61.1	−38*	+1
Closed panel HMO (Males = 49; Females = 23)	90,702	62,653	56.2	47.6	−31*	−16***
Hospital (Males = 96; Females = 18)	101,218	77,720	56.3	50.6	−23*	−10

*$p \leq .001$, using t-test of differences.
**$p \leq .01$, using t-test of differences.
***$p \leq .05$, using t-test of differences.
****$p \leq .10$, using t-test of differences.

Income per hour. At this point in the analysis, a more comparable summary figure would be helpful. The AMA has occasionally produced reports in which comparisons are made between male and female physicians that are based on income per hour. In 1989, the income per hour for female physicians with 0–4 years of experience was about $22.00 per hour, while male physicians earned about $35.00 per hour. The highest income for both male and female physicians was in the 10–19 years of experience category, where female physicians earned about $38.00 per hour and male physicians earned $50.00 per hour, a 24 percent differential (AMA 1989). Bobula (1980), using AMA data from 1978, also showed that female physicians earn less per hour than male physicians.

Although the AMA does not precisely describe how their income per hour figure is calculated, we decided to include this analysis on our data set because of the attractiveness of a simple summary number that might include both the productivity and income differentials that seem to exist. Our calculations are based on the assumption that physicians work 52 weeks a year. Although this is clearly not true, it is not necessary to introduce another calculation correcting this when our primary emphasis is on the possible differences between men and women. There seems to be little difference between male and female physicians in terms of weeks worked per year (AMA 1989). If this assumption were not true, and physicians worked fewer weeks per year, their income per hour would be higher.

Figure 5.3 shows the income per hour for four specialties (controlling for age), and Table 5.13 shows income per hour for males and females for several relevant variables. For every variable, female physicians make substantially less per hour than male physicians. The income/hour differential ranges from 13 percent less for female internists to 32 percent less for female OB/GYNs; from 14 percent less for female physicians involved in a hospital-based practice to 40 percent less for female physicians involved in solo practice, and from 7 percent less for female physicians over 55 years of age to 39 percent less for those in the 45–54 year-old range. Women physicians make less than men physicians, regardless of age, specialty, or practice arrangement.

We must confess to astonishment at the magnitude of the differences in income of male and female physicians. After these analyses were completed, we returned for a more extensive review of the literature. One of the first analyses of incomes of female and male physicians was done by Bobula (1980), using AMA data from 1978. He described the income differences by using hourly income and examined several variables that might affect income: specialty, type of practice, and several productivity measures, including hours worked per week and number of weeks worked per year. He also compared trends over time by analyzing data from 1972 in comparison with 1977. For most specialties, although

Figure 5.3   Physicians' Income per Hour by Specialty and Gender

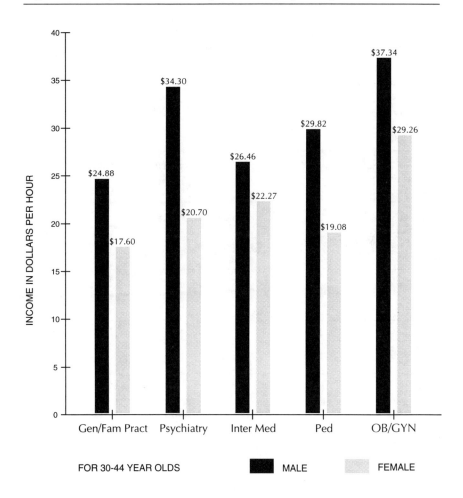

women's hourly income was closer to men's in 1977 than it had been in 1972, there was still a considerable difference. For example, in 1977, females in internal medicine made 30 percent less per hour than males; 25 percent less in OB/GYN; and about 20 percent less than their male colleagues in general/family practice, pediatrics, and psychiatry. After several corrections, he could not explain 17 percent of the income difference, and he concluded that the differences appeared to be due to gender.

Multivariate analyses of income differences between male and female physicians have been presented with the primary interest in determining how much of the income differential can be explained by an econometric model, and whether the observed differences in income

Table 5.13   Income per Hour for Several Variables

I. Specialty Group	Income/Hour		Percentage Differential
	Males	Females	
General/Family Practice	22.98	17.96	−22
Internal Medicine	25.82	22.46	−13
Pediatrics	26.94	19.25	−29
OB/GYN	39.82	26.92	−32
Psychiatry	33.05	27.08	−18
All others	34.56	28.84	−17

II. Practice Arrangement	Income/Hour		Percentage Differential
	Males	Females	
Solo practice	30.37	18.27	−40
Group of three or more	37.71	23.09	−39
Closed panel HMO	31.04	25.29	−19
Hospital	34.55	29.58	−14

III. Age	Income/Hour		Percentage Differential
	Males	Females	
30–44	33.13	24.63	−26
45–54	36.85	22.48	−39
55+	31.88	29.70−	−7

IV. Specialty Group	Income/Hour			
	30–44 years old		45–54 years old	
General/Family Practice				
Males	24.68	(−29%)	23.65	(−24%)
Females	17.50		18.04	
Internal Medicine				
Males	25.45	(−12%)	27.32	
Females	22.27		—*	
Pediatrics				
Males	29.62	(−36%)	23.17	(−20%)
Females	19.08		18.50	
OB/GYN				
Males	37.46	(−28%)	40.87	
Females	26.83		—*	
Psychiatry				
Males	34.30	(−40%)	32.68	(−15%)
Females	20.70		27.75	

*Based on fewer than five female physicians.

are due to differences in productivity or to discrimination. The first systematic econometric analysis, by Kehrer (1976), used data from a 1973 AMA study specifically designed to study the income differential between male and female physicians. Her main finding was that she could account for some, but not all, of the 40 percent income differential between male and female physicians. Additionally, she claimed that male and female physicians seem to respond differently to financial incentives: men appear to respond positively and women negatively to higher earnings, a situation that is termed a "backward-bending supply hypothesis." According to this theory, once a physician achieves a certain earnings level, it requires a substantial amount of extra money to induce the physician to work more hours rather than pursue leisure time. Mitchell (1984) tested this backward-bending supply hypothesis directly using 1978–1979 data collected by the National Opinion Research Center for the Health Care Finance Administration. Her results support Kehrer's findings that women are less responsive to increases in hourly earnings. Mitchell uses this finding as the primary explanation as to why women work fewer hours.

Langwell (1982) replicated Kehrer's model using 1977 data from the AMA's Twelfth Periodic Survey of Physicians, which included an oversample of female physicians. Langwell calculated what she termed "productivity differentials" for male and female physicians, primarily based on number of patients seen per week. Her results indicate that women physicians in 1978 saw 38 percent fewer patients than male physicians and received only 22 percent less income than male physicians. Langwell concluded that the income differences between men and women physicians were all related to these productivity differences and not to any sort of discrimination. Oshfeldt and Cullter (1986) also attempted an econometric analysis based on Kehrer's model but, unlike Langwell, made several adjustments in the specifications of the model in order to make it more accurate. This analysis was based on AMA SMS data from 1981–1982, and they concluded that there is a 12–13 percent unexplained income differential between male and female physicians. They argue that this differential is smaller than what has been noted previously primarily because of the more accurate specifications of the model.

The research utilizing these econometric models mainly has a technical focus on developing econometric models that can account for an increasing proportion of the income differential. The models themselves, whether improved as Oshfeldt and Cullter (1986) would argue or unimproved, all specify a variety of what are termed either "practice characteristics" or "personal characteristics." These include variables such as specialty, practice arrangements, and age as part of the model. Oshfeldt and Cullter (1986) noted that if there were any patterns of discrimination affecting any of these variables, it would be inappropriate to include the variable as part of the "personal characteristics" of the model. Indeed, many have argued that specialty choice, residency training, and type of practice are not individual variations but instead are the expressions of the systematic differences that seem to exist throughout medicine with respect to male and female physicians.

It seems to us, after reviewing the wealth of research that has been conducted on women in medicine, including the technical econometric approaches, and after carefully analyzing our own female respondents, that it is time to address a new level of research questions. This new research agenda seems urgent, since the income discrepancies between male and female physicians are getting worse, not better, despite the apparent convergence of many other practice characteristics. According to AMA figures, in 1978 women worked 14 percent fewer hours than male physicians and earned incomes that were 30 percent less. In 1987–1988, women physicians worked only 8 percent fewer hours but they earned 40 percent less than what male physicians earned (Bobula 1980; AMA 1989). As women in the medical work force grow in number, these sorts of gender differentials will have increasingly damaging effects.

Where to Go from Here?

The topic of women and money is troublesome for American society. When all labor categories are considered together, women earn less than men. Although the gap is narrowing, the process is very slow; in 1986 women earned $.64 for every $1.00 a male earned, and in 1991 women earned $.68 for every $1.00 a male earned (Gordon 1991), which translates to a gain of about one cent a year. Education is traditionally viewed as the way to increase income-earning potential, but it seems to help males more than females, and time does not seem to help. For example, in 1980 a male college graduate with ten years experience earned 31 percent more than a high school graduate, and 86 percent more in 1988. Women with college degrees and ten years of professional experience earned 37 percent more than women with high school degrees in 1980, and 60 percent more in 1988 (American Society for Training and Development 1991).

Even at the highest educational levels, income differences seem to persist. The most recent National Science Foundation survey found that female Ph.D. scientists earn between 20 and 25 percent less than their male colleagues (Silverman 1991). In the academic arena it is so well known that female faculty earn less than male faculty, that the American Association of University Professors (AAUP) has suggested a regression analysis technique to identify those women whose salaries need to be adjusted. The Association of American Medical Colleges (AAMC) has recently modified this model and suggests that it be used routinely within medical schools to correct salary inequities (Donoghue 1988).

That women in medicine earn less than men in medicine should not be surprising, given the overall income differences between men and women that obviously exist in American society. It is, however, important to move beyond mere description of the differences to learn more about exactly where these differences are likely to occur, and if possible, why. For example, the literature indicates that women physicians make an average income of almost 40 percent less than men physicians. There have been several explanations given for the differential, and we explored these in our data set. It is said that women make less money because they are more likely to be in lower-paid specialties—true, of course, but specialty does not explain the full income difference. Table 5.6 shows that, within the same specialty groups, women physicians make between 25 percent and 44 percent less than male physicians. A second explanation is that women earn less money because they are more likely to be involved in lower-paid practice arrangements. Although this is also somewhat true, the income differential still exists between men and women physicians within the same practice arrangement. A third explanation depends on time: women are likely to be younger and thus have fewer years of experience, which will produce lower incomes. Although this is true, both our data and the AMA data demonstrate the same 30–40 percent income differential between men and women in the same age group.

The final explanation concerns productivity, with several investigators suggesting that women earn less money because they are less productive. Although women do work fewer hours per week, it is much less than the income differential. Women in our sample work between 6 percent and 23 percent fewer hours per week for an income differential of 23–41 percent (Table 5.11). We tried to refine this notion of productivity even further by looking at the relationship between income per hour and specialty, practice arrangement, and age. As Table 5.13 shows, the income differentials persist, although they are somewhat lower— somewhere between 20 percent and 40 percent. We do not have enough women to do multivariate analysis, although when economists do a regression analysis on national data sets, the gender differential is lessened and, in some cases, disappears (Kehrer 1976; Langwell 1982; Ohsfeldt and Cullter 1986). We submit that these findings result from economic models that include specifications of variables characterized as "personal characteristics" that are actually related to barriers for female physicians, including specialty choice and practice arrangements.

Future research needs to concentrate on national samples of actively practicing physicians. The national sample—or at least a larger regional sample than we were able to achieve—would ensure a sufficient representation of women in all specialty groups. Our sample, for example, lacked enough women for us to analyze the surgical specialties, or the specialties of radiology and anesthesiology. All of these latter are higher-income specialties.

More standardization needs to be developed for the productivity measure. Although hours per week is certainly acceptable, probably using the hours spent in direct patient care is a more appropriate measure, since these are the income-generating hours. There was no specification in the studies we reviewed as to whether hours worked per week referred to total hours or direct care hours. On a related note, it is also important to include in the productivity estimate some measure of how many weeks a year physicians practice. There is very little information available about this figure.

Although multivariate models can—and should—be used to attempt to discover the relative importance of what are interconnected variables, it is extremely important that these models be accurately specified, acknowledging the complex social environment. More research needs to be done on why women seem to be overrepresented in some specialties and some practice arrangements. It is not enough to dismiss gender-based differentials due to women being younger or working less, since neither age nor productivity fully explains the income differences.

The suggestions outlined above address the more technical aspects of research on women in medicine, with a particular focus on measurement. We would also like to briefly address some of the more important content areas that need to be addressed in further research on women physicians. Perhaps the most salient comment is to admit that very little is actually known about female physicians, which Bowman and Gross (1986) have also suggested. First, most of the knowledge base about female physicians has been developed using information gathered when women were, in fact, a very small minority in medicine. We have included several examples where recent research has been too dependent on earlier research, much to the detriment of being able to analyze the complex medical-social environment in which female physicians find themselves working today.

Second, most of the knowledge base about female physicians has been developed by comparing them to male physicians. Models of specialty choice and location decision—as well as many practice patterns characteristics—all have been developed using information about male physicians and then applied to female physicians, without knowing whether the same factors are appropriate to female physicians. There is one area in which significant investigation has occurred using female physicians: productivity. There is pretty good evidence that women exhibit a different productivity pattern over their whole lifetime than men physicians (Kletke, Marder, and Silberger 1990; Heins et al. 1977). If this is true for productivity, it may be true for other areas of importance including specialty choice or location decisions, both of which are related to important policy areas.

This book is predicated upon the assumption that it is important to understand better the perceptions of physicians—a theme we will more fully develop in the next two chapters. It is very important to address the perceptions of female physicians separately from the perceptions of male physicians. There is much evidence to support separate investigations, and very little to suggest otherwise. In our preliminary analysis of several questionnaire items relating to level of satisfaction, there seemed to be systematic differences between male and female physicians, which will be detailed in the next chapter. There are some very intriguing results from the analysis of expectations presented in Table D.5. When using only those physicians (both male and female) who classify themselves as being at what they defined "at full professional capacity," there were the lowest differences between male and female physicians in terms of hours worked per week (which was our measure of productivity), although fewer women reported themselves to be at "full professional capacity."

Somewhere around 20 percent of the income difference between male and female physicians seems to be related only to gender. Interpretation of the importance of this difference can no longer be left as a matter of personal or political perspective. As Eisenberg, Lorber, and others have noted, women are an increasingly important part of the American physician supply. We cannot afford to alienate this important resource. The new research agenda not only needs to include technical refinements to sample size, productivity measures, and appropriate specification of variables for statistical analysis; it also needs to recognize the changed social environment of women and new research questions, only a few of which are mentioned here. The research questions that are prevalent in the older literature must be discarded in favor of research questions that more accurately reflect the medical work environment of the 1990s.

References

Allen, D. I. "Women in Medical Specialty Societies: An Update." *Journal of the American Medical Association* 262 (Dec. 1989): 3439–43.

AMA Center for Health Policy Research. *Socioeconomic Monitoring System 1988 Core Survey*. Chicago: AMA, 1989.

American Medical Association. "Physician Characteristics and Distribution in the U.S." 1986 Edition. Chicago: AMA, 1987a.

American Medical Association. *Women in Medicine Project: Data Source*. Chicago: AMA, 1987b.

American Medical Association. *Women in Medicine Project: In the Marketplace*. 2nd edition. Chicago: AMA, 1987c.

American Medical Association. *SMS Report*. Vol. 3, No. 6. Chicago: AMA Center for Health Policy Research, Nov. 1989.

American Society for Training and Development. *America and the New Economy*. Alexandria, VA: American Society for Training and Development, 1991.

Baucom-Copeland, S., E. T. Copeland, and L. L. Perry. "The Pregnant Resident: Career or Conflict?" *Journal of the American Medical Women's Association* 38 (1983): 103–5.

Bickel, J. "Women in Medical Education: A Status Report." *New England Journal of Medicine* 319 (Dec. 24, 1988): 1579–84.

Bobula, J. D. "Work Patterns, Practice Characteristics, and Incomes of Male and Female Physicians." *Journal of Medical Education* 55 (Oct. 1980): 826–33.

Bowman, M., and M. L. Gross. "Overview of Research on Women in Medicine— Issues for Public Policymakers." *Public Health Reports* 101 (1986): 513–21.

Clare, F. L., E. Spratley, P. Schwab, and J. K. Iglehart. "Trends in Health Care Personnel: Data Watch." *Health Affairs* (Winter 1987): 90–103.

Cohen, M., L. A. Woodward, and B. N. Femier. "Factors Influencing Career Development: Do Men and Women Differ?" *Journal of American Medical Women's Association* 43 (1988): 142–54.

Crozier, D. A., and J. K. Iglehart. "Trends in Health Manpower: Data Watch." *Health Affairs* (Winter 1986): 122–31.

Curry, L. "The Effect of Sex on Physician Work Patterns." In *Proceedings of the 22nd Annual Conference on Research in Medical Education*. Washington, DC: Association of American Medical Colleges, 1983, pp. 144–48.

Dennis, T., I. Harris, R. Petzel, R. Lofgren, E. Rich, R. McColister, J. Foley, and J. Lifto. "Influences of Marital Status and Parental Status on Professional Choices of Physicians About to Enter Practice." *Academic Medicine* 65 (Dec. 1990): 775–77.

Donoghue, G. D. "Eliminating Salary Inequities for Women and Minorities in Medical Academia." *Journal of American Medical Women's Association* 43 (1988): 28–29.

Dykman, R. A., and J. M. Stalnaker. "Survey of Women Physicians Graduating from Medical School 1925–1940." *Journal of Medical Education* 32 (1957): 3–38.

Eisenberg, C. "Medicine Is No Longer a Man's Profession or, When the Men's Club Goes Coed It's Time to Change the Regs." *New England Journal of Medicine* 321 (Nov. 30, 1989): 1542–44.

Gillis, K. D., and R. J. Willkie. "Employment Patterns of Physicians, 1983–1989." In M. L. Gonzalez and D. W. Emmons, eds., *Socioeconomic Characteristics of Medical Practice 1989*. Chicago: AMA Center for Health Policy Research, 1990.

Gordon, S. "How Women Are Battling Inequalities in the Workplace." *Boston Globe*, March 31, 1991.

Grunebaum, A., H. Minkoff, and D. Blake. "Pregnancy Among Obstetricians. A Comparison of Birth Before, During and After Residency." *American Journal of Obstetricians and Gynecologists.* 157 (July 1987): 79–83.

Heins, M. "Women in Medicine: Two Points of View on Medicine and Motherhood." *Journal of the American Medical Association* 249 (1983): 209–10.

Heins, M., S. Smock, L. Martindale, J. Jacobs, and M. Stein. "Comparison of the Productivity of Women and Men Physicians." *Journal of the American Medical Association* 237 (June 1977): 2514–17.

Hojat, M., J. S. Gonnella, J. J. Veloski, and S. Moses. "Differences in Professional Activities, Perceptions of Professional Problems and Practice Patterns Between Men and Women Graduates of Jefferson Medical College." *Academic Medicine* 65 (Dec. 12, 1990): 755–61.

Jussim, J., and C. Miller. "Medical Education for Women: How Good an Investment?" *Journal of Medical Education* 50 (1975): 571–80.

Kehrer, B. H. "Factors Affecting the Incomes of Men and Women Physicians: An Exploratory Analysis." *Journal of Human Resources* 11 (Fall 1976): 26–45.

Kletke, P. R., W. D. Marder, and A. B. Silberger. "The Growing Proportion of Female Physicians: Implications for U.S. Physician Supply." *American Journal of Public Health* 80 (March 1990): 300–305.

Langwell, K. M. "Factors Affecting the Incomes of Men and Women Physicians: Further Explorations." *Journal of Human Resources* 17 (1982): 261–75.

Levinson, W., S. W. Tolle, and C. Lewis. "Women in Academic Medicine: Combining Career and Families." *New England Journal of Medicine* 321 (Nov. 30, 1989): 1511–17.

Lisokie, S. "Why Work Fewer Hours." *Journal of American Medical Women's Association* 41 (May-June 1986): 87–89.

Lorber, J. "More Women Physicians: Will it Mean More Humane Health Care?" *Social Policy* (Summer 1985): 50–54.

Lorber, J. "A Welcome to a Crowded Field: Where Will the New Women Physicians Fit In?" *Journal of American Medical Women's Association* 42 (1987): 149–52.

Maheux, B., F. Dufort, F. Beland, A. Jacques, and A. Levesque. "Female Medical Practitioners: More Preventive and Patient-Oriented?" *Medical Care* 28 (Jan. 1990): 87–92.

Marder, W. D., P. R. Kletke, A. B. Silberger, and R. J. Willke. *Physician Supply and Utilization by Specialty: Trends and Projections.* Chicago: AMA, 1988.

McDonald, L. L. "Women Physicians and Organized Medicine." *Western Journal of Medicine* 149 (1988): 777–78.

Mitchell, J. B. "Why Do Women Physicians Work Fewer Hours Than Men Physicians?" *Inquiry* 21 (Winter 1984): 365–68.

Moore, F. D., and C. Priebe. "Board-Certified Physicians in the United States 1971–1986." *New England Journal of Medicine* 324 (Feb. 21, 1991): 536–43.

Ohsfeldt, R. L., and S. D. Cullter. "Differences in Income Between Male and Female Physicians." *Journal of Health Economics* 5 (1986): 335–46.

Pennell, M. Y., and J. E. Renshaw. "Distribution of Women Physicians." *Journal of American Medical Women's Association* 28 (1973): 181–86.

Potter, R. L. "Resident, Woman, Wife, Mother: Issues for Women in Training." *Journal of the American Medical Association* 38 (1983): 98–102.

Powers, L., R. D. Parmelle, and H. Weisenfelder. "Practice Patterns of Women and Men Physicians." *Journal of Medical Education* 44 (June 1969): 481–85.

Relman, A. S. "The Changing Demography of the Medical Profession." *New England Journal of Medicine* 321 (Nov. 30, 1989): 1543–47.

Roback, J. G., L. Randolph, and B. Seidman. *Physician Characteristics and Distribution in the U.S.* Chicago: Department of Physician Data Services, Division of Survey and Data Resources, American Medical Association, 1990.

Sayres, M., G. Wyshak, G. Denterlein, R. Apfel, E. Shore, and D. Federmann. "Pregnancy During Residency." *New England Journal of Medicine* 314 (1986): 418–23.

Schaller, J. G. "The Advancement of Women in Academic Medicine." *Journal of the American Medical Association* 264 (Oct 10, 1990): 1854–55.

Schloss, E. P. "Beyond GEMENAC—Another Physician Shortage from 2010 to 2030?" *New England Journal of Medicine* 318 (April 1988): 920–22.

Silberger, A. B., W. D. Marder, and R. J. Willkie. "Practice Characteristics of Male and Female Physicians." *Health Affairs* 6 (1987): 104–9.

Silverman, E. R. "Gender Gaps in All Categories." *The Scientist* (Aug. 19, 1991): 20–21.

Sinal, S., P. Weavil, and M. G. Canep. "Survey of Women Physicians on Issues Related to Pregnancy During a Medical Career." *Journal of Medical Education.* 63 (July 1988): 531–38.

Sloan, F. A. "Physician Supply Behavior in the Short Run." *Industrial & Labor Relations Review* 28 (July 1975): 549–69.

Weisman, C. S., D. M. Levin, D. M. Steinwachs, and G. A. Chase. "Male and Female Physician Career Patterns: Specialty Choices and Graduate Training." *Journal of Medical Education* 55 (1980): 813–25.

Williams, P. B. "Recent Trends in the Productivity of Women and Men Physicians." *Journal of Medical Education* 53 (May 1978): 420–22.

Chapter 6

Physician Perceptions of Medical Practice: Can They Be Measured?

Measuring Career Satisfaction

> Surprisingly few studies have been conducted on the topic of job sat-
> isfaction: those that do exist generally have included the measure as a
> concern secondary to some other primary research aim or have neglected
> some of the complexities involved in measuring the concept. (Lichenstein
> 1984, 61)

This observation remains as true today despite several efforts to measure physician satisfaction during the last ten years. It is not that the importance or desirability of measuring physician satisfaction is going unrecognized: physician satisfaction is a variable that is often alluded to in studies and increasingly is explicitly measured. However, the measurements have usually been specific to a particular practice site and have lacked generalizability. The lack of a generalizable measure has impeded the ability to explore the correlations between physician satisfaction and other variables such as practice arrangement, specialty, age, gender, and productivity.

One of the assumptions basic to the development of this book is that it is important to increase the knowledge base about physicians' perceptions of their role in the medical care delivery system. We have included personal anecdotes and comments by some of the study respondents that have added context to some of the more empirical results. We have also included analysis of responses to questions designed to provide information relating to physicians' perceptions about specific areas of interest, particularly concerning income. Both of these qualitative levels of information provide interesting and valuable information. This chapter focuses on taking the next step: to begin the process of attempting to capture physician perceptions in a more quantitative manner.

This chapter begins with a brief summary of the alternate theoretical views that are currently utilized to conceptualize physician perceptions, followed by a discussion of some important methodological considerations in terms of relating measurements to theoretical constructs. Our model of scale development will be discussed next, followed by a lengthy section presenting some of the most important results from the data gathered in western Massachusetts. The chapter concludes with two more general sections: one considering how satisfied physicians seem to be and the last presenting recommendations for future research in the process of developing a measurement instrument for physician satisfaction.

Conceptualizing Physician Perceptions

Physician perceptions are conceptualized in one of two ways. The first is to focus on the stress that is inherent in the role definition of physicians. The second way is to focus on those factors within a practice environment that cause physicians to be relatively satisfied or dissatisfied. The assumption of this second conceptual framework is that level of satisfaction or dissatisfaction is primarily related to the work environments, organizations, or practice arrangements of physicians, rather than to the inherent role designation of physicians. These are two distinctly different ways of thinking about physician perceptions and, as might be expected, the findings that result from these two approaches are quite different.

Stress inherent in the role of physicians

McCue (1982) has helped to articulate the general framework for studies exploring the stress inherent in the role of the physician. The article identified six distinct sources of stress, including "working with intensely emotional aspects of life governed by strong cultural codes for behavior, e.g., suffering, fear, sexuality, and death; inadequate training for fundamental professional tasks, e.g., handling 'problem patients'; and demands from society or patients that cannot be reasonably met, e.g., the need for certainty when current medical knowledge allows only approximation" (p. 459). Linn et al. (1985b) followed this line of research by attempting to determine how many of McCue's observations could be documented empirically, using a scale specifically constructed to measure stress. Several of McCue's observations were supported, including the intensity of stress involved in having to deal with the intensely emotional aspects of patients' lives; having to deal with problem patients; and having activities at home interrupted by work responsibilities.

Other research has consistently supported two particular sources of stress perceived by physicians. The first and most ubiquitous is the pressure of time. It is hard to find any study about physicians that does not include some mention of time pressures (Linn et al. 1985b; Makin, Rout, and Cooper 1988; Mawardi 1977). Frequently, time pressures are conceptualized as conflicts between the demands of work, home, family, and leisure (Linn et al. 1985b, 1986; Reidel and Reidel 1979). Recognition of time pressures are not new: in the classic 1963 community survey of Canadian physicians, Clute (1963) discovered that conflicting demands on a physician's time were primary concerns. Others have written extensively and very personally about this subject (Hilfaker 1985; Payne and Firth-Cozens 1987; Natelson 1990; Friedson 1989).

A second particular source of stress that appears repeatedly in the literature is related specifically to patients. The term "problem patient" is often used to include two distinct groups of patients: those for whom a clear diagnosis and treatment is difficult, as well as those patients who have problems that are easily diagnosed but not easily treated (McCue 1982; Linn et al. 1985b; May and Revicki 1985). The challenge of treating complex problems is one of the most satisfying activities for physicians, and the challenge is viewed positively. However, in many situations the challenge becomes unmanageable: the patient may be correctly diagnosed but treatment options are not successful, or there may not be effective treatments available. This challenge is an interesting and complex variable that needs more investigation.

Some research utilizing the conceptual framework of stress focuses on the consequences of working for long periods of time under perceived high levels of stress. These consequences include what is termed the "impaired physician," which often refers to some sort of substance abuse but which may also include mental and emotional health, particularly depression (Linn et al. 1986; May and Revicki 1985; Krakowski 1982; Gerrity, DeVellis, and Earp 1990). Another consequence is "professional stress syndrome," which occurs when physicians (or other professionals) continue to work in the stressful situation with no relief. It can lead to what is usually called "burnout" involving a variety of negative behaviors (Payne and Firth-Cozens 1987; Pfifferling 1980; Scheiber 1983; Gardner and Hall 1981; Maslach 1976, 1982; Scully 1980; Shubin 1978; Emener 1979; Sargent 1987; Rosemark 1986; Sargent et al. 1986).

Physicians do learn to adapt to—or at least cope with—the high levels of stress inherent in their patient responsibilities. Reames and Dunstone (1989) conducted in-depth interviews to identify stresses and document ways in which physicians cope with them. Physicians in this study who identified themselves as "satisfied" attributed this to their own personal "attitudinal adjustments," part of which involved a process of redefining the problem. May and Revicki (1985) developed a model of the professional stress syndrome among family physicians and identified ways physicians cope with stress levels. Others have explored ways physicians either cope with—or buffer themselves from—stress, including looking at ways in which organizations, the family structure, or specific programs may help buffer physicians from perceptions of high level of stress (LaRocco, House, and French 1980; Shore 1987; Numerof and Abrams 1981; Reuben et al. 1984; Borenstein and Cook 1982; Talbot et al. 1987).

Satisfaction and dissatisfaction as the conceptual framework

The typical view of stress is that it arises from high levels of dissatisfaction, and some of the research supports the relationship between stress and low levels of satisfaction (Makin, Rout, and Cooper 1988; Clarke et al. 1984). However, others point out that stress levels are not related to level of satisfaction (Linn et al. 1986). It is important to recognize the well-developed theoretical models relating to satisfaction and dissatisfaction. These two concepts are not simply at the opposite ends of the same continuum (Herzberg, Mausner, and Snyderman 1959). Stress is more appropriately viewed as a third and separate concept—and as another way of analyzing physician perceptions. '

Only recently have there been serious efforts made to address how satisfied health care professionals are with their jobs. The major group studied is nurses, probably because their high turnover rates are so costly to organizations. There is a substantial body of literature on nurses' level of work satisfaction, summarized in a book describing what is now considered to be the definitive scale to measure occupational satisfaction of nurses and which is also used to change the work environment of nurses to decrease nursing turnover (Stamps and Piedmonte 1986).

Despite many indications of high levels of dissatisfaction, most of the research focusing on nurses emphasizes satisfaction, not dissatisfaction. This is not the case with physicians; the focus is much more likely to be on dissatisfaction of physicians. Part of this focus may arise from the increasingly common reports of dissatisfaction in the mass media, which provide unsettling conclusions about medicine and the motivation of physicians. Many of these reports arise from results of surveys of physicians by trade journals. For example, a survey of physicians conducted by *Physician's Management* (Feb. 1991, 8–11) presents a profile of a "profession at odds with itself." In other words, "doctors love their work but hate the business." Respondents indicated dissatisfaction with long work hours, and a majority say they work harder than they did three years ago. In this survey, 63 percent indicate they would not recommend that their children choose medicine as a career. Similar results were obtained by another survey conducted by a professional magazine, in which respondents were very dissatisfied with what they termed the "hassle factor" of medicine (*Boston Globe*, April 12, 1991, p. 34).

Although it is not wise to generalize from surveys conducted by professional magazines, which often poll only their own readers, some national polls have produced results that are very similar. For example, a recent Gallup poll indicated that 40 percent of physicians would not choose to enter medical school again (*Boston Globe*, May 21, 1990, p. 15). This result was particularly striking since it is in contrast to the result for lawyers, only 19 percent of whom would not choose to enter law school again. The AMA does periodic surveys of physicians: the picture that emerges is one of anxiety. Physicians seem to believe increasingly that an oversupply of physicians does exist and that the increased competition will lead to income restrictions. Also mentioned is the declining perception of satisfaction from medical practice due to the increasing restriction of professional and clinical autonomy from various levels of regulation. As before, over half of the respondents in these national surveys would not recommend medicine to a young person as highly as they would have ten years ago (American College of Hospital Administrators 1984; Freshnock 1984; Harvey and Shubat 1989).

A cynical response to these generally negative perceptions is that physicians are unhappy with any external regulation on their practice. An even more generalized response is to note that any professional group has trouble with change and external regulation, and all observers would agree that medicine has changed significantly in the last ten to fifteen years, especially with respect to the increased external regulations. However tempting this response might be, it is not helpful because it does not permit the examination of the nature of the unhappiness. Without a more solid knowledge base about what dissatisfies—and satisfies—physicians in their work, it is too easy to convert the results of these national surveys into a professional or political agenda. Several researchers have attempted to examine physician satisfaction and dissatisfaction more carefully, and we summarize some of their work here.

Physician satisfaction is most frequently included as one variable in a study whose major objective is something else. In the late 1980s and early 1990s, the most common approach is to study physician satisfaction in the context of a larger study whose primary analysis concerns organizational or administrative issues. This orientation is a continuation of the way research was conceptualized beginning in the mid- to late 1970s, when organizational issues were being considered systematically. One of the most often cited articles in terms of the effect of organizational setting on physician satisfaction was Mechanic's 1975 study, in which the major objective was to determine how a prepaid setting affected physicians. Data on a variety of characteristics were presented, including sociodemographic attributes, size of community, income, and workload, among others, for both prepaid and nonprepaid settings, which, at that time, were termed "traditional" sites. Mechanic also included a couple of measures related to satisfaction: one called "social orientation to medical care" and a series of items that provided a more direct measure of satisfaction with medical care. Breslau, Novack, and Wolf (1978) continued this line of investigation but focused more directly on satisfaction, both of physicians and nonphysician personnel. In both of these studies satisfaction was considered to be a dependent variable, and the nature of the organization was considered to be the independent variable. In both studies, the level of satisfaction of physicians was found to be less in the more highly structured organizations. This conclusion has permeated the literature as an unspoken assumption for many years, although in today's medical practice climate, both articles seem unfairly biased against more organized practice settings.

A more recent study grows out of this line of reasoning and also shows an evolution of the use of satisfaction as a measure, by relating the decision to leave a prepaid group practice to the level of satisfaction of the physician with the group practice experience (Mick et al. 1983). This study divided physicians into those who left a prepaid group practice and those who stayed and compared the level of satisfaction in the two groups. The results were rather nebulous, and the authors conclude with an observation that perhaps turnover is more complicated than merely being an expression of dissatisfaction.

Only very recently has research questioned the assumption that physicians who work in organized group practices are less satisfied. Schulz et al. designed a scale modeled on the work of Lichenstein (1984) and Stamps (Stamps et al. 1978; Slavitt et al. 1978) and administered it first in a mental health setting in Germany, and then to HMO physicians in Dane County, Wisconsin (Schulz and Schulz 1988; Schulz, Girard, and Sheckler 1992). Unlike previous studies, this research indicates that increasing organizational size and management constraints do not relate to a perception of diminished clinical autonomy or to a lower level of satisfaction. In both of these articles, there is some suggestion that physicians may feel somewhat protected or buffered by the organizations in which they work.

The most common use of physician satisfaction measures in the context of an organizational analysis is in an academic medical environment. Many studies actually focus on the stress that is unique to physicians in training, often conceptualized as learning about the "uncertainty" of medicine (May and Revicki 1985; Fox 1957; Schwartz 1978; Thomas 1975;

Crapen 1980; Linn 1981). Two particular studies focused on satisfaction, using this as a variable to assess the effect of organizational changes on the interns and residents. In both studies, physician satisfaction increased with those organizational arrangements that reinforced continuity of care (Linn et al. 1985a; Lofgren and Mladenovic 1990).

Another group of studies provide examples of research whose major objective is to identify or describe variables that seem related to physician satisfaction. By far, the largest and most consistent category of variables related to physician satisfaction are those pertaining to patients —in most cases, specific to the physician-patient relationship (Linn et al. 1985b, 1986; Mawardi 1979; Reidel and Reidel 1929; Mechanic 1975; Kravitz, Linn, and Shapiro 1990). In some cases, more specific aspects of dealing with patients are emphasized: for example, receiving respect and appreciation from patients (Mawardi 1979; McCranie, Hornsby, and Calvert 1982), helping patients (Charles et al. 1987), or even more specifically, helping patients with diagnosable conditions (Grol et al. 1985). Sometimes, explicit mention is made of the diversity of patients (Linn et al. 1985b; Kravitz, Linn, and Shapiro 1990); in other cases, distinctions are made between types of physicians, such as rural physicians valuing physician-patient relationships more highly than nonrural physicians (Hassinger et al. 1980).

Related to patient care is the subject of work load, most commonly expressed as patient volume. The relationship between physician satisfaction and patient volume is not as consistent as it seems to be for the centrality of the physician-patient relationship. Some studies demonstrate that physician satisfaction seems related to patient volume (Reidel and Reidel 1979; Kravitz, Linn, and Shapiro 1990), but for most studies there seems to be no relationship (Linn et al. 1985a). The most important predictor of physician satisfaction seems to be not the number of patients seen, but the efficiency with which they are seen (Linn et al. 1985a).

Some aspects of satisfaction seem to be related to certain characteristics of physicians, although these are not often included in research models. For example, increasing age seems to be closely related to an increased level of satisfaction, not only for physicians but also for most other workers (Kravitz, Linn, and Shapiro 1990). Sometimes characteristics of physicians may partially determine what is more likely to provide satisfaction. For example, physicians practicing in nonrural areas, who are more likely to be specialists, are also more likely to gain satisfaction from the technical aspects of their jobs (Hassinger et al. 1980); those who are "disease oriented" view medicine differently than those who are "patient oriented," and their level of satisfaction is different (Linn 1981). Physician characteristics are such an important variable that Schulz and Schulz (1988) put them as a significant variable in their model.

One difficulty in attempting to summarize those factors that provide satisfaction to physicians is the variation in the way investigators conceptualize, and thus measure, satisfaction. In some studies, for example, the word "satisfaction" is never used; rather, the word "dissatisfaction" is used. In some studies, the terms are "most satisfied," "moderately satisfied," and "least satisfied." The difference between "least satisfied" and "dissatisfied" is perhaps only a semantic one, but it makes a systematic content analysis difficult. Of course, part of the problem lies in the nature of the area being investigated, since some variables may produce satisfaction or dissatisfaction or both. Perhaps the best examples are variables relating to patients. Patient care also has the potential to produce serious levels of dissatisfaction. The British studies are careful to acknowledge that a significant contributor to physician satisfaction is a low level of emotional involvement with patients (Makin, Rout, and Cooper 1988; Cooper, Rout, and Faragher 1989). U.S. physicians also may be extremely dissatisfied with aspects of patient care: sometimes the patients are too sick (Clarke et al. 1984); are not sick enough, but demand services (Reidel and Reidel 1979); have undiagnosable or psychosomatic/psychosocial problems; or do not cooperate with therapy (Mawardi 1979; Krakowski 1982). Fears of malpractice suits, or even physical violence from patients, also produce a profound sense not only of dissatisfaction, but also of anxiety (Charles et al. 1987; Mawardi 1979). There seems to be some evidence that increased contact with patients during the internship year not only decreases levels of satisfaction, but also causes more negative views of patients in general (Sparr et al. 1988). The positive aspects of both the challenge and intellectual stimulation of medicine and the rewards of the physician-patient relationship obviously have limits for most physicians.

Which measurements to use?

The diversity of topics covered in the many articles concerned with physician satisfaction and perception of stress is impressive. However, after reading them, one is left not with a sense of a "body of knowledge," but with a sense of frustration. The frustration arises not so much from the inconsistency and contradictory nature of the findings, although that is frequently the case. More discomforting is the conceptual confusion: although some studies are clearly oriented in the stress framework and some are clearly oriented in analyzing satisfaction and dissatisfaction, many actually include questions that address both. Another conceptual confusion is about whether satisfaction, dissatisfaction, or stress is an independent or dependent variable. Within this literature, there are examples of each. For those studies that include an organizational analysis, satisfaction is generally viewed as a dependent variable, varying with the organizational arrangement. For those studies with a descriptive objective, satisfaction is frequently discussed as if it were the independent variable.

Finally, in too many of the studies, some conclusions jump too far ahead of the knowledge base. An example of this is the statement: "These findings suggest that improving physician and patient satisfaction may have economic as well as psychological and social benefits" (Linn et al. 1985a, 811). This, of course, is technically true; after all, the word "may" is clearly conditional. But it is so intuitively appealing that empirical evidence is not pursued. It is too tempting to accept the several conclusions of these studies without a sharp realization that it is important to devote time to the development of a measurement instrument. The first step in this development process is to be conceptually clear. This is not really a question of which is better, since each alternative approach is different and thus answers a different set of questions, each one valuable. Both feelings—that of being stressed or of being either satisfied or dissatisfied—are based on personal perceptions. There is some evidence that perceptions of stress are able to be buffered, either by an organization or family or friends, although they cannot be eliminated (LaRocco, House, and French 1980). Within this understanding, perceptions of satisfaction or dissatisfaction may be seen to be a dependent variable, occurring as a result of a physician characteristic (such as age, gender, or specialty), or organization or practice arrangement.

We feel that two lines of investigation exist here and should be pursued separately. Research into the inherent stress present in a physician's role responsibilities will ultimately lead to a better understanding of physicians and may enable the prediction of negative behaviors that may be associated with unrelieved levels of stress. A separate area of investigation is to focus on those factors that provide satisfaction and dissatisfaction. Identification of these factors should help prevent burnout by providing insights on how best to control the stress inherent in a physician's role. The satisfaction framework allows the investigation of the effect of organizations on physician perceptions.

We have chosen to anchor our work in the satisfaction/dissatisfaction framework. This choice has been primarily influenced by practical considerations related to the prediction of serious health care reform. Most of the reforms suggested involve physicians working in organizations; it is important to have a better sense of those factors that physicians perceive to be satisfying so that these organizations are more likely to be successful. The secondary reason for choosing to orient our work around the concepts of satisfaction and dissatisfaction concerns measurement. Although it is certainly difficult to measure perceptions of satisfaction, it is much harder to measure physician perception of stress. Evidence indicates that there is considerable diversity among physicians in both their perception of stress and their tolerance of stress. Finally, it is our belief that understanding what satisfies and dissatisfies physicians will provide the tools to help prevent—or at least mediate—perceptions of stress.

Currently, it is impossible to summarize the general level of satisfaction or dissatisfaction of physicians, partly because of the obvious diversity of factors that provide satisfaction and dissatisfaction. However, another very important consideration lies in the way in which satisfaction and dissatisfaction are measured. Many methodological problems exist.

Methodological Issues

The type of measurement used to quantify physician satisfaction, dissatisfaction, or stress arises from the way in which the investigator conceptualizes the nature of the problem. It is very hard to separate out methodology—including study design, sample selection, and measurement—from conceptual framework, findings, and results. In the previous section, we focused on conceptual framework and results, and in this section we focus on methodological issues, with a particular emphasis on measurement. Some findings and observations relevant to analyzing the measurement used are discussed here.

As with all efforts to develop measurements, there is a range from more qualitative to quantitative measures; there is also a diversity of measures with respect to generality or specificity, with some studies being so specific for one particular setting as to constitute a case study approach. The theoretical orientation also affects the nature of the measure: for example, some studies involve the development of a scale to measure uncertainty or stress, while others focus on satisfaction. Our primary emphasis will be on the development of a measurement instrument for perception of satisfaction or dissatisfaction. This section will be organized by methodological approach rather than content, beginning with the more qualitative methods, including personal interviews and general questionnaires. More quantitative methods, usually questionnaires, will be addressed next, and this section will conclude with a description of the scales that have been developed.

Measurement by qualitative methods

Qualitative methods are generally viewed as being most appropriate to the beginning of the research process, although this is not always true. In some cases, a qualitative method may be viewed as a more appropriate methodology, even if more quantitative measures exist. Development of a quantitative measure for perceptions of satisfaction is extremely difficult; as a result, there are several studies that utilize more qualitative approaches. Two recent studies provide interesting examples of a qualitative approach. In one, Reames and Dunstone (1989) interviewed 19 physicians primarily to determine how physicians define and solve problems facing the profession of medicine. This study had as its objective an abstract problem—how physicians view their own profession. The population selected was not representative—19 respondents selected by the authors as physicians who are not highly dissatisfied, but who are able to articulate problems facing medicine. The data collection method consisted of a taped personal interview in which each respondent was asked to define the nature of problems facing physicians, the way in which the respondent was coping with these, and general perceived levels of satisfaction. Even though the very nature of this research limits the generalizability, the insights into the medical profession are interesting.

A second example of a qualitative approach is that of Hassinger et al. (1980), who interviewed 121 practicing physicians in rural and metropolitan areas to determine if rural and nonrural physicians gain satisfaction from different factors. In this case, physicians were asked to respond to the question, "How satisfied are you with your present work situation?" with response categories ranging from "very satisfied" to "very dissatisfied." This study, along with several others from the same time period, showed that rural physicians tend to be most satisfied with the quality and continuity of physician-patient relationships, while metropolitan physicians tend to be more satisfied with the technical side of medicine.

Both of these studies used Mawardi's (1979) work, one of the most frequently cited articles on physician satisfaction, as the rationale for a qualitative methodology. In her longitudinal study, she interviewed physicians graduating from Case Western Reserve during the first decade (1956–1965) following a major curriculum revision. Although she also used a modification of a scale (the Brayfield job satisfaction blank), she depended heavily upon the results of the personal interviews to determine the satisfaction and dissatisfaction of the respondents. It was Mawardi who first noted that physicians seem to be more satisfied with the nature of the physician-patient relationship and less satisfied with time pressures, a theme that has been continued over time.

The move from interviews to semistructured questionnaires

Four studies represent what may be considered a second state of measurement development, the use of a semistructured questionnaire, rather than an interview, in an effort to provide more structure to the information gathered from the respondent. Two of the best examples of this approach are from the same period of time.

Perhaps the most influential in the long run has been Mechanic (1975), whose primary objective was to determine the effect of organized practice styles on a variety of physician characteristics. The study used a large national sample from AMA collected data, which included a questionnaire. The questionnaire gathered data on a wide variety of physician characteristics, including physician satisfaction. Physician satisfaction was measured by nine items asking about specific facets of satisfaction, along with one separate global item. The nine items included variables such as amount of time with each patient, opportunities for professional contacts, amount of income, office facilities, community status and esteem, and amount of leisure time, among others. Mechanic also had two other measures: "attitude toward various aspects of medical practice" and "social orientation to medical care." In the former, physicians were asked to agree or disagree with statements such as the following: "One should not become a doctor unless he is willing to sacrifice his own needs to the general welfare" and "Given the conditions of general practice, the doctor is not really in a position to make many of the assessments he is called upon to make"; and to agree or disagree with items such as: "Doctors working on a salaried basis" or "Federal financing of the organization of medical care." For the questionnaire on social orientation to medical care, physicians were asked to respond to several items regarding patient care, including level of agreement with responsibility for psychological care, or level of frustration with "unnecessary visits." The general findings of this study sound out of step with today's world of organized general practice, as, for example, the statement: "The data suggest that the patient load characteristic of general practice in prepaid groups encourages a more assembly line practice which is less responsive to patients than the pattern characteristic of fee-for-service practice" (p. 189). The specific data regarding level of physician satisfaction are mixed.

A similar approach, although on a smaller scale, was used by Reidel and Reidel (1979) in analyzing the results of the Ambulatory Care Project in Connecticut. In this study personal interviews and questionnaires were used to gather a wide variety of information on some 200 physicians practicing in the state of Connecticut. Level of satisfaction was determined by use of open-ended questions, such as "most gratifying aspect of medical practice" or "percent of patient population that physician knows well" or "skill which physician feels has been most developed since school," among others. Once again, the results are rather ambiguous, difficult to summarize, and not very generalizable.

More sophisticated questionnaires

The next step in the development of a measurement instrument is to develop a questionnaire more focused than the ones just described. The items appear to be related, but little or no statistical testing is done on the structure of the instrument itself, which differentiates it from a scaling approach. The advantage of a more focused questionnaire is that the results may be much more easily summarized and, one would hope, the items included are somewhat more generalizable than those in semistructured questionnaires. More sophisticated questionnaires are not prevented from being used for site-specific studies, as the three examples we will note here show.

McCranie, Hornsby, and Calvert (1982) developed a 76-item questionnaire based on Mechanic's 1975 work. The 76 items were divided into three sections. The first set of items covered the degree of satisfaction physicians had with different aspects of their practices, as well as with their career and work in general. In this section, physicians were asked to rate on a seven-point scale, from "very satisfied" to "very dissatisfied," items such as "the hospital privileges I have"; "the respect I receive from my patients"; and "the time I have for leisure and relaxation," among others. The second set of items asked the physicians about problems, including "having to take care of medical problems beyond my training"; "interference of external regulations and/or agencies in the physician-patient relationship"; and "having too many patients to see." The third section of items concerned other related attitudes about medical training, practice characteristics, and demographic items. This questionnaire was distributed to a national sample of residency-trained family physicians, drawn from the AMA's Masterfile and the American Academy of Family Physicians list of diplomates. This study, which is often cited, indicated fairly high levels of general satisfaction among family physicians, with several specific areas of dissatisfaction noted, including practice time pressures, paperwork, and perceived interference of external regulations or agencies in the physician-patient relationship.

When Mick et al. (1983) were assessing the differences between physicians who left group practices and those who stayed, they used a questionnaire that included items organized into two groups. One they labeled as "attitudes toward professional work," which included items such as "making a lot of money," "having opportunities to be helpful to others and to society," and "having prestige in the community." The second group of items included what they termed "prepaid group practice characteristics," such as freedom from supervision, freedom from excessive bureaucratic regulations, and working with intellectually stimulating colleagues. Although they did not label these as measures of physician satisfaction, others have included similar items in questionnaires that are so designated. Their findings are set completely in the context of the physician's decision to leave or stay in a prepaid group practice, and are not as useful for our purpose as some of the other studies that are more general in focus.

Lofgren and Mladenovic (1990) used a questionnaire specifically designed to measure physician satisfaction with an organizational change in a teaching hospital clinic. It was a self-administered questionnaire that contained 15 statements measuring three dimensions of satisfaction: educational experience, organization and function of the clinic, and quality of care. By using a five-point response mode and by treating the questionnaire as a scale, they were able to use one summary number to represent physician satisfaction on a pretest and on a posttest, before and after the organizational change. This study was able to show that the physicians' level of satisfaction increased on all three components as a result of the clinic reorganization.

As studies use more structured types of questionnaires, more features of scales appear. For example, it is common to utilize an attitude-scale-type response mode to structured questions, often using either a five- or seven-point scale. In some cases, the items are themselves grouped into similar clusters and responses to groups of items may be summed together to create one summary score. However appealing this level of quantification is, these are not scales. The definition of a scale does not lie in the response mode; rather it lies in the construction, which should involve not only reliability analysis, but also validity analysis. Meeting the statistical criteria for scale development ensures having a measurement that meets the accepted standards for reliability and validity, which allows for more sophisticated statistical analysis of the results. If a group of items can be defined as measuring one concept, then one summary number may be used to represent that concept, either as an evaluation of organizational effectiveness or in exploring correlations between variables.

For example, the questionnaire used by McCranie, Hornsby, and Calvert (1982) contains 17 items that measure what they term "ratings of satisfaction with various aspects of physicians' careers and practices." Included in this set of items are statements relating to hospital privileges, respect from patients, adequacy of training, physical resources, opportunity for professional contact, organization and management of practice, time for leisure and relaxation, as well as financial costs of the practice. This set of items obviously covers a wide variety of what are probably different aspects of physician satisfaction. In order to be able to use one summary number, the investigator must first have confidence that the items that are being added together in fact all measure the same thing. It is very likely that the 17 items used by McCranie, Hornsby, and Calvert are measuring different things.

Scale construction is an effort to discover the underlying scale struc- ture, which is to search for what is actually being measured, or to dis- cover the validity of the scale. Scale development usually occurs in those fields where there is a general agreement about the concepts being measured, since theoretical agreement is necessary before such structured measurements can be developed. Ideally, a scale will be general enough to be highly usable; although others may refine the scale, redefining the concepts or constructs is not usually necessary. Such has not been the case in the effort to measure physician satisfaction. The first disagreement is conceptual: the difference between considering stress or satisfaction to be the theoretical framework. Even within each of these concepts, there seems to be little agreement: there are three different scales to measure physician stress (Makin, Rout, and Cooper 1988; Linn et al. 1986; May and Revicki 1985; Revicki and May 1983), and eight different scales used to measure physician satisfaction, which are described below.

Scales to measure physician satisfaction

One of the first, and still most thorough, efforts at constructing a scale to measure physician satisfaction was completed by Lichenstein (1984). He first elaborated a conceptual framework for measuring physician satisfaction, drawing heavily on the prior work by Stamps and Pied- monte in developing a scale to measure nurse satisfaction (Stamps et al. 1978; Slavitt et al. 1978). Lichenstein conceptualized job satisfaction as lying within the conceptual framework of discrepancy theory, which requires the respondent to compare an ideal work situation to the current situation. He also recognized the multidimensionality of job satisfaction and identified seven separate facets of physician job satisfaction. Finally, he made the important observation that global satisfaction should be measured separately, rather than being viewed as the sum of the re- sponses to the various facets, as is the usual case in scale development. He developed a satisfaction scale and field-tested it on a national sample of physicians, all of whom were working within a prison setting. A factor analysis produced six discriminable facets of job satisfaction, requir- ing 33 items. These facets were satisfaction with resources, self-directed autonomy, other-directed autonomy, patient relationships, professional relationships, and status. A seventh facet of four items measured global satisfaction. He used the scale to predict physicians' estimates of the likelihood of terminating their current employment and found that the satisfaction scale predicted 38 percent of the variance in physicians' in- tentions to leave. This work is primarily important today in terms of setting a model for scale development. The results themselves are of less relevance, since the scale was designed for use with one specialized group of physicians, those who work within a prison setting. Additionally, it is recognized today that turnover is far more complicated than an expression of dissatisfaction (Mick et al. 1983).

One particular investigator who has pursued the development of a scale to measure physician satisfaction in several settings is Lawrence Linn, whose work in this area built on Lichenstein's (Linn et al. 1985a, 1985b). The initial job satisfaction scale he developed was composed of 13 items with an alpha reliability of .85. The 13 items were not further divided into subscales, and no factor analysis was reported to confirm the structure of the scale. The items include such topics as "contact with other physicians," "salary/income," "ability to meet needs and demands of patients," and "degree of status and prestige associated with your job," among others. The collection of these items was treated as a scale in that total mean values were developed. The scale was then used to investigate relationships with other scales, including a nine-item work/social conflict scale that had items such as "I am able to leave my personal concerns behind when I am at work"; "I miss social obligations because of my job"; and "I feel torn between the demands of my work and my personal life." Linn also developed a set of items describing job-related problems or stressors, which were factor analyzed to produce five factors: clinical competence and interpersonal relations; coming to terms with realities of medical practice; anxiety about the future; time pressures; and dealing with difficult patients. All three of these scales were used, along with a life satisfaction scale and a health status scale to compare the health status, job stress, and life satisfaction of a group of academic and clinical faculty.

In later research, Linn and associates refer to some 11 separate job satisfaction scales they have developed, but they include in their published work the results of only two of these: a global satisfaction scale, which has an alpha reliability coefficient of .76, and a comparative satisfaction scale, which explores the comparisons of job experiences of physicians in several settings (Linn et al. 1985a, 1986). The other 11 scales developed were social/personal relations, patient population, educational/teaching climate, organization/administration, facilities/resources, status/prestige, interdisciplinary content, attitude toward general internal medicine, salary, concept of group practice, and system of academic medicine. In one study, Linn et al. used the scales to assess the work satisfaction and career aspirations of internists working in a teaching hospital group practice (Linn et al. 1986). In the other study, he used the scales to analyze the organization of medical group practices, with the objective of determining whether physician satisfaction and patient satisfaction can be affected by organizational arrangements. The results indicated that both patient and physician satisfaction scores increase with increased continuity of care (Linn et al. 1985a). This particular organizational change—the increase of continuity of care—is the most common use of physician satisfaction measures.

There are three physician satisfaction scales in the literature that have been developed and used in an international setting: one of these was then utilized in the United States. Although the findings may not be directly relevant to the United States physicians, the methodology and content of the scales are of interest. The first one is from Canada, a country to whom the United States is looking with some interest in terms of the health care system, and Linn is one of the investigators involved (Kravitz, Linn, and Shapiro 1990). The study itself was situated in Ontario, involving a probability sample of more than 1,000 physicians. Part of the objective of the study was to determine whether job satisfaction was related to the involvement of physicians with the 1986 physician strike in Ontario. They used as a measure of satisfaction the 13-item scale developed by Linn et al. (1985b) and added 3 more items. A factor analysis was performed, indicating the existence of four satisfaction facets: resources for providing high-quality care, psychological and material rewards of practice, patient interactions, and social and intellectual work environment. The statistical characteristics were acceptable for these subscales, including the factor loadings for each item. Item correlations ranged from .40 to .62; Cronbach's alpha was .85 for the total scale, and the alpha levels for the four subscales ranged from .64 to .74. The statistical analysis of the results of this study were more sophisticated than most other studies using a measure of physician satisfaction, due in part to the confidence in the physician satisfaction measure. A multiple regression model showed that participation in the Ontario physicians' strike was primarily related to those aspects of satisfaction under direct influence of the government, but not to those aspects that are mainly a product of the specific work environment.

A slightly different approach to scaling was done in the Netherlands, using a sample of general practitioners (Grol et al. 1985). A 24-item questionnaire was constructed using four positive feelings (contentedness, challenge, self-esteem, and well-being) and four negative feelings (lack of time, frustration, tenseness, and doubts). These eight feelings were used to rate three aspects of work: helping patients with physical complaints that are diagnosable; helping patients with psychosomatic or psychological complaints; and extra nonpatient activities, such as continuing education or consulting. A factor analysis produced two separate factors: the degree to which general practice is experienced as positive and the degree to which general practice is experienced as being negative.

The reliability coefficients for both factors is good: .76 and .80. This scale was then used to describe the satisfaction of general practitioners and also to relate some quality issues, including referral and prescribing behavior. Although the structure of the scale and the results are specific to medical care in the Netherlands, the results are interesting because of their link to physician behaviors, which is of ultimate interest. Of particular interest was the finding that the more negative a general practitioner felt, the more likely a patient visit was to involve drug prescription.

Of perhaps more relevance to the U.S. interest in the relationship between the organizational setting and physician satisfaction is an article by Schulz and Schulz (1988) involving a German study that took place in the mental health system. This presents a conceptual framework that draws heavily on job redesign and considers that perceived professional autonomy is an intervening variable between physician and institutional characteristics and physician satisfaction. The effort to develop a scale to measure physician satisfaction draws heavily on Lichenstein's work, and their original scale was constructed around Lichenstein's six facets. Subsequent factor analysis produced three factors that accounted for 43 percent of the variance: satisfaction with resources, satisfaction with autonomy and status, and satisfaction with professional relations. Following Lichenstein's lead, they also added a fourth component, one that specifically measures overall satisfaction. The statistical parameters of the scale are well within the acceptable range for scaling: Cronbach's alpha coefficients are .74 to .85 for the four components. The scale has been used in samples of psychiatrists in Germany, Great Britain, and most recently in a large sample of physicians practicing in a managed care environment in Wisconsin (Schulz, Girard, and Sheckler 1992). Of the several interesting findings in both studies, perhaps the most interesting is that, unlike other earlier studies, increasing organizational size and management constraints did not relate to diminished perceived clinical autonomy. In fact, large organizations were related to perceptions of higher clinical autonomy, which in turn seems to be related to higher levels of physician satisfaction.

Model of Scale Development

After reviewing the studies summarized above, two conclusions seem apparent. The first relates to the nature of the conceptual framework used, since measurement instruments are determined first by theoretical frameworks. Although there is a substantial body of knowledge on the stress associated with a physician's responsibility and with burnout, it is not the most useful theoretical framework to guide the development of a measurement instrument that will be applicable in a variety of practice settings. This is not a rejection of the *notion* of stress. Indeed, it is obviously true that physicians have many stresses that are an inherent part of their job. However, it seems that these stresses vary by both specialty and practice arrangement; physicians also vary considerably in their personal perception and individual tolerance of stress. It is also obvious from the literature that some amount of stress is challenging. All of this ambiguity contributes to measurement problems. Also, it is our position that it is important to control stress so that the phenomenon of burnout may be prevented, which is only possible by developing an understanding of what satisfies and dissatisfies physicians in their work environments. Therefore, we feel that a more useful and more general theoretical framework is to develop a measurement that enables the assessment of those factors that provide satisfaction to physicians, as well as those factors that contribute to dissatisfaction.

The second conclusion is pertinent to the level of measurement that has been used in the studies that have addressed physician satisfaction. As is obvious from the preceding section that focused on methodology, information about physician satisfaction has been gathered in many ways, ranging from qualitative methods, including personal interviews and semistructured questionnaires, to more quantitative methods, including more structured questionnaires and even some attempts to create some part of an attitude scale to measure physician satisfaction. Much of this literature uses measures of physician satisfaction as if the scale level had been attained—particularly those studies that attempt to measure the effect of organizational structure on physician satisfaction, although the tendency is not limited to that group of studies.

This observation indicates that there is a need in the field for a scale-level measure for physician satisfaction. The questions being addressed by researchers are substantial; the measures of other variables are steadily becoming more sophisticated. Because of the general knowledge base and because of the perceived need in the field, it seems appropriate to pursue the development of a scale-level measurement for physician satisfaction.

An obvious first question in this situation is to determine whether any of the existing scales are appropriate as they are, or can be used as a base from which to develop a new scale. We reviewed all the scales that exist in the published literature, both for perceptions of stress and perceptions of satisfaction or dissatisfaction. Although the three scales that exist for measurement of stress and/or uncertainty are interesting and provide several important insights (Makin, Rout, and Cooper 1988; May and Revicki 1985; Garrity, DeVellis, and Earp 1990), they are not appropriate because of their emphasis on stress.

We also carefully reviewed the several scales that have been developed to measure physician satisfaction (Linn et al. 1985a, 1985b; Makin, Rout, and Cooper 1988; Reidel and Reidel 1979). Linn and associates are responsible for three of these, but they do not all meet our definitions of a scale: the items are not constructed as a scale and the underlying factor structure is not always assessed by factor analytic techniques. Additionally, Linn and associates have worked in the area of measuring stress, and, in fact, most of the scale construction work has actually been accomplished in that area, rather than in measures of satisfaction.

The two approaches that seem most appropriate are those taken by Lichenstein (1984) and by Schulz and associates (Schulz and Schulz 1988; Schulz, Girard, and Sheckler 1992), who follow the conceptual framework of Lichenstein. Both of these approaches are careful to describe the theoretical framework being used; both utilize a multidimensional approach to measurement; and both follow carefully the requirements for scale construction. Schulz and associates, in particular, relate physician satisfaction to the organizational arrangements for medical care, a significant and ongoing concern in the United States, and the single most common way in which physician satisfaction is incorporated into studies.

Neither of these scales is appropriate to use as they are, however. Lichenstein developed his scale to measure physician satisfaction of physicians involved in the prison health care system, and he notes the limitations of this approach. Schulz and associates at first limited their work to psychiatrists; the more recent study includes all specialties, but only physicians working in a managed care setting. Both scales do provide a basis upon which to build.

There are three other scales that are sometimes used to provide a measure for physician satisfaction. The first is the Warr-Cook-Wall job satisfaction scale, which has high reliability and was developed for a British population (Makin, Rout, and Cooper 1988; Cooper, Rout, and Faragher 1989; Warr, Cook, and Wall 1979). The advantages of this particular scale are its shortness (14 items), reliability, and ease of use. The disadvantage of this measure is that it was originally developed for a variety of British occupations, so almost one-third of the items are not really appropriate for physicians, such as satisfaction with "your immediate boss" or "your job security." This scale is frequently used, particularly in British studies, but it is almost always used in conjunction with other scales or measures of satisfaction.

Two other scales which frequently appear in the literature as providing a measure for physician satisfaction are the Brayfield job satisfaction blank and the job description index (Mawardi 1979; Brayfield and Roth 1951; Breslau, Novack, and Wolf 1978; Hulin, Smith, and Kendal 1963). These two scales share two important characteristics. The first is age:

the Brayfield job satisfaction blank was developed in 1951 and the job description index (JDI) was developed in 1963. The second characteristic is that both were developed to measure level of job satisfaction of blue-collar workers. Like the Warr-Cook-Wall scale, therefore, some adjustments must be made in order to utilize the scale for physicians. Both the Brayfield scale and the JDI—but especially the JDI—are reliable and valid measures of job satisfaction, but the further away from blue-collar workers and the more time passes, the less appropriate these become (Lichenstein 1984). The most recent uses of these two scales are by Breslau, Novack, and Wolf in 1978 (JDI) and Mawardi in 1979 (Brayfield scale). These two studies are extensively quoted in the literature, both for content and methodology.

As a result of this survey of the literature, it seems that none of the existing scales are entirely appropriate for measuring physician satisfaction. The advantages of developing a new measure for physician satisfaction include the ability to control the scale construction process so that the conceptual model is appropriately followed. Also, the development of a new scale will permit a general enough construction to be maximally usable in a variety of situations. Previous experience in scale construction gives us the analytic and experiential tools to develop such a scale (Stamps and Piedmonte 1986).

The scale development process is tedious and lengthy, involving repeated administrations of a scale and revisions based on each new data set. In this study, the process of scale development can be started but not finished. The process has four basic parts: the conceptual framework, the important constructs to be included in a scale, the statistical framework, and practical considerations, including the ability of others to utilize the scale.

Conceptual framework

As noted previously, the conceptual framework used to develop a scale-level measurement is the general construct of satisfaction. In addition to this framework that provides definition to the content, we would also like to address two aspects related to the type of measurement instrument to be developed within the content area of physician satisfaction. First, as others have suggested, we feel that the most appropriate measurement is one that is multidimensional. Physician satisfaction is a complex phenomenon, one that is perceptual in nature. It is important to distinguish between like dimensions or constructs in an effort to determine separately all the parts that may constitute a definition of physician satisfaction. Secondly, as suggested by Lichenstein (1984), it is important to consider global or general satisfaction as a separate component, rather than a summation of the total scale items, as is so common. Although the statistical definition of a scale may be achieved, it is far more likely that a physician satisfaction scale will be a combination of subscales, which may not be subject to summing for one total score.

Identification of the components

As might be expected, several common facets or components of satisfaction are represented in the group of studies summarized in this chapter. Patient relationships are almost always considered to be important to include, since they are such an important contributor to physician satisfaction (Lichenstein 1984; Linn et al. 1986; Clarke et al. 1984; Mick et al. 1983; Kravitz, Linn, and Shapiro 1990; Charles et al. 1987). The organization and management of the medical practice itself, and professional relations with colleagues and other clinical personnel are frequently included as part of the measure, as is satisfaction with the resources necessary for patient care (Lichenstein 1984; Linn et al. 1985a, 1985b, 1986; Clarke et al. 1984; Breslau, Novack, and Wolf 1978; Schulz and Schulz 1988; Lofgren and Mladenovic 1990; Kravitz, Linn, and Shapiro 1990). Factors related primarily to individual physicians are also obviously important, including autonomy and status and psychological and monetary rewards, as well as a challenging/intellectually stimulating environment (Lichenstein 1984; Linn et al. 1986; Clarke et al. 1984; Breslau, Novack, and Wolf 1978; Mick et al. 1983; Schulz and Schulz 1988; Kravitz, Linn, and Shapiro 1990). Several studies also include a separate overall measure of satisfaction (Lichenstein 1984; Linn et al. 1986; Clarke et al. 1984; Schulz and Schulz 1988; McCranie, Hornsby, and Calvert 1982). Despite their importance, less frequently included as part of the measure are time pressures, paperwork demands, and quality of care (Grol et al. 1985; Lofgren and Mladenovic 1990).

After reviewing these studies and holding discussions with many practicing physicians, we observed that two specific components have not been included in previous research. The first are those personal factors that physicians find satisfying about the location of their medical practice. These factors—such as climate, geography, presence of family and friends, educational opportunities for family, and recreational opportunities—are frequently included in location studies but have not been included in the satisfaction paradigm. Although some may classify these factors as external to the practice setting, we feel that they may substantially influence practice location, which seems related to satisfaction.

A second component that may influence practice location and that certainly does influence perception of satisfaction is the physician's thoughts about the medical practice climate of the state in which he or she is located. This component is closely related to the notion of external regulations and perceived clinical autonomy. Our extensive interviews with physicians indicate that the medical practice environment concept is one that includes professional review, as well as federal and state regulations. Although some federal and professional regulations are constant, states increasingly are able to affect the medical practice environment. The physician's perception of this environment is an important determinant of the level of perceived clinical autonomy.

The questionnaire distributed to the physician respondents contains 35 items arranged into what were initially identified as relevant components of satisfaction, based on the work of others as well as our interviews. They are shown in Appendix B, item sets Q-3 and Q-5.

Statistical framework

Attempting to achieve a scale-level measurement means that both reliability and validity must be assessed. For reliability analysis, we used item-total correlations to assess how related each individual item is to a particular scale and Cronbach's alpha as a measure of the degree of association of all items defining a certain scale. There is some discussion in the field about guidelines for both of these statistics (Green and Lewis 1986; Thurston and Chave 1929; Lickert 1932). Higher correlations are better in the sense that higher scores are indicative of closer relationships. Correlations of .30 are viewed as being too low to be acceptable; .40 and .50 indicate modest reliability and suggest a scale in a developmental stage; while correlations of .60, .70, and .80 are viewed as approaching requirements for standardization. We decided to use .40 as the minimum acceptable item-total correlation and .60 as the minimum acceptable Cronbach's alpha.

Validity is most commonly assessed by one of the factor analytic techniques, which helps to determine the actual underlying factor structure and to identify what is really being measured. To ignore questions related to validity invites criticism and limits the usefulness of an attitude scale (Stamps and Finkelstein 1981). We utilized principal components analysis with a varimax rotation factor matrix with Kaiser normalization (Nie et al. 1975), and we compared this to a maximum likelihood analysis with a promax rotation (SAS Institute 1985; Nunnally 1978). Items were evaluated as having a strong and unambiguous relationship with only one factor if their loading on that factor was greater than .40 while their loading on other factors was less than .20.

Table 6.1 shows the results of the reliability and validity analyses. There are six separate scales or indexes. Each is acceptable statistically, and several appear to be robust measures.

Table 6.1 Six Indexes Used to Measure Satisfaction of Physicians

Index 1   Personal   Index Mean: 21.3   s.d. = 2.8   Range: 5–25

	Item Mean	s.d.	Item-Total Correlation	Factor Loading
1. Climate/geographic features	4.3	.68	.61	.63
2. Presence of family and/or friends	4.2	.76	.64	.68
3. Opportunities for social life	4.2	.75	.74	.80
4. Recreational & sports opportunities	4.3	.66	.73	.78
5. Quality of educational opportunities	4.0	.87	.51	.51

Cronbach's alpha: .84

Index 2   Resources for Practice   Index Mean: 19.3   s.d. = 2.9   Range: 5–25

	Item Mean	s.d.	Item-Total Correlation	Factor Loading
1. Professional interaction with other physicians	4.2	.74	.54	.58
2. Opportunity for contact with medical school	3.5	1.05	.48	.55
3. Availability of hospital facilities	4.2	.77	.57	.67
4. Availability of appropriate subspecialties	3.9	.97	.51	.57
5. Availability of good social welfare, home care, or nursing home services	3.4	.99	.46	.47

Cronbach's alpha: .78

Index 3   Review of Profession   Index Mean: 5.6   s.d. = 1.8   Range: 2–10

	Item Mean	s.d.	Item-Total Correlation	Factor Loading
1. Utilization reviews	2.9	1.02	.71	.82
2. Professional review organizations	2.7	1.03	.71	.70

Cronbach's alpha: .83

Index 4   Satisfaction with Medicine as a Profession   Index Mean: 16.4
      s.d. = 4.4   Range: 5–25

	Item Mean	s.d.	Item-Total Correlation	Factor Loading
1. My current income is satisfactory for the amount of work I do. (s.a. = 5)	3.0	1.2	.55	.54
2. I stay in medicine mainly because I am not sure what else I can do. (s.d. = 5)	3.2	1.3	.51	.58

Continued

Table 6.1 Continued

Index 4   Satisfaction with Medicine as a Profession   Index Mean: 16.4
         s.d. = 4.4   Range: 5–25

	Item Mean	s.d.	Item-Total Correlation	Factor Loading
3. If I had the decision to make again I'd still go into medicine. (s.a. = 5)	3.5	1.2	.49	.61
4. I am seriously thinking about leaving clinical practice altogether. (s.d. = 5)	3.5	1.2	.51	.62
5. All things considered, I am satisfied with my medical practice. (s.a. = 5)	3.3	1.1	.69	.81

Cronbach's alpha: .77

Index 5   Regulatory Climate of Massachusetts   Index Mean: 8.8
         s.d. = 3.0   Range: 5–25

	Item Mean	s.d.	Item-Total Correlation	Factor Loading
1. Ban on balance billing	1.6	.92	.68	.77
2. Retroactive medical malpractice premium	1.2	.53	.67	.74
3. Tort system of medical malpractice	1.5	.77	.56	.61
4. Mandatory Medicaid	2.4	1.26	.53	.58
5. Base medical malpractice premiums	2.1	1.05	.47	.51

Cronbach's alpha: .70

Index 6   Massachusetts as a Good Place to Practice   Index Mean: 9.4
         s.d. = 2.9   Range: 4–20

	Item Mean	s.d.	Item-Total Correlation	Factor Loading
1. It is my impression that a lot of physicians are dissatisfied specifically with medical practice in Massachusetts. (s.d. = 5)	1.5	.67	.55	.83
2. I am likely to leave the state of Massachusetts to practice medicine elsewhere. (s.d. = 5)	3.4	1.08	.49	.57
3. I don't really think practicing medicine in Massachesetts is any different from anywhere else. (s.a. = 5)	2.0	.98	.61	.42
4. I am generally satisfied with Massachusetts as a place to practice medicine (s.a. = 5)	2.4	1.15	.67	.61

Cronbach's alpha: .79

The first scale measures those personal factors relating to the location of the practice. This has five items, a Cronbach's alpha of .84, and item-total correlations and factor loadings for each item that are well above the minimum acceptable level. The second scale assesses perception of resources for a medical practice. It is also a five-item scale with a Cronbach's alpha of .78. The item-total correlations and factor loadings are slightly lower than those in the first scale, but are still acceptable. The third scale is very strong statistically, but only has two items, both of which are concerned with professional review. The fourth scale is a five-item measure of global or general satisfaction. The Cronbach's alpha is high, and the reliability and validity analyses are all certainly within the acceptable range.

The remaining two scales are specific to physicians in this study. Both contain items that are pertinent to Massachusetts. One is concerned with specific regulations of Massachusetts, and the last scale focuses on perceptions of Massachusetts as a place in which to practice medicine. Both of these have acceptable reliability and validity estimates.

Practical considerations

The final guideline for scale development relates to practicality: any attitude scale needs to be able to be utilized by others. The ease of utilization naturally concerns the scoring procedure, but also requires consideration of how an attitude scale might be utilized. As is obvious from the earlier sections of this chapter, most studies of physician satisfaction fall into one of two categories. The first category has a primary objective of increasing the knowledge base about physicians in order to better understand (or perhaps even predict) their behavior. Studies in this category usually require at least a regional, if not national, sample. The second category of studies utilizing a physician satisfaction scale is more organizational in nature: the emphasis is generally on how organizational changes affect physician satisfaction. The sample is frequently small and composed of physicians who have a similar practice arrangement, or work in the same organization.

The first type of study—a national or regional one—requires a scale that can be generalizable, while the second requires a scale that is more specific. Although these two types of needs may seem mutually exclusive, they are not. Physicians have many external factors that significantly affect their ability to do their work. These external factors include state and federal regulations, the nature of the patients, and the type of practice setting, among others. Our goal is to create a measurement instrument that includes factors related to general concerns of physicians, as represented by four of the scales, as well as specific attributes of a particular medical practice environment, in this case the state of Massachusetts, as represented by the last two scales.

Limitations

Within the six separate scales, one index (professional review) has only two items, which is clearly not sufficient to be considered a scale even though these two items are very closely related to one another. Two of the scales are of specific interest to the particular practice climate of Massachusetts; as such, they might be less generalizable to other settings. The other four scales are more generalizable, although clearly further research is needed to see if these issues are equally appropriate to other settings.

At this moment, these six scales should not be treated as subscales to one overall scale, but as six separate indexes. This unity may be achieved with additional administrations of a set of scales similar to these, but for the present these scales should be treated as multidimensional measures of physician satisfaction, with one of the scales being a measure of overall satisfaction.

Each of the individual items represented on one of the six scales may contribute to a physician's satisfaction or dissatisfaction. The scales are scored in such a way that a higher score indicates a higher level of satisfaction, which implies that satisfaction and dissatisfaction are on a continuum, rather than being distinct concepts. Although it is important to understand that theoretically satisfaction and dissatisfaction are not on a continuum, it is very hard to create a practical measurement instrument representing this conceptualization.

Despite these limitations, these six indexes provide a valuable starting place for development of a measure of satisfaction that will be appropriate for all practicing physicians.

Results

This section is organized to include several examples of results that may be obtained by utilizing a measure for physician satisfaction. The first example is that of a descriptive use in which several variables are examined, including gender, years in medical practice, age, practice arrangement, and specialty. The second example is more analytic and examines the relationship between satisfaction and income, productivity, and gender; it concludes with a regression model that examines the relationship of several of these variables with satisfaction. The third component of this section focuses on the integrity of these indexes as a measure of physician satisfaction, including not only methodological issues, but also whether these indexes seem consistent with the other information that we have gathered about physician satisfaction.

Descriptive use of indexes

Four variables are commonly included when analyzing medical practice patterns. Two are usually categorized as demographic variables (gender and years in medical practice or age) while the remaining two relate to medical practice characteristics (practice arrangement and specialty).

Gender. The increasing number of women in the medical field has created many interesting—and sometimes controversial—observations and conclusions, as discussed in Chapter 5. Very little is known about what provides satisfaction to female physicians in their medical practices, and not much is known about what dissatisfies female physicians. This lack of knowledge is perhaps not surprising since not much is known either about what satisfies male physicians, although more attention has been paid to burnout of male physicians. Even today, with substantial increases in the number of women in medicine, few studies that focus on practicing physicians have enough women included in order to analyze them as a group. In those few studies that do have sufficient women in the sample and that attempt to measure satisfaction, the results are mixed: some studies seem to indicate that gender has little or no effect on satisfaction, while others note that female physicians seem less dissatisfied than male physicians (Kravitz, Linn, and Shapiro 1990; McCranie, Hornsby, and Calvert 1982; Cooper, Rout, and Faragher 1989).

Our study has enough women in the sample (106) to be able to examine them as a group, although we are also limited in the ability to completely analyze this subsample in as much detail as is desirable. By using these six indexes to analyze perceptions of male and female physicians, we have the opportunity to examine in some detail whether male and female physicians differ systematically with respect to job satisfaction.

Table 6.2 shows the scores resulting from the analysis of the six satisfaction indexes for the whole respondent group and separately for males and females. The first obvious detail to note relates to the number of female respondents. Although the percentage and actual number of women in medical school continues to increase, their presence as practicing physicians is still fairly limited in terms of overall proportion of any particular sample. As a result, it is fairly common for between 13 percent and 15 percent of a total physician sample to be female, which is true for our respondent group. Although the absolute number of female physicians in our study is too small to support many subdivisions, it is certainly sufficient to examine the effect of gender as a major analytic category.

There are statistically significant differences between male and female physicians for four of the six indexes. Women are less satisfied with the resources available for their medical practices, and more satisfied with the two indexes that measure perceptions of Massachusetts as a place in which to practice. The largest difference is in the regulatory climate of Massachusetts index: women physicians are far less dissatisfied than men physicians, although this index shows overall dissatisfaction for both male and female physicians.

Years in medical practice and age. Most professionals show a characteristic relationship between years of professional experience (or age) and level of occupational satisfaction, so that there is generally an increased level of satisfaction with one's job as one ages and gains more professional experience. Those few studies that have directly assessed this relationship for physicians have shown supporting findings; the best example is Kravitz, Linn, and Shapiro (1990), whose data consistently demonstrate that increased age is related to increased levels of satisfaction. Physicians in our study generally demonstrate a similar pattern, with some interesting exceptions. Table 6.3 shows the statistical relationship between the scores on the six satisfaction indexes, and age and years of professional experience in Massachusetts. For the resources index, male physicians seem more satisfied as age and professional experience increase, although not female physicians. Both male and female physicians are more satisfied with Massachusetts as a place in which to practice medicine as age increases, but years of experience has no effect on this index. Also fitting the general expectations is the relationship between years of professional experience and satisfaction with the personal aspect of the medical practice: there seems to be higher satisfaction with these personal factors as years of experience increase, both for males and females.

However, increasing age and professional experience does not seem to lead to increased satisfaction with the regulatory climate of Massachusetts. Older male physicians are more dissatisfied with the regulatory climate of Massachusetts, and both male and female physicians are less satisfied as their years of professional experience in Massachusetts increase. For the more global index of satisfaction with medicine as a field, increased years of professional experience lead to less satisfaction for both male and female physicians. It seems that increasing experience leads to increased satisfaction with personal factors and resources related to a specific medical practice, but not necessarily with the regulatory climate. As physicians age and their practice becomes mature, they seem

Table 6.2 Level of Satisfaction for Males and Females

	Personal Mean Score† (range 5–25)	Resources Mean Score (range 5–25)	Review Mean Score (range 2–10)	Satisfaction with Medicine Mean Score (range 5–25)	Massachusetts Regulatory Climate Mean Score (range 5–25)	Massachusetts as a Good Place to Practice Mean Score (range 4–20)
Total sample (N = 777)	21.3	19.3	5.6	16.4	8.8	9.4
Males (n = 673)	21.4	19.4	5.6	16.3	8.6	9.3
Females (n = 104)	20.8	18.5	5.9	17.3	10.0	9.9
t-Test	3.07	9.59**	1.39	3.90***	18.44*	4.24***

*p ≤ .001, using *t*-test of differences.
**p ≤ .01, using *t*-test of differences.
***p ≤ .05, using *t*-test of differences.
****p ≤ .10, using *t*-test of differences.
†There are slight differences in sample size for each of the mean scores, since not everyone responded to each item.

Table 6.3 Relationship between Age, Years of Experience, and Satisfaction for Male and Female Physician Respondents

	Personal Mean Score (range 5–25)	Resources Mean Score (range 5–25)	Review Mean Score (range 2–10)	Satisfaction with Medicine Mean Score (range 5–25)	Massachusetts Regulatory Climate Mean Score (range 5–25)	Massachusetts as a Good Place to Practice Mean Score (range 4–20)
Age						
30–44 (n = 431)	21.1	19.0	5.6	16.7	9.0	9.2
Male (n = 346)	21.2	19.1	5.6	16.6	8.8	9.1
Female (n = 85)	20.8	18.6	5.8	17.2	10.1	9.9
45–54 (n = 192)	21.6	19.4	5.5	16.4	8.4	9.1
Male (n = 179)	21.7	19.5	5.5	16.3	8.3	9.0
Female (n = 13)	20.5	17.9	5.8	16.8	9.2	10.2
55+ (n = 163)	21.4	20.1	5.8	15.8	8.6	10.1
Male (n = 157)	21.4	20.2	5.8	15.7	8.5	10.0
Female (n = 6)	22.8	17.7	6.7	18.5	10.8	10.4
ANOVA *t*-test						
Overall	2.19	8.18*	1.38	2.48	3.74***	5.77**
Male	1.80	7.96*	1.24	1.91	1.86	6.89*
Female	1.39	0.41	0.76	0.29	0.55	0.14

Continued

Table 6.3 Continued

	Personal Mean Score (range 5–25)	Resources Mean Score (range 5–25)	Review Mean Score (range 2–10)	Satisfaction with Medicine Mean Score (range 5–25)	Massachusetts Regulatory Climate Mean Score (range 5–25)	Massachusetts as a Good Place to Practice Mean Score (range 4–20)
Years Experience in Massachusetts						
0–3 (n = 87)	20.8	18.6	6.0	17.5	9.9	9.5
Male (n = 58)	20.8	18.5	6.0	17.5	9.5	9.5
Female (n = 29)	20.8	18.7	5.8	17.4	10.8	9.7
4–10 (n = 285)	20.9	19.0	5.6	16.6	9.0	9.2
Male (n = 232)	21.1	19.2	5.5	16.4	8.8	9.0
Female (n = 53)	20.5	18.4	5.8	17.5	9.9	10.0
11+ (n = 415)	21.6	19.2	5.6	16.1	8.4	9.5
Male (n = 393)	21.6	19.7	5.6	16.1	8.3	9.4
Female (n = 22)	21.8	18.2	6.0	16.4	9.3	10.0
ANOVA t-test						
Overall	6.08**	6.21**	1.47	3.39***	10.82*	1.0
Male	4.03***	5.67**	1.80	2.29	5.35**	1.87
Female	1.47	0.14	0.19	0.70	1.27	0.15

*$p \leq .001$.
**$p \leq .01$.
***$p \leq .05$.
****$p \leq .10$.

less satisfied with the regulatory climate specific to Massachusetts, perhaps because their resentment increases as they become older or perhaps because a mature practice is subject to a greater degree of regulatory intervention, particularly from the state. In any case, the most helpful insight to those in Massachusetts is that the current level of dissatisfaction that does exist among Massachusetts physicians is not primarily among younger physicians, but apparently is far more prevalent among older, more experienced physicians.

Female physicians demonstrate a pattern remarkably similar to that of male physicians, with the primary difference lying in the index measuring perception of resources available for the practice.

Of perhaps even more interest is the observation that there is not as strong a relationship between increasing age and professional experience and increased satisfaction, as might be predicted from the literature for both male and female physicians. These results also reinforce the notion that level of satisfaction is a complicated variable. The insights gained by measuring satisfaction via six separate indexes are much greater than previous attempts to have a single scale attempt to capture the dimensions.

Practice arrangement. As shown in Chapter 2, the organizational characteristics of medical practice have been of significant interest to those who investigate physician satisfaction. When physicians are presented with a variety of factors that measure level of satisfaction, they consistently demonstrate the least satisfaction with the organizational and administrative arrangements of their practices. As Linn et al. (1986) have noted, physicians have greatest dissatisfaction over what they view as the part of their practice over which they have the least control. For most studies, this dissatisfaction is conceptualized as something related to administration. It is a common conceptual focus to therefore assume that physicians are less satisfied in more organized, more complex medical practices, as we noted in the beginning of this chapter, despite some current research to the contrary (Mawardi 1979; May and Revicki 1985; Schulz and Schulz 1988; Schulz, Girard, and Sheckler 1992; McCranie, Hornsby, and Calvert 1982).

The subject of which practice setting is most satisfying to physicians is more complicated than perhaps originally thought. Not only is the measurement of physician satisfaction a continuing problem, but so also is the observation that organizational arrangements themselves are more diverse and complex than many investigators acknowledge. Added to this complexity is the recognition that it is important to separate out the notion of external influences of all types from those specific administrative controls exercised on physicians in any particular practice setting. We attempted to differentiate the larger constraints from the more specific practice-related constraints by addressing issues related to regulation in the indexes.

The advantage of using six separate indexes to provide a profile of satisfaction is shown by the analysis of the relationship between practice setting and satisfaction for males and females (Table 6.4). For each practice setting, there is a different pattern of what satisfies male versus female physicians. For example, in group practice settings, female physicians are more satisfied than males with components measured by these indexes: review, satisfaction with medicine, and both Massachusetts-specific indexes. In the hospital setting, however, female physicians are more satisfied than male physicians in only two areas—satisfaction with medicine and the Massachusetts regulatory climate.

Although HMOs are the practice environment where women are most highly represented, HMOs are not necessarily a more satisfying practice arrangement for women. Women physicians practicing in HMOs have a lower score on every index except one (review) than males practicing in an HMO setting, although these differences do not always attain statistical significance. For all practice settings, women generally have lower scores on the personal and resources indexes, and higher scores on the two indexes that measure perceptions of Massachusetts as a place to practice medicine as well as the index that measures general satisfaction with medicine as a profession.

The practice arrangement that seems most dissatisfying in general is solo practice, both for men and women, followed by group practice. The hospital setting is generally more satisfying as a practice environment, and the HMO setting seems the most satisfying of all, in spite of the lower incomes in this practice setting.

Specialty. Despite the importance of specialty as one of the most important variables to account for, only two studies have analyzed level of satisfaction by specialty, and both are very limited. One is a survey done by a professional trade journal (*Physician's Management*, Feb. 1990), which concluded that family practitioners were more satisfied than any other specialty. The other is an extremely interesting qualitative study in which the primary care physicians seemed to be the most satisfied (Reames and Dunstone 1989).

This dearth of comparative studies results because most research that includes physician satisfaction focuses on one particular specialty or similar specialties. For example, primary care physicians are often the focus of studies, especially those that include an analysis of prepaid group setting versus nonprepaid group setting, since primary care physicians are more likely to be in a prepaid practice setting. Most of the results of these studies emphasize the practice setting rather than

Table 6.4 Relationship between Practice Arrangement and Satisfaction, by Male and Female Respondents

	Personal Mean Score (range 5–25)	Resources Mean Score (range 5–25)	Review Mean Score (range 2–10)	Satisfaction with Medicine Mean Score (range 5–25)	Massachusetts Regulatory Climate Mean Score (range 5–25)	Massachusetts as a Good Place to Practice Mean Score (range 4–20)	Percentage Satisfied with Income
Group practice							
Total (N = 261)	21.8	19.8	5.5	15.9	8.2	8.7	
Male (n = 239)	21.9	19.9	5.4	15.8	8.1	8.7	58.9
Female (n = 21)	20.9	19.2	6.1	16.8	8.7	9.0	57.1
Solo practice							
Total (N = 225)	20.8	19.0	5.7	15.5	8.2	9.1	
Male (n = 205)	20.8	19.1	5.7	15.5	8.1	9.0	55.9
Female (n = 19)	20.4	17.3	5.1	16.2	9.2	9.7	63.2
Hospital							
Total (N = 114)	21.1	19.2	5.9	17.9	9.6	9.8	
Male (n = 96)	21.1	19.3	5.9	17.8	9.4	9.8	63.3
Female (n = 18)	21.1	18.5	5.7	18.4	10.5	9.5	66.2
HMO							
Total (N = 72)	21.2	19.2	5.8	18.5	11.1	11.2	
Male (n = 49)	21.5	19.4	5.8	18.8	11.2	11.3	83.3
Female (n = 23)	20.5	18.9	5.9	18.0	10.7	10.8	82.8
ANOVA							
Total	6.08*	3.72***	1.51	14.27*	23.18*	15.77*	
Male	6.52*	2.54	1.91	11.86*	19.78*	13.72*	
Female	0.21	1.17	1.24	1.37	1.55	1.76	

*p ≤ .001.
**p ≤ .01.
***p ≤ .05.
****p ≤ .10.

specialty (Mechanic 1975; Mick et al. 1983). Other specialties that have provided a primary focus for physician satisfaction studies have included family practitioners (May and Revicki 1985; McCranie, Hornsby, and Calvert 1982), internal medicine (Clute 1963; Linn 1981; Linn et al. 1985a), neonatologists (Clarke et al. 1984), psychiatrists (Schulz and Schulz 1988), and general practitioners (Makin, Rout, and Cooper 1988; Grol et al. 1985; Cooper, Rout, and Faragher 1989; Porter, Howie, and Levinson 1985); the latter two groups are studies from Europe and Great Britain. It is hard to compare the results from these several studies because the measures used to quantify physician satisfaction are so different.

Ours is the first study to systematically analyze physician satisfaction that has a large enough sample size to directly address the question of whether there are significant differences in level of satisfaction between specialties. The size of our sample enables us to investigate the satisfaction differences between nine different specialties (Table 6.5). The specialty that seems the most satisfied in a general sense is pediatrics, followed by general/family practitioners. Those physicians involved in a surgical specialty—or in general surgery—seem to be the most dissatisfied overall. The two greatest sources of dissatisfaction for general surgeons and surgical specialists are the two indexes that measure their perceptions of Massachusetts. Their scores on the index related to their general satisfaction with medicine as a field are also lower than those in other specialties.

Other specialties also demonstrate unhappiness with the two components that are specific to the state of Massachusetts, although general surgeons and the surgical specialists are by far the most negative. The most satisfied specialties with these two indexes are pediatrics, general/family practitioners, internal medicine, and psychiatry. Even among these relatively satisfied specialties, it should be noted that their scores are well below the midpoint of the range, indicating that these two indexes are describing degrees of relative dissatisfaction.

Other statistically significant differences occur in the more general indexes. For example, examination of the review index shows that several specialties, in addition to the surgical ones, are extremely negative—including internal medicine and psychiatry. This index is another one in which even the highest scores (pediatrics, anesthesiologists, radiologists, OB/GYN, and general/family practitioners) are only slightly above the midpoint. Scores well above the midpoint are seen for all specialties for the index measuring satisfaction with resources for the practice. The lowest score (psychiatry) is above the midpoint for the range, and the two highest scoring specialties (OB/GYN and pediatrics) are well above that.

Significant differences are also noted for the index that provides a general measure of satisfaction with medicine as a profession. These

Table 6.5 Relationship between Specialty and Satisfaction

	Personal Mean Score (range 5–25)	Resources Mean Score (range 5–25)	Review Mean Score (range 2–10)	Satisfaction with Medicine Mean Score (range 5–25)	Massachusetts Regulatory Climate Mean Score (range 5–25)	Massachusetts as a Good Place to Practice Mean Score (range 4–20)
General/family practice (n = 83)	21.5	19.1	6.0	17.4	9.5	10.9
Pediatrics (n = 74)	21.6	20.0	6.5	18.4	10.3	11.1
Internal Medicine (n = 125)	21.2	19.4	5.1	15.7	9.4	9.7
OB/GYN (n = 49)	20.6	20.1	6.0	15.2	8.1	9.1
Psychiatry (n = 59)	21.9	17.0	5.4	18.0	9.4	9.5
Anesthesiology (n = 33)	21.5	19.2	6.2	15.3	8.5	8.5
General Surgery (n = 44)	20.6	19.8	5.6	14.5	7.6	7.9
Surgical Specialties (n = 126)	21.0	19.9	5.2	15.0	7.5	7.9
Radiology (n = 41)	22.0	18.4	6.2	18.2	8.7	9.8
ANOVA F-Ratio	1.78	7.24*	6.03*	8.41*	8.27*	13.81*

*$p \leq .001$.
**$p \leq .01$.
***$p \leq .05$.
****$p \leq .10$.

scores are not as high as those on the resource index, but the two lowest (general surgery and surgical specialties) are at about the midpoint of the range. Those specialties that seem most positive about medicine as a field include radiology (the highest-income specialty), psychiatry, and pediatrics, followed by general/family practitioners.

The scores on the index measuring satisfaction with personal factors are the highest across all specialties. Interestingly enough, there are no statistically significant differences between specialties for this index. In general, all the specialties show a similar pattern in the ordering of the indexes in terms of satisfaction. For every specialty except psychiatry, the two factors that are most closely related to their own practice (personal factors and resources available for their medical practice) show the highest level of satisfaction. The lowest levels of satisfaction are exhibited for the two components that measure the level of satisfaction with Massachusetts as a place in which to practice, with the index measuring specific regulations in the state of Massachusetts being the most negative. The index measuring perceptions of general professional review is also relatively dissatisfying. General satisfaction with medicine as a field shows moderate satisfaction for all specialties: lower than the first two indexes but much higher than the remaining three indexes.

Table 6.6 shows the rankings of the specialties with respect to each of the six indexes. This table demonstrates the importance of considering each of the components of satisfaction separately for each specialty. Rather than a common overall pattern, what emerges here is an observation that level of satisfaction varies considerably for each specialty.

We know from Chapter 5 that gender seems to be closely related to specialty and we wanted to examine whether there were any differences for male and female physicians within the same specialty. There are five specialties in which we have sufficient women to be able to do this analysis, shown in Table 6.7. There are several interesting and statistically significant differences between male and female physicians. For example, although there were no differences across all specialties with respect to satisfaction with personal factors related to a medical practice, there are when male and female physicians are considered separately. Female pediatricians and female surgeons are less satisfied with the personal aspects of their medical practice than their male colleagues, while female OB/GYNs are more satisfied than their male colleagues.

Female physicians in each of the five specialty groups are more satisfied with the regulatory climate of Massachusetts, although this difference is greatest for those women in general/family practice and in OB/GYN. For the index measuring satisfaction with Massachusetts as a place in which to practice, female physicians in all specialties except OB/GYN and pediatrics are more satisfied than males, with those in the

Table 6.6   Ranking of Level of Satisfaction for Nine Specialties for the Six Indexes of Satisfaction

Personal Index *(range 5–25)*	*Resources for Practice* *(range 5–25)*	*Satisfaction* *with Medicine* *(range 5–25)*
1. Radiology (22.0)	1. OB/GYN (20.1)	1. Pediatrics (18.4)
2. Psychiatry (21.9)	2. Pediatrics (20.0)	2. Radiology (18.2)
3. Pediatrics (21.6)	3. Surgical Specialties (19.9)	3. Psychiatry (18.0)
4. General/Family Practice (21.5)	4. General Surgery (19.8)	4. General/Family Practice (17.4)
5. Anesthesiology (21.5)	5. Internal Medicine (19.4)	5. Internal Medicine (15.7)
6. Internal Medicine (21.2)	6. Anesthesiology (19.2)	6. Anesthesiology (15.3)
7. Surgical Specialties (21.0)	7. General/Family Practice (19.1)	7. OB/GYN (15.2)
8. General Surgery (20.6)	8. Radiology (18.4)	8. Surgical Specialties (15.0)
9. OB/GYN (20.6)	9. Psychiatry (17.0)	9. General Surgery (14.5)

Review *(range 2–10)*	*Massachusetts* *Regulatory Climate* *(range 5–25)*	*Massachusetts as a* *Place to Practice* *(range 4–20)*
1. Pediatrics (6.5)	1. Pediatrics (10.3)	1. Pediatrics (11.1)
2. Radiology (6.2)	2. General/Family Practice (9.5)	2. General/Family Practice (10.9)
3. Anesthesiology (6.2)	3. Internal Medicine (9.4)	3. Radiology (9.8)
4. OB/GYN (6.0)	4. Psychiatry (9.4)	4. Internal Medicine (9.7)
5. General/Family Practice (6.0)	5. Radiology (8.7)	5. Psychiatry (9.5)
6. General Surgery (5.6)	6. Anesthesiology (8.5)	6. OB/GYN (9.1)
7. Psychiatry (5.4)	7. OB/GYN (8.1)	7. Anesthesiology (8.5)
8. Surgical Specialties (5.2)	8. General Surgery (7.6)	8. General Surgery (7.9)
9. Internal Medicine (5.1)	9. Surgical Specialties (7.5)	9. Surgical Specialties (7.9)

surgical specialties showing the biggest difference. Female physicians also seem more positive about the index measuring general satisfaction with medicine as a profession, with the biggest difference again being in OB/GYN. From this table, it seems that female physicians practicing in general/family practice and OB/GYN are generally the most satisfied.

Analytic use of indexes: income, productivity, and satisfaction

The previous section focused on using the six indexes that measure physician satisfaction descriptively, that is, to identify those components that satisfy or dissatisfy physicians in their work environments. Another important possible use of these indexes is in a more analytic sense—to

Table 6.7 Relationship between Satisfaction and Specialty for Male and Female Physicians

Specialty	Personal Mean Score (range 5–25)	Resources Mean Score (range 5–25)	Review Mean Score (range 2–10)	Satisfaction with Medicine Mean Score (range 5–25)	Massachusetts Regulatory Climate Mean Score (range 5–25)	Massachusetts as a Good Place to Practice Mean Score (range 4–20)
General/Family Practice						
Male (n = 70)	21.5	19.4	6.0	17.4	9.2	10.6
Female (n = 13)	21.2	17.5	5.9	17.4	11.4	11.7
Pediatrics						
Male (n = 52)	22.2	20.3	6.5	18.4	10.2	11.4
Female (n = 22)	20.2	19.6	6.5	18.2	10.7	10.3
Internal Medicine						
Male (n = 104)	21.2	19.3	5.1	15.6	9.2	9.6
Female (n = 20)	21.5	19.5	5.5	16.5	10.3	10.0
OB/GYN						
Male (n = 36)	20.4	20.3	5.8	14.4	7.6	9.2
Female (n = 12)	21.2	19.4	6.8	17.6	9.4	9.0
All surgical (includes general surgery and surgical specialties)						
Male (n = 115)	21.2	20.1	5.5	14.9	7.4	7.7
Female (n = 12)	20.5	18.5	4.5	15.5	7.5	9.0
ANOVA						
Male	2.70***	2.29	6.22*	9.36*	11.06*	22.22*
Female	0.49	1.13	1.92	0.84	1.14	1.89

*p ≤ .001.
**p ≤ .01.
***p ≤ .05.
****p ≤ .10.

pursue some basic research questions, which partially depend on having a quantification for the variable of physician satisfaction. For example, there are several assumptions about physician behavior and its determinants underlying the various public policy decisions that have been devised to modify physician behavior. One of the primary assumptions about physician behavior is that income is the main motivator. It is also commonly thought that higher income professionals are more satisfied with their jobs. In industrial settings, productivity is related to income, and this premise also infiltrates the medical field. Female physicians as a group are also subject to several common stereotypes, including ideas that women physicians are more satisfied than males and that money is not as important to female physicians as to males, as was discussed in Chapter 5.

There is an obvious need to be able to investigate the relationships between income, productivity, and level of satisfaction, both for male and female physicians. In this section, we would like to draw on the analysis of income productivity that was presented in Chapter 4 and relate it to analysis of satisfaction, as measured by the six indexes. Income is not commonly included as a variable in physician studies, except perhaps as a descriptive variable. A few studies have tried to discover how satisfied physicians are with their incomes, but results are not consistent. For example, Breslau, Novack, and Wolf (1978) compared level of satisfaction with income between physicians and nonphysicians, and showed, not surprisingly, that physicians in all settings were more satisfied with their income than nonphysician medical workers in all settings. Their mean scores on the component that measured satisfaction with income/pay were higher than the scores on the other two components (satisfaction with work and with co-workers). In a later study in Ontario, Kravitz, Linn, and Shapiro (1990) found that about 15 percent of the physicians in their study were dissatisfied with their incomes, and in their qualitative study, Reames and Dunstone (1989) observed that those who seemed most concerned about money were the subspecialists.

The relationship between income and satisfaction is probably mediated somehow by the number of hours of work it takes to produce a certain income level (Mechanic 1975). For example, in Mick's study, those who had left the prepaid group practice setting earned significantly more money but also worked more hours per week, although they denied that maximizing their income was the reason for their leaving the prepaid group practice (Mick et al. 1983).

The paucity of information about physician income and also about physician productivity encouraged us to collect adequate information to be able to measure both, presented in Chapter 4. Because of several findings that were counterintuitive, we decided to add the concept of satisfaction to the analysis. The first direct assessment was very simply to divide the whole respondent group into two halves—those who make over $100,000 and those who make under $100,000. We compared the responses of these two groups to one item: "All things considered, I am satisfied with my medical practice." There was no statistically significant difference between the two groups.

Table 6.8 provides a more precise analysis of this general finding by using four income levels and the six satisfaction indexes. Three of the five components are significantly related to income, but not always in the expected direction. For example, satisfaction with the two components specific to Massachusetts goes down as income goes up. Also statistically significant is the relationship between income and the index measuring satisfaction with resources available for the practice, but the pattern is not as clear: those in a relatively lower-income group show less satisfaction than those in the higher-income groups. There seems to be no relationship with the other indexes and income level. When we examined this by gender, the statistically significant results were true only for male physicians. For female physicians, income and level of satisfaction does not seem to be closely related.

We also looked at physicians' perceptions of income through responses to two specific items on the questionnaire. One item asked respondents to rate the "income of my practice"; 62 percent rated their income as either satisfactory or very satisfactory, while 30 percent indicated that the income of their practice is not satisfying. The second item, "My current income is satisfying for the amount of work I do," is more specific; predictably, only 47 percent note agreement or strong agreement, while 45 percent indicate disagreement. This pattern is fairly typical of responses to general versus specific attitude statements. We then correlated the scores from the six satisfaction indexes to the responses to these two items. As Table 6.9 shows, those who express higher levels of satisfaction with their income also seem to have higher levels of satisfaction, as measured by each of the six indexes. This finding supports some of our previous observations that perception of adequacy of income is a more important determinant of level of satisfaction than is the actual amount of money received. Perception of adequacy of income is related to expectations, and expectations undoubtedly arise from observation of what other physicians in the same peer group are receiving as well as the definition of peer group being used by a physician. For example, McCarty (1988) argues that low incomes are one reason that there is a decline in internal medicine as a specialty. In response to several letters to the editor protesting this conclusion, McCarty noted, "Fifth, they say that money doesn't matter. False. It only doesn't matter to those who have it. It matters a great deal to those who are being shortchanged."

Table 6.8 Relationship of Income to Six Satisfaction Indexes

Income	Personal Mean Score (range 5–25)	Resources Mean Score (range 5–25)	Review Mean Score (range 2–10)	Satisfaction with Medicine Mean Score (range 5–25)	Massachusetts Regulatory Climate Mean Score (range 5–25)	Massachusetts as a Good Place to Practice Mean Score (range 4–20)
$60,000 or less (n = 103)	21.6	19.2	5.9	16.2	9.4	10.2
$61–100,000 (n = 244)	21.4	18.9	5.8	16.4	9.2	9.8
$101–140,000 (n = 210)	21.0	19.3	5.7	16.2	8.7	9.1
$141,000 or > (n = 184)	21.3	19.9	5.4	16.8	8.0	8.7
F-Ratio†	1.14	4.50**	2.34	0.47	6.68**	8.21*

*$p \leq .001$.
**$p \leq .01$.
***$p \leq .05$.
****$p \leq .10$.
†F ($Pr > F$).

Table 6.9 Relationship of Responses to Two Questionnaire Items and Six Satisfaction Indexes

Response	Personal Mean Score (range 5–25)	Resources Mean Score (range 5–25)	Review Mean Score (range 2–10)	Satisfaction with Medicine Mean Score (range 5–25)	Massachusetts Regulatory Climate Mean Score (range 5–25)	Massachusetts as a Good Place to Practice Mean Score (range 4–20)
Income of my practice is satisfying given amount of work I do						
Strongly Agree/Agree						
Total (N = 358)	21.7	19.3	5.8	18.9	9.7	10.6
Male (n = 303)	21.8	19.5	5.8	18.9	9.5	10.6
Female (n = 55)	21.4	18.6	5.9	18.7	10.6	10.6
Undecided						
Total (N = 63)	21.1	19.4	5.9	17.4	9.2	9.7
Male (n = 50)	21.2	19.4	5.8	17.3	9.2	9.9
Female (n = 13)	20.7	19.0	6.2	18.0	9.7	9.1
Disagree/Strongly Disagree						
Total (N = 347)	20.9	19.2	5.4	13.7	7.9	8.1
Male (n = 312)	21.0	19.3	5.4	13.6	7.7	7.9
Female (n = 35)	20.1	17.8	5.7	14.6	9.2	9.1
ANOVA Results						
Total	8.67**	0.26	5.66***	180.86*	33.54*	81.60*
Male						
Female						

Income of my practice

Very Satisfactory/Satisfactory						
Total (N = 482)	21.6	19.6	5.8	17.9	9.3	10.1
Male (n = 414)	21.6	19.7	5.8	17.9	9.2	10.1
Female (n = 68)	21.2	19.0	5.9	18.2	10.6	10.2
Undecided						
Total (N = 58)	20.8	18.4	5.7	16.8	9.4	9.6
Male (n = 48)	20.8	18.7	5.6	16.9	9.2	9.8
Female (n = 10)	20.8	16.8	5.8	16.3	10.4	8.8
Unsatisfactory/ Very Unsatisfactory						
Total (N = 239)	20.8	18.9	5.3	13.5	7.6	7.9
Male (n = 212)	21.0	19.1	5.2	13.3	7.4	7.7
Female (n = 25)	19.8	17.6	5.7	15.1	9.6	9.5
ANOVA Results						
Total	6.31**	6.79**	5.58**	100.56*	27.39*	52.93*
Male	4.83**	4.22***	5.32**	91.68*	28.86*	55.51*
Female	2.13	3.36***	0.12	6.95*	0.24	1.51

$*p \leq .001.$
$**p \leq .01.$
$***p \leq .05.$
$****p \leq .10.$

McCarty's observation arises from using all physicians as the relevant peer group. In our study, physicians may be using a more narrow peer group—other HMO physicians, other women physicians, or perhaps other primary care physicians. In this case, the discrepancy between expected and actual income is much smaller than if, for example, primary care physicians are comparing their incomes to radiologists. This observation may help explain why in our study 83 percent of physicians in HMO settings are satisfied with their incomes, even though these incomes are much lower than those received by physicians in other practice settings. The same process may be operating in both female physicians and those physicians in lower-income specialties. In both of these examples, what the other members of the peer reference group (other women physicians or other general practitioners, for example) receive may be very similar. Of course, it may also be that income for physicians is one of those factors that produces dissatisfaction if not present in sufficient amount, but is not a strong satisfier. Then, only physicians who are dissatisfied with income—for whatever reason—would talk about money, as McCarty (1988) and Herzburg, Mausner, and Snyderman (1959) suggest.

Responses to these two income items offer an interesting glimpse into some differences between male and female physicians. Of the nearly two-thirds that indicated their income is satisfactory or very satisfactory (Table 6.9), women are less satisfied than men with both components measuring satisfaction with their individual practice (personal factors and resources for their practice). They are less dissatisfied than men with the regulatory environment in Massachusetts, and they also find more satisfaction than men do in general perceptions about medicine as a profession. Differences between male and female physicians are more pronounced among those who are not satisfied with their income. Of this group, women are less satisfied with personal factors related to their practice and they are less dissatisfied with the regulatory environment, the state medical practice environment, and medicine as a field.

Even with the more specific perceptions of income mediated by amount of work, were the proportion satisfied with their income declines, the pattern of male and female physicians remains similar. Among those who are satisfied with their income, women are less dissatisfied with the regulatory environment and less satisfied than their male colleagues with both components measuring satisfaction with their personal medical practice. For those who are dissatisfied with income, women are less satisfied with resources for their medical practice and less dissatisfied with the regulatory environment and with the state medical practice environment.

This analysis indicates to us that there is a lot that is not yet understood about how money motivates professionals—in this case, physicians. These data are not consistent with many of the assumptions noted in Chapter 5 that are made about money. What we have learned suggests that perception about money (most likely based on expectations and perceptions of what peers are receiving) seems to be a more important determinant of satisfaction than the actual amount of money.

Noticeably absent in this analysis is another variable that is thought to be important in determining income, and that is some measure of productivity. We turn our attention now to that.

Productivity. Productivity is a difficult variable to measure in many fields, and in the medical profession it is especially problematic. The simplest measure is hours worked per week, which we used as well as a modification to differentiate between professional activities involving direct patient care and those involving what are usually classified as indirect patient care activities, including research, administration, teaching, and continuing education. The analysis of these data have provided some interesting insights into the relationship of income and productivity (Chapter 4). In this section, we focus on how satisfied physicians are with their productivity (as measured by hours per week) and also how satisfied they are with what they perceive to be their work load (as measured by whether they view themselves to be at what we have termed "full professional capacity").

Table 6.10 shows the correlation between level of satisfaction as measured by the satisfaction indexes and hours worked per week, for the total sample as well as separately for males and females. Dissatisfaction seems to increase as hours worked per week increases, as shown by the negative correlations. The only exception to this is in the second index—resources. Correlations for female physicians are in the same direction, but their responses are less often statistically significant, primarily because of the smaller sample size. Appendix Table D.12 shows the correlations between actual hours worked per week—both direct care and total hours—and the scores on the satisfaction indexes. As can be seen from this table, the only significant correlations are in terms of total hours worked per week. The r values are all positive in direction for those who work fewer total hours per week; mixed at 31–60 hours per week; all negative at 61–90 hours per week; and mixed again for 91 or more hours per week—the highest number of total hours worked per week.

A purely economic analysis might suggest that working more hours should produce more income; higher incomes should produce higher levels of satisfaction. However, it is not always true that working more hours always produces more satisfaction. At some income level, people choose leisure time over money. Based on our data and on the literature presented in both Chapter 4 and 5, there seems to be a curvilinear relationship between satisfaction and hours worked per week, rather than a direct relationship.

Table 6.10 Correlations of Scale Scores with Average Hours Worked per Week, by Gender

	Personal Mean Score (range 5–25)	Resources Mean Score (range 5–25)	Review Mean Score (range 2–10)	Satisfaction with Medicine Mean Score (range 5–25)	Massachusetts Regulatory Climate Mean Score (range 5–25)	Massachusetts as a Good Place to Practice Mean Score (range 4–20)
All active physicians, r	−.113**	.083***	−.069	−.166*	−.118**	−.154*
Males, r	−.117**	.090***	−.052	−.155*	−.077***	−.161*
Females, r	−.138	−.020	−.148	−.198	−.024***	−.076

*p ≤ .001.
**p ≤ .01.
***p ≤ .05.
****p ≤ .10.

This measure of productivity is based on self-reports of actual hours worked per week. In analyzing income in Chapter 4 and in examining the relationship of income and satisfaction, it seemed that perception of income is a more useful variable than actual income. In order to measure perception of work load—or productivity—we asked respondents to indicate whether they felt their current medical practice was such that they were operating at what might be termed "full professional capacity." The respondents were also asked to indicate whether they were satisfied with their current work load. Table 6.11 explores these relationships.

This table shows that those who view themselves as practicing at what they define as their full professional capacity are more satisfied than those who view themselves as not at full capacity. This relationship holds for males and females across all six indexes, but it is particularly strong for the index that measures satisfaction with medicine as a profession. Interestingly, those who feel they are not practicing at full capacity do in fact work fewer hours per week than those who report being at full capacity—52 hours per week in comparison to 59 hours per week. Although 52 hours per week is considered a longer-than-average workweek by most occupational standards in the United States, it is less than average for physicians as a group, since 58 hours per week is both the national average and the average for all physicians in this study. Perhaps even more intriguing is the analysis of those who indicate that they are not working at full capacity. When this group is asked whether they are satisfied with their work load, they are fairly evenly split between being satisfied and not satisfied. Those who feel they are working at less than full capacity and are dissatisfied tend to work more hours (56.4 per week) than those who are satisfied with working fewer hours per week (48.4 hours per week). In fact, there is little difference in actual hours worked per week between those who define themselves to be at full capacity (working 59 hours per week) and those that define themselves to be at less than full capacity and unhappy about this work load (working 56.4 hours per week).

The rest of Table 6.11 is designed to explore gender differences in level of satisfaction and this notion of perceived capacity. There is a big difference between male and female physicians in terms of whether they view themselves to be at full capacity: 81 percent of male respondents view themselves as at full capacity, while only 61 percent of female physicians have this perception. There do not seem to be large differences in terms of level of satisfaction between male and female physicians, independent of perceived work load. For example, when comparing women who indicate they are at full professional capacity with men who are also at full professional capacity, the pattern of satisfaction is similar. Those who view themselves as not operating at their

Table 6.11 Relationship of Perception of Productivity and the Six Satisfaction Indexes

	Personal Mean Score (range 5–25)	Resources Mean Score (range 5–25)	Review Mean Score (range 2–10)	Satisfaction with Medicine Mean Score (range 5–25)	Massachusetts Regulatory Climate Mean Score (range 5–25)	Massachusetts as a Good Place to Practice Mean Score (range 4–20)	Hours Worked per Week
Yes, Practicing at Full Capacity							
Total (N = 597)	21.4	19.4	5.7	16.8	8.9	9.4	
Male (n = 535)	21.5	19.5	5.6	16.8	8.8	9.4	59.2
Female (n = 62)	20.8	18.9	6.0	17.6	9.8	9.9	
No, Not Practicing at Full Capacity							
Total (N = 163)	20.9	18.8	5.6	15.1	8.5	9.2	
Male (n = 123)	20.9	19.1	5.6	14.5	7.9	8.9	51.6
Female (n = 40)	21.0	17.6	5.6	16.8	10.4	9.9	
ANOVA							
Total	4.86***	6.18**	0.25	20.95*	2.60	0.94	
Male	5.98**	1.67	0.05	25.52*	10.25**	2.28	4.81***
Female	0.22	3.58	1.15	0.93	0.80	0.00	

Not at Full Capacity, Satisfied							
Total (N = 93)	21.5	19.2	5.7	17.0	9.6	10.0	
Male (n = 60)	21.3	19.8	5.7	16.6	9.0	10.0	
Female (n = 33)	21.8	18.3	5.8	17.6	10.7	10.2	48.4
Not at Full Capacity, Not Satisfied							
Total (N = 83)	20.1	18.4	5.4	13.1	7.5	8.0	
Male (n = 73)	20.2	18.6	5.4	12.9	7.2	7.8	
Female (n = 10)	19.1	16.2	5.4	14.6	9.6	9.5	56.4
ANOVA Results							
Total	8.91**	3.22	1.42	46.36*	21.03**	25.38*	
Male	4.30***	4.78***	0.79	30.09*	14.31**	21.28*	
Female	4.80*	2.64	6.02*	0.53	0.34	0.77	13.37**

*p ≤ .001.
**p ≤ .01.
***p ≤ .05.
****p ≤ .10.

full professional capacity but are satisfied with this are more likely to have higher scores on the six satisfaction indexes, for both men and women. The strongest difference lies in the index designed to measure general perceptions about medicine as a profession. Both men and women who are satisfied with a lower work load have much higher scores on this index—the biggest numerical difference of any of the analyses of these indexes.

Whether one chooses to have a smaller work load is probably important and raises issues that are also discussed in Chapter 5. The effect of being dissatisfied with one's lower work load is different between men and women: women are less satisfied with the two indexes measuring satisfaction with their personal practices (personal and resources), but are more satisfied with the index that measures general satisfaction as well as the two that measure perceptions toward Massachusetts. This analysis demonstrates the importance of examining perceptions—of both income and productivity—as well as actual figures. As with other results in this chapter, this result also reinforces the notion of treating satisfaction as a multidimensional variable.

Summary. This section has focused on presenting and analyzing the results obtained from measuring level of satisfaction by the six satisfaction indexes and examining the relationship between satisfaction and several variables, primarily through bivariate and univariate analyses. Not all of these variables are independent, and it is clearly useful to do a multivariate analysis. The technical details of this regression analysis can be found elsewhere (Stamps and Cruz, unpublished); the general results will be summarized here.

High levels of satisfaction with the personal factors index are best predicted by being male, having a lower income, working fewer hours, and being in a group practice setting. Specialty does not seem to affect this particular index, nor does age.

Physicians who are more highly satisfied with the resources available to their practice are more likely to be older, involved in primary care, practicing in either a group practice or an HMO, and earning slightly more money. Men and women do not seem to have strong differences with respect to this index, and hours worked per week also does not seem to affect satisfaction with resources.

The weakest index of the six is the one that attempts to measure perception of professional reviews within medicine, as might be predicted by its brevity, if nothing else. Throughout all of the analyses in this chapter, this index does not provide much differentiation. In the regression model, a high level of satisfaction is only predicted by being in a hospital setting and even that association is weak.

The level of satisfaction with medicine as a profession is predicted by having a higher income, but working fewer hours per week. Interestingly enough, being in some specialty other than surgery is also predictive, even though surgeons obviously have higher incomes. Also positive for this index is practicing in an HMO, which involves a lower income. Despite what the literature suggests, neither age nor gender predict level of satisfaction with this index. The pattern of correlations for this index reveals the complexity of physician satisfaction: a high income is satisfying, but so is a lower work load. Surgery—a high income and high work load specialty—seems particularly dissatisfying. Practicing in an HMO setting—clearly the lowest income practice—is related to higher levels of satisfaction, as shown repeatedly in all the results.

The two indexes measuring level of satisfaction with practice in Massachusetts show some very interesting similarities. First of all, as is obvious from the previous analysis, the scores on these two are consistently lower: these indexes represent factors that physicians find dissatisfying. Higher levels of satisfaction for the more specific of these two—the regulatory climate in Massachusetts—is best predicted by being in an HMO, practicing in primary care, and working fewer hours. Age and gender do not seem to affect this index; income level does not directly affect it either, although income is clearly represented through practice setting and specialty. A similar pattern occurs for the more general index, measuring satisfaction with the practice climate of Massachusetts. Satisfaction is predicted by being in primary care, working fewer hours, and practicing in an HMO. Also important here is age: increasing age is related to increased satisfaction.

We also included in the regression model the income variable that asks physicians to rate the acceptability of their income, given the work load. Satisfaction with this variable is best predicted by higher income and fewer hours worked. Once again, practicing in an HMO setting was important. Gender was significant: men were far more likely to be satisfied with income than women.

These results raise many interesting issues, not only for Massachusetts as a specific region, but also for more research into what physicians find satisfying and dissatisfying about their medical practices. Perhaps the most appropriate way of summarizing the results is to observe that a general summary is not possible. Not only are the patterns distinct for each of the six indexes, but also the patterns are distinct for different physician characteristics. Within each index, it is appropriate to generalize about primary care physicians, or physicians practicing in a certain practice arrangement, for example. It is not appropriate to summarize the level of satisfaction for "all physicians," however. For only one variable is there less variation than expected—gender. In terms of level of satisfaction, female physicians are more similar to male physicians than we anticipated, raising the possibility that the convergence theory discussed in Chapter 5 may be descriptive of the medical field.

Are the six satisfaction indexes a good measure?

Physician satisfaction is a complicated topic; it is complicated from a conceptual perspective and it is complicated from a measurement perspective. Although qualitative measures are a valuable and viable methodology for capturing physician satisfaction, the need for a more quantitative measure cannot be ignored. If a quantitative measure is to be developed, then care should be taken that it be as accurate as possible.

The first issue generally addressed in evaluating the credibility of a measure is statistical. As can be seen from Table 6.1, the statistical analysis of these six indexes ranges from acceptable to strong. The Cronbach's alpha measure ranges from .70 to .84; item-total correlations and factor loadings are all well within the suggested ranges, with only a few items falling below .50.

Equally important to the integrity of any measure is some sense of what is usually called "face validity." Using Tables 6.1 and 6.2 is helpful in addressing this issue. Of the six indexes, two are specific to the medical practice climate in Massachusetts—one concerning the regulatory climate in Massachusetts and the other, more broad, focusing on satisfaction with Massachusetts as a place in which to practice. The scores on these two indexes are lower than all the others and remain so throughout all the analyses presented in this chapter. The mean score for the whole sample on the regulatory climate index (8.8) is well below the midpoint for the possible range of that scale (15.0), and the mean score for the index of Massachusetts as a place to practice (9.4) is somewhat below the midpoint (12.0) for the range of that scale.

Two indexes are concerned with factors related to a physician's own individual medical practice. The personal factors index has a mean score of 21.3—well above the 15.0 midpoint—while the resources index mean score of 19.3 is also above the midpoint, but not as dramatically so. This result demonstrates that physicians are able to differentiate between factors that affect their own practices and those of a state environment. Also, physicians differentiate between personal and lifestyle issues and professional concerns for adequate resources for their medical practices.

One index was specifically created to measure general level of satisfaction, following those in the literature who feel that this should be a separate component rather than a summation of a total scale score. Scores on this index were lower than on the two practice-related ones; average score for the whole sample is 16.4, which is only slightly above the midpoint. The results presented in this chapter support the need for a specific measure of general or global satisfaction.

The fourth general index concerns professional review. It was created in order to capture a more general level of review and regulation than that measured by the Massachusetts-specific index. Only two items clearly belong in this index, as indicated by the statistical analysis. The presence of only two items certainly indicates a weak index if only for brevity, and, in fact, the performance of this index throughout the results presented here is unremarkable. The average scores are at about the midpoint of the range, which is interesting in contrast to the remarkably negative view of the regulatory climate specific to Massachusetts. The smallness of the variation in the scores on this index may indicate a certain level of acceptance of national review and regulation on the part of physicians. The fact that the scores on this index are always relatively higher than those for Massachusetts-specific regulatory climate indicates that physicians do differentiate between federal/national and professional review and more state-level control. We feel that this particular index needs to be strengthened and perhaps reconceptualized in order to capture the broader policies that govern the medical profession.

Throughout the analysis of these six indexes, we made many attempts to combine all six into some sort of scale that would provide a single summary figure to represent physician satisfaction. Many of these efforts produced a neutral summary number—one that was obviously balanced by the positive perceptions of a physician's own medical practice versus the negative perceptions of Massachusetts as a particular place in which to practice. After a careful review of these efforts as well as the results presented in this chapter, it seems that physician satisfaction may be too complex to be represented in one summed scale. At the least, the scale should be weighted by expectations, as is the Index of Work Satisfaction (Stamps and Piedmonte 1986). However, at the present time, there is not enough information to weight the components. Therefore, a more profitable line of investigation is to pursue creating indexes, each of which measures one particular aspect of physician satisfaction. After gaining experience in using and revising them, it may be appropriate to make the effort to combine them.

Internal reliability and validity: A check. In addition to the statistical analysis and the face validity analysis, it is very common to see if there is consistency between summary scores and responses to a questionnaire item. Tables D.13 and D.14 show this analysis, using responses to two items indicating general satisfaction: "All things considered, I am satisfied with my medical practice" and "I am generally satisfied with Massachusetts as a place to practice." For both items, a positive response (strongly agree/agree) is related to a higher score on each of the six indexes. The index that shows the strongest relationship is the one measuring general or global satisfaction with medicine, and the weakest trend is for the two indexes measuring perceptions of a physician's own practice. The relationship between the scores for the two Massachusetts-specific indexes and the responses to the item concerning Massachusetts are interesting (Table D.14). Those who strongly agree/agree that they are generally satisfied with Massachusetts as a place to practice have higher mean scores on the two Massachusetts indexes than occurred in analyzing any other variable. This is relative since even these scores place them only slightly above the midpoint (for the Massachusetts Practice Index) and substantially below the midpoint (for the Massachusetts Regulatory Climate Index).

For all six indexes, those who agree or strongly agree have higher scores than those who are undecided; those who are undecided have higher scores than those who strongly disagree/disagree. The consistency of response provides a positive sense of face validity.

Relation of index scores to frequency distribution. As important and valuable as these quantitative index scores are, they do not provide a complete picture of the level of satisfaction. In order to set the context for the index scores, it is useful to also examine the frequency distributions of the responses to the items composing the indexes. To provide one example of this, we will briefly describe the relationship of the index scores and responses to questionnaire items for two groups of physicians: those practicing in an HMO setting and those practicing in a solo practice setting. We have chosen these two groups because their satisfaction scores are quite different, implying that HMO physicians as a group have higher professional satisfaction than those in solo practice—particularly noteworthy because the early studies (especially Mechanic 1975 and Breslau, Novack, and Wolf 1978) indicated that physicians are much less satisfied when they practice in an organized setting. Also, physicians in solo practice make about twice as much money as physicians in HMOs, although HMO physicians perceive their incomes more positively than solo practitioners.

For the personal/lifestyle index, the vast majority of physicians in both practice sites demonstrate relatively high levels of satisfaction, as reflected by the scores (21.2 for HMO and 20.8 for solo practice physicians). The frequency distribution analysis certainly supports these numerical values since at least 85 percent of physicians in both practice settings are either satisfied or very satisfied with each item in this index but one. Only on the item related to educational opportunities for their families is the level of satisfaction lower, and then it is still at 75 percent. The major difference between these two groups is that there are a greater percentage of HMO physicians who respond "very satisfied" to the items.

Resources index scores show that there is no difference in level of satisfaction with this component. Responses to the items measuring this index are very similar and mostly positive. The lowest level of satisfaction is found—for both groups—to be in their interactions with medical school colleagues.

Although both groups of physicians have low levels of satisfaction with the regulatory climate in Massachusetts, the index scores show that physicians in solo practice are significantly more dissatisfied than HMO physicians (Table 6.4). As might be expected, both groups exhibit general dissatisfaction on many of the items contained in the index, although solo practice physicians are generally more negative in their responses. For example, among HMO physicians, the greatest source of dissatisfaction is with the retroactive way in which malpractice premiums are assessed, with 60 percent very dissatisfied. Solo practitioners are even more dissatisfied, with 92 percent very dissatisfied. One item on which there is a large discrepancy is the possibility of Massachusetts moving to a mandatory Medicaid participation program—HMO physicians are much less negative about this than solo practitioners. They are also far more likely to be undecided—35 percent of HMO physicians versus only 9 percent of solo practitioners.

In general, although both groups of physicians are negative about the five specific items that are being used to measure satisfaction with the Massachusetts regulatory environment, those in the solo practice environment are more extreme in their dissatisfaction than those who practice in HMO settings. HMO physicians are also more ambivalent, as demonstrated by their higher percentage response to the undecided option.

The perception of Massachusetts as a specific place to practice is another index that exhibits low levels of satisfaction, with solo practitioners being much more dissatisfied. For example, about half of HMO physicians are generally satisfied or very satisfied with the Massachusetts practice environment, while only 23 percent of those in solo practice express this. Solo practitioners are more likely to believe that there are other dissatisfied physicians in Massachusetts. Although a small majority of HMO physicians (54 percent) feel that practicing medicine in Massachusetts is different from other states, a larger proportion of solo practice physicians (80 percent) see the medical practice climate as being different.

One item asks for a prediction of behavior in this component: "I am likely to leave the state of Massachusetts to practice medicine elsewhere." HMO physicians are more strongly committed to staying in Massachusetts: 56 percent either disagree or strongly disagree with this statement, while 43 percent of the solo practice physicians disagree or strongly disagree. It is useful to be very specific in analyzing this item: 20 percent of HMO physicians and 13 percent of solo practice physicians are strongly committed to staying in Massachusetts, as evidenced by their "strongly disagree" response to this item. Only 4 percent of HMO physicians and 8.6 percent of solo practice physicians are very likely to leave, as demonstrated by their "strongly agree" response. About 30 percent of both groups are undecided.

The general satisfaction with medicine component measures, among other things, the likelihood of a physician's leaving medicine altogether. There is a strong difference between HMO physicians and those involved in a solo practice in terms of their response to this particular item: only 13 percent of HMO physicians agreed or strongly agreed that they were "seriously thinking about leaving medical practice altogether," while 34 percent of those in solo practice either agreed or strongly agreed with this statement. Certainly, a much higher percentage disagreed—46 percent of HMO physicians in fact strongly disagreed, and 28 percent of solo practice physicians strongly disagreed.

The overall scores on this particular index indicate moderate satisfaction, but also demonstrate that HMO physicians are much more satisfied with medicine as a profession than are those in solo practice (18.5 versus 15.5). Over half of both groups would go into medicine again and about half are generally satisfied with their medical practice, but HMO physicians are more positive about both items. Those in solo practice are more likely to express strong disagreement or be undecided when asked whether they are satisfied with their medical practices.

This component also measures level of satisfaction with income. A much higher percentage of solo practice physicians are either dissatisfied or very dissatisfied with their income (37 percent) than in the HMO group (14 percent). For those in an HMO setting, the level of dissatisfaction with income is present, but it is not the item that generates the most dissatisfaction. This result is especially interesting since the incomes of solo practice physicians are almost twice as much as HMO physicians, although a higher proportion of HMO physicians view themselves as satisfied with their income.

In all cases, the scores on the indexes provide useful summary figures, and the frequency distribution analysis provides the appropriate context for the interpretation of these figures.

How Satisfied Are Physicians?

The results presented in this chapter obtained by using the six indexes as a measure for satisfaction provide several new insights about physicians—what they think about medicine in general as well as what they think about their own particular practice setting. An obvious question is whether these physician respondents are unique so that these findings are therefore only useful to the western Massachusetts area. In general, on the overall measures where comparisons are possible, this respondent group is not significantly different from national profiles, including variables such as income, specialty distribution, practice arrangements, hours worked per week, age and years of professional experience, and proportion of women in practice.

Of course, no comparisons of physician satisfaction can yet be made, given the lack of research on this topic. That can be only determined by replication studies in other regions. From such replication a data base could be developed that would help better determine what satisfies, and motivates, physicians, as well as what dissatisfies them.

Until that time, there are three types of comparisons that can be made, although the strength of the comparisons is obviously limited by noncomparable measurement. Within this limitation, we explore these comparisons since they help set the stage for future research.

General level of physician satisfaction

The first general category of comparative results arises from the studies that have been conducted on physician satisfaction. We examined the details related to specific variables in the first part of this chapter, but we did not address the general conclusions.

The focus of the published literature is generally on those factors that cause physicians to be dissatisfied, so it is easy to concentrate on the negative aspects of the physician's role. We evaluated eleven studies that provided some measure of level of satisfaction and also tried to summarize results by an overall conclusion. Of these eleven, only two characterized their overall findings as physicians being relatively dissatisfied with their jobs. One of these was Reames and Dunstone (1989), whose thoughtful study has too small a sample size to be generalizable, and the other was Lichenstein (1984), whose conceptual framework and scale are sophisticated, but applied only to a sample of physicians working in one particular setting, that is, in prisons. These physicians had very high levels of dissatisfaction with several aspects of their jobs.

However, in the other nine studies, the levels of satisfaction for the majority of the physicians sampled was moderately high. These nine studies cover a period of time from 1978 to 1991; they include several types of measures but generally employed scales. They are primarily U.S. studies, although one study is from Canada and one is from Great Britain. Additionally, these studies had several objectives; not all had a primary objective of measuring physician satisfaction. For example, Mechanic's (1975) early study had as its primary objective the determination of differences between physicians working in a prepaid group setting and those working in a nonprepaid group setting. He could find no strong relationship between practice setting and level of satisfaction, and all groups reported generally high levels of satisfaction, although the measures were not specific to satisfaction. Another example from the same time period is by Breslau, Novack, and Wolf (1978) who were comparing levels of satisfaction between physicians and nonphysician professionals in group and nongroup settings. As with Mechanic, their hypothesis of lower satisfaction in more organized settings was not supported: in fact, physicians in both practice settings had high levels of satisfaction.

Three studies used scales; in all three, physicians scored around the midpoint or slightly above the midpoint, demonstrating moderate to moderately high levels of satisfaction among the majority of respondents (Linn et al. 1986; McCranie, Hornsby, and Calvert 1982; Cooper, Rout, and Faragher 1989). Two studies showed that, although the majority of physicians were satisfied with their professional lives, about 15 percent were dissatisfied (Clarke et al. 1984; Kravitz, Linn, and Shapiro 1990).

These studies all reinforce the need to divide satisfaction into its component parts. For example, in the Kravitz, Linn, and Shapiro (1990) study, which found about 15 percent of the physicians surveyed to be dissatisfied, there were some specific aspects of their medical practice that had between one-fourth and one-third of respondents dissatisfied. In our study, physicians had high levels of satisfaction with personal aspects and resources related to their own practice; moderate levels of satisfaction with a global or general measure of medicine as a profession; and very low levels of satisfaction for the regulatory environment of Massachusetts and the medical practice climate in the state.

Several of our conclusions are supported by the literature on physician satisfaction. First, it is important to measure satisfaction in terms of components or aspects. Components more accurately reflect the nature of job satisfaction and therefore provide more precise ways of summarizing results. This concept is very clear in the analysis of our results: patterns and trends are not consistent across all six indexes. Second, it is desirable to develop a quantitative measure so that comparisons can be easily made between groups of physicians. The interpretation of the measures should be relative—moderate or high level of satisfaction, for example— but without quantification such comparisons are not possible. Third, it is important to have a distinct measure for global or general satisfaction as one component of satisfaction, as Lichenstein (1984) suggested. The alternative—to add up a total score—is not meaningful since positive and negative responses may very well average, as they did with our overall scale scores. Finally, it is clear from these results that satisfaction is the appropriate theoretical construct, not dissatisfaction. As long as the measure includes the various specific components or facets, there will be sufficient information to differentiate between what satisfies and dissatisfies physicians.

Comparison of physician satisfaction to other health care professionals

A second type of comparison question relates to how physicians' level of satisfaction compares to the level of satisfaction of other health professionals. This comparison is more complicated because of the problem of modifying measurement tools to be appropriate to more than one health professional group. Breslau, Novack, and Wolf (1978) compared level of satisfaction of physicians and nonphysicians in group and nongroup settings, using the job description index. They showed that physicians were more satisfied with only one aspect of their work, income; with the other major dimensions of work, nonphysicians were just as satisfied as physicians.

The Stamps-Piedmonte index of work satisfaction was initially developed using hospital-based nurses. In the early development phases, the scale was modified for use with ambulatory physicians (Stamps et al. 1978), and Lichenstein (1984) used it to develop his physician satisfaction scale. In the later development phases, this scale was modified for use with emergency medical technicians (Stamps and Shopnick 1981), and also for many different types of nursing professionals (Stamps and Piedmonte 1986; Slavitt et al. 1978). The scale was ultimately validated for hospital-based nurses, with a caution for uses for other types of nursing professionals until a normative data base had been developed for hospital-based nurses.

In fact, it was partly this experience with premature application of an attitude scale to other groups of health professionals that convinced us to develop a separate measurement of level of satisfaction for physicians. The six indexes described here are quite different in structure from the Stamps-Piedmonte Index of Work Satisfaction. As more research is encouraged in occupational satisfaction of health professionals, we may discover enough similarities that more comparable satisfaction scales may be developed. Until then, caution must govern modification of satisfaction scales for health professionals other than those for whom the scale was originally designed. This limitation obviously constrains the ability to make comparisons between different types of health professionals.

Within these constraints, one comparison is possible, and that is between four individual items that are common to the Stamps-Piedmonte Index of Work Satisfaction and the questionnaire given to physicians.

Table D.15 shows the responses to these items. When asked a simple question about income or salary, physicians are far more likely than nurses to be satisfied. Interestingly, when both physicians and nurses are asked to consider income in terms of amount of work, the percentage satisfied drops considerably. For both groups, between 15 percent and 19 percent fewer are satisfied when asked to consider the amount of money they earn in the context of their work load. However, physicians are still more satisfied than nurses with their income. Physicians are also far more satisfied with professional interactions with their peers than nurses are.

One would expect physicians to be much more satisfied with their careers than nurses, given the differences in professional autonomy and income, but level of responsibility and stress may diminish the high levels of satisfaction felt by physicians. It is a little unsettling that only about 60 percent of either nurses and physicians would go into their respective fields again if they had the choice. Most nurses are clear about the alternative: only 11 percent are uncertain, while fully 30 percent would not go into nursing again. Physicians are more ambivalent: 20 percent are undecided, while only 20 percent would clearly avoid the field given a second chance.

Of course, the numerical values from the Index of Work Satisfaction and the six satisfaction indexes are not comparable. However, it is interesting to consider the overall distribution of scores. The overall unweighted scores for nurses are far below the midpoint of the possible range of scores, about equivalent to what physicians score on the three indexes about which they are more negative—the review index and the two indexes that are concerned with Massachusetts. On the other three indexes, physicians seem far more satisfied than nurses are.

How do physicians compare to other, nonhealth professionals?

There is, of course, a final comparative question: Are physicians unique in their perception of level of satisfaction? This area clearly needs serious research effort, since we know very little about professional level workers—what motivates them, what satisfies them, or what rewards provide them with incentives. As noted previously, most of what is known in either occupational sociology or economics is based on blue-collar workers.

There are some preliminary comparisons, but they are almost all focused on the idea of leaving the profession. A popular comparison is with lawyers: in 1984, about 27 percent of practicing American lawyers indicated that they would seriously consider leaving their profession (Smith 1984). A similar national survey of lawyers conducted in 1990 identified that the most dissatisfied lawyers were women, younger attorneys, and attorneys of color; about 16 percent indicate dissatisfaction and 19 percent said they would choose another profession (*Boston Globe,* May 21, 1990, p. 15).

The studies we have reviewed seem to indicate a similar proportion of physicians who identify themselves as being dissatisfied—somewhere around 15 percent. In our study, 25 percent of the total sample indicated that they were "seriously thinking about leaving medical practice altogether," although this proportion varied significantly with practice setting; 35 percent of those in solo practice agreed with this statement. However, there are several studies in which larger percentages of physicians have said they would choose another profession if they could—40 percent in a national Gallup poll (*Boston Globe,* May 21, 1990, p. 15), although other studies have put this figure at 20 percent or 27 percent (Linn et al. 1985b; McCranie, Hornsby, and Calvert 1982). Another commonly used measure is the proportion of physicians who would not recommend medicine to their own children—63 percent in two separate surveys (Charles et al. 1987; *Physician's Management,* Feb. 1990).

Naturally, these types of findings are dramatic and often receive publicity through media coverage. However, the results of these surveys do not shed much light on determining whether physicians are unique among other professionals in terms of expectations, perception of rewards, and satisfaction. This knowledge is important because the U.S. economy is becoming increasingly specialized. Some research in Great Britain has been devoted to gathering information on level of satisfaction of a variety of professionals in British society, but it is not applicable to the U.S. setting (Cooper, Rout, and Faragher 1989).

Of course, even if physicians are discovered to be significantly more dissatisfied than other professional groups, this does not necessarily mean immediate remedial action of some sort. As Kravitz, Linn, and Shapiro (1990) have pointed out:

> Furthermore, there are many social goals at least as worthy as preserving physician satisfaction for its own sake. Nonetheless, as policy makers consider new approaches to improving access and controlling health care costs in the U.S., they should be cognizant of the effects such strategies may have upon physician satisfaction, and of the potential for social disruption that such dissatisfaction may imply. (p. 510)

Where to Go from Here?

Developing a valid and reliable scale-level measurement for a variable as individualistic as level of satisfaction is a demanding task, one that not only requires careful research but also appropriate circumstances. The circumstances that are required certainly exist. The first is the attainment of a certain basic level of knowledge. There is considerable research about physicians, although it suffers from a lack of conceptual clarity and standardization of operational terms so comparability has been limited. The second circumstance is a perceived need for a summary measure, which is revealed in many of the published articles summarized in this chapter. In several instances, results from questionnaires were being used as scale-level measurement. Although many investigators would agree on the need for a scale to measure physician satisfaction, there are many points of disagreement, indicating a need for further research. We conclude this chapter by presenting two distinct areas in which research needs to be conducted to address several important questions.

The first general area of needed research lies in clarifying the conceptual framework. The first step is one we suggested at the beginning of the chapter, concerning the theoretical framework in which scale development takes place. At the present moment, there are two orienting concepts: the inherent stress within a physician's role and the identification of factors that contribute to physician satisfaction or dissatisfaction. They are two separate lines of research and should be so pursued. Although it is tempting to investigate the overlap that exists, it is more appropriate to develop separate measures for each. Linn's work on developing a scale is somewhat limited in applicability because of his efforts to measure both satisfaction and stress (Linn et al. 1985b, 1986; Kravitz, Linn, and Shapiro 1990).

We have chosen to anchor our efforts at scale development in the orienting framework of satisfaction. Despite several examples of research into physician satisfaction, there is still a lack of agreement in terms of conceptualizing satisfaction, extending as far as whether level of satisfaction is a dependent or independent variable. There is a serious need for more theoretical research on satisfaction as a variable and what it seems to be related to. Lichenstein (1985) began this with an admirable review article, but there has been little work since.

Schulz and associates presented a model in which satisfaction is treated as a dependent variable and perceived clinical autonomy is viewed as an intervening variable (Schulz and Schulz 1988; Schulz, Girard, and Sheckler 1992). The results from our study do not support this conceptualization. In our study, we treated satisfaction as a dependent variable, but more appropriate intervening variables are certain physician characteristics that seem to influence the expectations of a physician, including age, gender, and specialty.

Several researchers have considered the relationship between satisfaction and other variables. A particularly common approach is to consider satisfaction as an outcome of some organizational reconfiguration, especially efforts to increase continuity of care (Linn et al. 1985a, 1985b, 1986; Numerof and Abrams 1981; Linn 1981). Other research considers the relationship of satisfaction and physician behavior, which is of obvious interest and importance. Much of this research considers satisfaction as an independent variable and the behavior the dependent variable. An example is provided by the common assumption in research on physicians moving their practices, that relocation is associated with—if not caused by—physician dissatisfaction. Actually, physicians seem to relocate at the same rate as other workers: about 20 percent move every year, and there is a general movement toward the Sunbelt (Steiber 1982). Urban/rural location differences are also frequently framed as being related to satisfaction, although it is consistent with our results and others to consider this a choice based on physician characteristics, particularly specialty and geographic area in which the physician has personal experience. Although we analyzed the relationship between level of satisfaction and perception of whether one's practice is rural, there were no significant findings.

Two other physician behaviors have been investigated in terms of their relationship to satisfaction level. The first is turnover, particularly physicians leaving a group practice arrangement, although the findings were inconclusive (Mick et al. 1983). One particularly extreme physician behavior that seems to be related to level of dissatisfaction is willingness to participate in a strike (Kravitz, Linn, and Shapiro 1990; *AJPH* 79: 1218–19).

Of even more interest is the possible relationship between level of satisfaction and quality of patient care, an area of investigation that is current in other countries as well as the United States. The notion that prescribing behavior or utilization of diagnostic tests may be related to factors other than medical assessment of the patient has been explored, with interesting and intriguing findings (Makin, Rout, and Cooper 1988; Gerrity, DeVellis, and Earp 1990; Pfifferling 1980; Scheiber 1983; Numerof and Abrams 1981; Grol et al. 1985; Greene et al. 1989).

These studies indicate that the level of interest in physician satisfaction is high, and there is a desire to investigate the relationship of physician satisfaction to several variables, including patient satisfaction and quality of care. Although these studies are interesting and many times the results are particularly intriguing, research of this type is premature because of the limitation of the measures for physician satisfaction.

The second broad area in which research is needed is in the vital area of measurement development. Without more serious and systematic efforts at scale development, research into physician satisfaction and related variables will continue to be fragmented and debatable. Effort needs to be devoted to the development of a scale to measure physician satisfaction. Based on our review of other research and our own results, it seems that the most appropriate way to achieve a scale to measure physician satisfaction is to continue the approach of refining several focused scales or indexes, each of which measures one dimension of physician satisfaction. They should each be given in repeated administrations and revised based on statistical analysis. After this phase of identifying and refining the dimensions, it may be possible to combine them into one scale to achieve the use of one summary number, which may be said to represent physician satisfaction. It may be possible to weight the various components, as with the Index of Work Satisfaction approach used with nurses (Stamps and Piedmonte 1986).

As part of this measurement development process, an additional question must be addressed: Is it possible to develop one scale—or set of scales—to measure satisfaction of all physicians, regardless of specialty or practice setting? Our model of scale development assumes that it is possible to develop one measure for all practicing physicians. Schulz and associates are using an alternative approach, which is to develop a scale specific to one practice setting; in their case, it is managed care (Schulz and Schulz 1988; Schulz, Girard, and Sheckler 1992). More research needs to be done to determine which of these models is most appropriate, bearing in mind the questions one is trying to answer.

Finally, one additional recommendation concerns the need to consider carefully how this scale might be used. If past literature is any guide to future research, a scale to measure physician satisfaction will be used in two ways: in studies that are large in scope—attempting to gather comparative data—and in organizational studies in which the objective is to determine the relationship of physician satisfaction and organizational arrangements. Consequently, a scale must be generalizable enough to be utilized in national or regional studies, but also specific enough to be utilized in a particular practice setting. We have attempted to meet this need by including four scales that address general concerns of physicians and two scales that address issues that are particular to the medical practice climate in which our research has been located.

Physicians are diverse, both in personal characteristics and in professional characteristics. This diversity affects the personal perception of what physicians find satisfying and dissatisfying in their professional roles. Capturing the complexity of these perceptions is challenging but worthwhile, since it will add an important measure for a significant variable. This chapter has presented what should be viewed as a beginning to a new way of measuring physician satisfaction.

References

American College of Hospital Administrators. *Health Care in the 1990's: Trends and Strategies.* Chicago: American College of Hospital Administrators, 1984.

Borenstein, D. B., and K. Cook. "Impairment Prevention in Training Years: A New Mental Health Program at UCLA." *Journal of the American Medical Association* 247 (May 21, 1982): 2700–2703.

Brayfield, A. H., and H. R. Roth. "An Index of Job Satisfaction." *Journal of Applied Psychology* 311 (1951): 307.

Breslau, N., A. H. Novack, and G. Wolf. "Work Settings and Job Satisfaction: A Study of Primary Care Physicians and Paramedical Personnel." *Medical Care* 16 (Oct. 1978): 850–62.

Charles, S. C., R. B. Warnecke, J. R. Wilbert, R. Lichtenstein, and C. DeJesus. "Sued and Nonsued Physicians: Satisfactions, Dissatisfactions, and Sources of Stress." *Psychosomatics* 28 (Sept. 1987): 462–68.

Clarke, T. A., W. M. Maniscalco, S. Taylor-Brown, K. J. Roghmann, D. L. Shapiro, and C. Hannon-Johnson. "Job Satisfaction and Stress among Neonatologists." *Pediatrics* 74 (July 1984): 52–57.

Clute, K. F. *The General Practitioner: A Study of Medical Education and Practice in Ontario and Nova Scotia.* Toronto: University of Toronto Press, 1963.

Cooper, C. L., U. Rout, and B. Faragher. "Mental Health, Job Satisfaction, and Job Stress Among General Practitioners." *British Medical Journal* 298 (Feb. 1989): 366–70.

Crapen, P. "Stress: Medical School's Perilous Rites of Passage." *New Physician* 29 (Nov. 1980): 18–23.

Emener, J. "Professional Burnout: Rehabilitation's Hidden Handicap." *Journal of Rehabilitation* 45 (1979): 55–58.

Fox, R. C. "Training for Uncertainty." In R. K. Merton, G. C. Reader, and P. L. Kendall, eds. *The Student Physician: Introductory Studies in the Sociology of Medical Education.* Cambridge, MA: Harvard University Press, 1957, pp. 228–41.

Freshnock, L. J. *Physician and Public Attitudes on Health Care Issues.* Chicago: American Medical Association, 1984.

Friedson, E. *Medical Work in America: Essays on Health Care.* New Haven, CT: Yale University Press, 1989.

Gardner, E. R., and R. C. Hall. "The Professional Stress Syndrome." *Psychosomatics* 22 (1981): 672–80.

Gerrity, M. S., R. F. DeVellis, and J. A. Earp. "Physicians' Reactions to Uncertainty in Patient Care: A New Measure and New Insights." *Medical Care* 28 (Aug. 1990): 724–36.

Green, L. W., and F. M. Lewis. *Measurement and Evaluation in Health Education and Health Promotion.* Palo Alto, CA: Mayfield Publishing Company, 1986.

Greene, H. L., R. J. Goldberg, H. Beattie, A. R. Russo, R. C. Ellison, and J. E. Dalen. "Physician Attitudes Toward Cost Containment: The Missing Piece of the Puzzle." *Archives of Internal Medicine* 149 (Sept. 1989): 1966–68.

Grol, R., H. Mokkink, A. Smits, J. V. Eijk, M. Beek, P. Mesker, and J. Mesker-Nietsten. "Work Satisfaction of General Practitioners and the Quality of Patient Care." *Family Practice* 2 (1985): 128–35.

Harvey, L. K., and S. L. Shubat. *Physician and Public Attitudes on Health Care Issues.* Chicago: American Medical Association, 1989.

Hassinger, E. W., L. S. Gill, D. J. Hobbs, and R. L. Hageman. "Perceptions of Rural and Metropolitan Physicians about Rural Practice and the Rural Community, Missouri, 1975." *Public Health Reports* 95 (Jan. 1980): 69–79.

Herzberg, F., B. Mausner, and B. Snyderman. *The Motivation to Work*. 2nd Edition. New York: John Wiley and Sons, 1959.

Hilfaker, D. *Healing the Wounds: A Physician Looks at His Own Work*. New York: Random House, 1985.

Hulin, C. L., P. C. Smith, and L. M. Kendal. *Cornell Studies of Job Satisfaction, II. Model and Method of Measuring Job Satisfaction*. Ithaca, NY: Cornell University Press, 1963.

Krakowski, A. J. "Stress and the Practice of Medicine II. Stressors, Stresses, and Strains." *Psychosomatics* 38 (1982): 11–23.

Kravitz, R. L., L. S. Linn, and M. F. Shapiro. "Physician Satisfaction under the Ontario Health Insurance Plan." *Medical Care* 28 (June 1990): 502–12.

LaRocco, J. M., J. S. House, and J. R. P. French. "Social Support, Occupational Stress, and Health." *Journal of Health and Social Behavior* 21 (Sept. 1980): 202–18.

Lichenstein, R. "Measuring the Job Satisfaction of Physicians in Organized Settings." *Medical Care* 22 (Jan. 1984): 56–68.

Lichenstein, R. (Review Article): "The Job Satisfaction and Retention of Physicians in Organized Settings." *American Sociological Review* 129 (Oct. 1985): 139–79.

Lickert, R. A. "A Technique for the Measurement of Attitudes." *Archives of Psychology* 140 (1932): 44–53.

Linn, L. S. "Career Orientations and the Quality of Working Life Among Medical Interns and Residents." *Social Science and Medicine* 15A, (1981): 259–63.

Linn, L. S., R. H. Brook, V. A. Clark, A. R. Davies, A. Fink, and J. Kosecoff. "Physician and Patient Satisfaction as Factors Related to the Organization of Internal Medicine Group Practices." *Medical Care* 23 (1985a): 1171–78.

Linn, L. S., J. Yager, D. Cope, and B. Leake. "Health Status, Job Satisfaction, Job Stress, and Life Satisfaction Among Academic and Clinical Faculty." *Journal of the American Medical Association* 254 (Nov. 15, 1985b): 2775–82.

Linn, L. S., R. H. Brook, V. A. Clark, A. R. Davies, A. Fink, J. Kosecoff, and P. Salisbury. "Work Satisfaction and Career Aspirations of Internists Working in Teaching Hospital Group Practices." *Journal of General Internal Medicine* 1 (Mar. 1986): 104–8.

Lofgren, R. P., and J. Mladenovic. "How Reorganizing a General Medicine Clinic Affected Residents' and Patients' Satisfaction." *Academic Medicine* 65 (Sept. 1990): 604–8.

Makin, P. J., U. Rout, and C. L. Cooper. "Job Satisfaction and Occupational Stress Among General Practitioners—A Pilot Study." *Journal of the Royal College of General Practitioners* 38 (July 1988): 303–6.

Maslach, C. "Burned Out." *Human Behavior* 5 (1976): 21–35.

Maslach, C. "Understanding Burnout: Definitional Issues in Analyzing a Complex Phenomenon." In W. S. Paine, ed. *Job Stress and Burnout*. Beverly Hills, CA: Russell Sage, 1982.

Mawardi, B. H. "Satisfactions, Dissatisfactions and Causes of Stress in Medical Practice." *Journal of the American Medical Association* 241 (April 1979): 1483–86.

May, H. J., and D. A. Revicki. "Professional Stress Among Family Physicians." *Journal of Family Practice* 20 (1985): 165–71.

McCarty, D. J. "Sounding Board." *New England Journal of Medicine* 318 (Feb. 18, 1988): 456.

McCranie, E. W., J. L. Hornsby, and J. C. Calvert. "Practice and Career Satisfaction Among Residency Trained Family Physicians: A National Survey." *Journal of Family Practice* 14 (1982): 1107–14.

McCue, J. D. "The Effects of Stress on Physicians and Their Medical Practice." *New England Journal of Medicine* 306 (Feb. 25, 1982): 458–63.

Mechanic, D. "The Organization of Medical Practice and Practice Orientations Among Physicians in Prepaid and Nonprepaid Settings." *Medical Care* 13 (March 1975): 189–204.

Mick, S. S., S. Sussman, L. Anderson-Selling, C. Delnero, R. Glazer, E. Hirsch, and D. S. Rowe. "Physician Turnover in Eight New England Prepaid Group Practices: An Analysis." *Medical Care* 21 (March 1983): 323–37.

Natelson, B. H. *Tomorrow's Doctors: The Path to Successful Practice in the 1990's.* New York: Plenum Press, 1990.

Nie, N. H., C. H. Hull, J. G. Jenkins, K. Steinhennor, and D. H. Bent. *Statistical Package for the Social Sciences.* New York: McGraw-Hill, 1975.

Numerof, R. E., and M. N. Abrams. "Before Impairment: Physician Stress and the Organization's Responsibility." *Health Care Management Review* (Fall 1981): 77–82.

Nunnally, J. C. *Psychomatic Theory.* New York: McGraw-Hill, 1978.

Payne, R., and J. Firth-Cozens. *Stress in Health Professionals.* New York: John Wiley and Sons, 1987.

Pfifferling, J. *The Impaired Physician: An Overview.* Chapel Hill, NC: The Center for Well-Being of Health Professionals, 1980.

Porter, A. M. D., J. G. R. Howie, and A. Levinson. "Measurement of Stress as It Affects the Work of the General Practitioner." *Family Practice* 2 (1985): 135–46.

Reames, H. R., and D. C. Dunstone. "Professional Satisfaction of Physicians." *Archives of Internal Medicine* 149 (Sept. 1989): 1951–56.

Reidel, R. L., and D. C. Reidel. *Practice and Performance: An Assessment of Ambulatory Care.* Ann Arbor, MI: Health Administration Press, 1979.

Reuben, D. B., D. H. Novack, T. J. Wachtel, and S. A. Wartman. "A Comprehensive Support System for Reducing House Staff Distress." *Psychosomatics* 25 (1984): 815–20.

Revicki, D. A., and M. H. May. "Development and Validation of the Physician Stress Inventory." *Family Practice Research* 2 (1983): 211–25.

Rosemark, E. H. "Residency Stress Leading to Suicide: A Mother's View." In R. H. Combs, D. S. May, and G. W. Small, eds. *Inside Doctoring: Stages and Outcomes in the Professional Development of Physicians.* New York: Praeger, 1986.

Sargent, D. A. "Preventing Physician Suicide." *Journal of the American Medical Association* 257 (1987): 2955–56.

Sargent, D., V. W. Jensen, T. A. Petty, and A. Raskin. "Preventing Physician Suicide: The Role of Family, Colleagues and Organized Medicine." In R. H. Combs, D. S. May, and G. W. Small, eds. *Inside Doctoring: Stages and Outcomes in the Professional Development of Physicians.* New York: Praeger, 1986.

SAS Institute, Inc. *SAS User's Guide: Statistics.* Version 5 Edition. Cary, NC: SAS Institute, 1985.

Scheiber, S. C. "Emotional Problems of Physicians: Nature and Extent." In S. C. Scheiber and B. B. Doyle, eds. *The Impaired Physician.* New York: Plenum Press, 1983, pp. 3–10.

Schulz, R., C. Girard, and W. E. Sheckler. "Physician Satisfaction in a Managed Care Environment." *Journal of Family Practice* 34 (1992): 298–304.

Schulz, R., and C. Schulz. "Management Practices, Physician Autonomy, and Satisfaction." *Medical Care* 26 (Aug. 1988): 750–63.

Schwartz, A. H. "Medical School and the Process of Disillusionment." *Journal of Medical Education* 12 (May 1978): 182–85.

Scully, R. "Stress in the Nurse." *Americal Journal of Nursing* 80 (1980): 912–15.

Shore, J. "The Oregon Experience with Impaired Physicians on Probation." *Journal of the American Medical Association* 257 (1987): 2931–34.

Shubin, S. "Burnout: The Professional Hazard You Face in Nursing." *Nursing* 8, (1978): 22–27.

Slavitt, D. B., P. L. Stamps, E. B. Piedmonte, and A. B. Haage. "Nurses' Satisfaction with Their Work Situation." *Nursing Research* 27 (March-April 1978): 114–20.

Smith, R. S. "A Profile of Lawyer Lifestyles." *American Bar Association Journal* 70 (1984): 50.

Sparr, L. F., G. H. Gordon, D. H. Hickam, and D. E. Girard. "The Doctor-Patient Relationship During the Medical Internship: The Evolution of Dissatisfaction." *Social Science and Medicine* 26 (1988): 1095–1101.

Stamps, P. L, and N. T. B. Cruz. "Development of a Measurement of Physician Satisfaction: An Index Approach." Unpublished.

Stamps, P. L., and J. Finkelstein. "Statistical Analysis of a Patient Satisfaction Scale." *Medical Care* 19 (Nov. 1981): 1108–35.

Stamps, P. L., and E. B. Piedmonte. *Nurses and Work Satisfaction: An Index for Measurement.* Ann Arbor, MI: Health Administration Press, 1986.

Stamps, P. L., E. B. Piedmonte, A. B. Haase, and D. B. Slavitt. "Measurement of Work Satisfaction Among Health Professionals." *Medical Care* 16 (April 1978): 337–52.

Stamps, P. L., and B. Shopnick. "Emergency Medical Technicians' Perception of Acceptance by Nurses and Physicians." *Journal of Ambulatory Care Management* 4 (Nov. 1981): 69–86.

Steiber, S. R. "Physicians Who Move and Why They Move." *Journal of the American Medical Association* 248 (Sept. 24, 1982): 1490–92.

Talbot, G. D., K. V. Gallegoes, P. O. Wilson, and T. L. Porter. "The Medical Association of Georgia's Impaired Physician's Program." *Journal of the American Medical Association* 257 (1987): 2927–30.

Thomas, C. B. "What Becomes of Medical Students: The Dark Side." *Johns Hopkins Medical Journal* 138 (Summer 1975): 353–75.

Thurston, L. L., and E. J. Chave. *The Measurement of Attitudes*. Chicago: University of Chicago Press, 1929.

Warr, P., J. Cook, and T. Wall. "Scales for the Measurement of Some Work Attitudes and Aspects of Psychological Wellbeing." *Journal of Occupational Psychology* 52 (1979): 129–48.

Chapter 7

Research and Reform:
Learning from Massachusetts

Why Study Physicians?

This book is concerned with creating a conceptual focus around which to organize research into physicians' behaviors, attitudes, and motivations. It is our contention that a better understanding of physicians is central to the development of successful health policy and health reform efforts. In order to increase the understanding of physicians, two avenues of investigation are necessary. The first is the need for increased information about physicians. At first thought, it would appear that a vast amount of information is available about physicians, practice patterns, medical organizations, and financial arrangements. Much of the information is descriptive, gathered and maintained by the AMA in a national data base that is very useful for comparative research and for identifying trends. However, the information collected is frequently not detailed enough to provide more than fairly general observations. Dependence on national data bases has resulted in a lack of specific information about the complexities of medical practice.

Two additional problems exist that limit the conclusions that can be drawn about physicians: terminology and time (both of which have been methodological themes throughout this book). Use of nonstandard operational definitions has seriously impaired the ability to compare the results of studies. Although this is true generally, perhaps the best example is found in Chapter 3, where we discuss research into enumerating physicians. Time is sometimes the reason why nonstandard operational definitions are used. In every chapter of this book, we have found that current research about physician practice patterns is frequently based on results from research in the 1960s and 1970s. Much of this framework does not apply to the medical care system of the 1990s. This problem was discussed in most detail in Chapter 5, but it is certainly not limited to the study of female physicians.

The second area of investigation that is important to pursue is studying perceptions of physicians. As pointed out in Chapter 6, very little is known about what motivates physicians, much less what satisfies or dissatisfies them. Very little information has been gathered about the physicians' world view—what physicians think about their own medical practice, the medical profession itself, or the health care delivery system in which they work. The physician view of the health care world has been pretty much discounted as a viable research topic. To attempt a substantial restructuring of the health care system without a basic understanding of the nature of the physicians' work and of what physicians think about their work is probably to invite failure.

There are several common misconceptions surrounding efforts to identify physician perceptions. Perhaps the most important is that physicians will not be willing or able to share their thoughts. The questioning of their ability is to discount the value of discovering someone's views: physicians certainly are able to voice their views about their profession. Physicians are also more willing to be questioned than is commonly thought. We have been much impressed with the desire of physician respondents in western Massachusetts to share their views with us. The nature of these comments, as one might suspect, has been diverse, and has ranged from the personal to the political.

Despite the diversity, however, one theme is very obvious throughout all of the comments: the increasing recognition of an "us versus them" mentality. Western Massachusetts physicians portrayed this in many ways. For example, a family practitioner chose to comment on terminology: "I hate being addressed as a 'health care provider' or a 'vendor' or just a 'provider.' I am a 'physician'. . . . " A gastroenterologist commented, "I enjoy medicine, but I have the feeling that government looks at us as thieves and corrupt professionals." When physicians are asked to identify the main problem, there is no unanimity of opinion. To many, of course, it is "the government," such as the family practitioner who said:

> Has anyone surveyed what happens financially to costs of services when government enters a service industry such as ours? . . . (1) staggering cost of service increases, (2) decreasing availability of service, (3) maldistribution of availability with the poor being shut out again, (4) death of medicine as a profession, (5) these were not the intention but this is the result.

Closely related to "government" being identified as the main problem is "paperwork" often used in conjunction with "overregulation." An internist summed it up by saying, "Federal overregulation is superimposed on state problems. Extra paperwork takes many hours away from patient care [explaining medical care is as time-consuming as doing it]." Another physician commented, "Generally speaking, I am unhappy being squeezed between overbearing regulations and paperwork, and financial considerations pressuring me to do less for patients and malpractice forcing me to do more."

Malpractice was frequently mentioned by physician respondents as one of the major problems facing them. As expected, they speak differently about malpractice than nonphysicians. An emergency room physician noted a way to improve malpractice:

> Improve the court system in which the M.D. is always seen as the 'guy with bucks' and before the verdict is guilty. . . . Secure a fair trial and no settlements out of court, which encourages people to pursue even ridiculous complaints. We should have the right to countersue in those unjustifiable and time-losing suits.

One physician shared a personal experience:

> Your questions don't really elicit or explore the factor of fear and lack of respect in doctors. Since I was accused of malpractice and taken through the months of tribunals for four years, fear and anxiety (with everybody looking over my shoulder to see if I did something wrong—much of it petty and outcome-affected, not really malpractice) have become a large part of medical practice. Very unsatisfying for someone who is wonderfully trained, capable and works his heart out.

Some physicians in our study have tried to work for reform, especially in the malpractice area. One general surgeon talked about the importance of no-fault malpractice:

> It is the only way to go to solve this problem—the tort system must be removed from it and a fee schedule set up that will go 100 percent to the patient that society can afford. The [lawyer's] power of being in the legislature has kept this golden goose going for longer than it should have. . . .

Not all physicians blame some outside force: several of the respondents pointed to problems within medicine. An anesthesiologist said:

> I think it is also fair to say that the medical profession does a very poor job in dealing with lousy and dishonest M.D.s. There are also some groups of physicians that have pretty much raped the system with their outrageous fees for short procedures and virtually no patient care in off-hours in the hospital.

Other physicians are unhappy with the nature of their work, especially primary care physicians. A typical comment from an internist:

> Some of my dissatisfaction with the practice of medicine is directed at the field of internal medicine. I feel that those of us in primary care medicine are over-worked, over-regulated and frustrated because we have so little free time.

Several physicians noted societal pressures as a major source of their frustration. An anesthesiologist said:

> The high costs in medicine should be blamed more on high costs of supplies and equipment as well as extremely high patient demand for "the latest" treatments whether of benefit or not to an individual. The litigiousness of our society is not much more of a problem in medicine than in many other areas.

Reading the many comments by respondents to our survey has demonstrated the existence of a very large gap between what physicians think about the health care system and what nonphysicians think about it. One physician termed this "war": "Neither side in 'the war' seems capable of working toward peace and healing." Regardless of whether this—or any other of the physicians' perceptions—is true, the perception of an adversarial arrangement between physicians and policymakers is not helpful. First, if physicians do not understand the need for regulation, they will simply get more defensive. Second, if policymakers do not understand the view of physicians, they are in danger of enacting regulations that may have negative consequences.

There is much discussion about reforming the health care system. Although significant reform may be necessary, we are concerned that changes are being suggested without the necessary research to anticipate the consequences. Lost in the efforts to change the system is what Alan Sager (1988) has referred to as the need for a new "social compact" with physicians. This social compact implies that the needs of physicians, patients, and society need to be explicitly stated—as much as possible—and a system to reinforce the desired behaviors of both physicians and patients be developed. The needs of physicians, patients, and society must be balanced, a process that is highly dependent on cooperation and compromise and that must be based on more accurate knowledge. This book is a contribution to the creation of a more complete knowledge base about physicians—both their behavior and their perceptions about their role in the health care delivery system.

Learning from Massachusetts

This book has presented data gathered from actively practicing physicians in the western part of the state of Massachusetts. Although the data have a regional flavor, the information gathered has been dictated by national concerns. Massachusetts, as a state, does have several unique restrictions on physicians, but the broad issues are the same as are of concern nationally. The areas that we have included in this book have two striking similarities. First, policy decisions have been justified on the basis of mostly descriptive information. Second, there are so many important methodological problems in the collection, analysis, and interpretation of the research that we are much troubled by the move from research to regulation. In each case, we have first reviewed the literature and presented a synthesis and critique of what is known, and then compared the regional data we have collected. In this section, we would like to summarize some of the more important methodological suggestions that have arisen from our research in Massachusetts.

Supply

One of the most basic of questions that permeates almost all research on physicians is the question of enumeration of physicians. Although there is a high degree of sophistication in this area, our review demonstrated a critical lack of comparability—not just in method of enumeration, but also in conceptualization. Decisions about whom and what activities to count can only be made in the context of a clear operational definition of supply. This lack of clarity permeates the published literature; it also contributed significantly to the acrimonious situation in Massachusetts, the political backdrop of this research.

Two specific recommendations that affect other areas of research arise from this chapter. The first is a suggestion about specialty nomenclature. The variable of specialty is one of the most important when researching physicians, regardless of whether one is considering medical practice patterns, income, productivity, or reimbursement patterns. Yet, there is an amazing lack of comparability with respect to measuring this important variable. Some researchers use board-certified titles, others ask for a functional description of the specialty in which the majority of the practice falls. Perhaps the worst problem is in combining specialties into larger categories for analysis. One of the more important policy analyses occurs around the concept of primary care physician. Yet, there is a large variation in the literature about what specialties are properly combined into primary care. Unfortunately, one of the specialties involved (internal medicine) has a large number of practitioners, so the difference between including and excluding it as a primary care specialty is very large. It is critical that more comparable nomenclature be developed and used; our preference is to utilize more functional descriptions and to include internal medicine specialists in the primary care designation.

The second specific recommendation that arises from our research in physician supply is more conceptual. Most policy decisions about physicians are focused on actively practicing physicians, yet much research includes all physicians, without designating their practice status. Table 3.1 shows the difference this makes in terms of enumerating physicians. Differences of this magnitude are unacceptable, especially when the research is being translated into policy. Our suggestion is to more clearly delineate actively practicing physicians as the group in which we are interested—not just for supply but also for other investigations. The use of what we have termed the "direct-care equivalent" physician in enumerating physicians and in identifying physicians to be included in studies will help standardize research.

Income and productivity

When we began our research, some of the nonphysicians questioned the necessity of gathering information about physician incomes, arguing that "everybody knows" what determines a physician's income. The physicians with whom we talked during the development of the research project and the questionnaire presented another view, however. From them, we could see that physician income is a much more complicated variable than it appears, and our results in this area are consistent with this view.

The empirical findings arising from the survey of western Massachusetts physicians are generally consistent with the national trends within medicine, although physicians in western Massachusetts do make substantially less money than in other regions of the country. In western Massachusetts, the top-income specialties are radiology, surgical specialties, and anesthesiology. The four bottom-income specialties are psychiatry, internal medicine, pediatrics, and general/family practice. There is a $88,400 differential between the top-income specialty (radiology) and the bottom-income specialty (general/family practice).

Physicians were more willing to share information about income with us than we predicted. Some physicians chose to add more information, as one general surgeon who delineated his monthly expenses (including car loan payments, food, clothing, and electric bills) and added the following comments:

"Too tired to enjoy anything, small house, few luxuries, angry wife, alien-ated children, patients don't even say thank-you, why am I doing this? No net worth, no securities at age 40, wife now gets up at 5:30 a.m. and teaches special education (four years of college and two post) for $13,000 per year. You think docs complain?"

It is obvious from several respondents' comments that income is far more complex to physicians than it is to most researchers and policymak-ers. Income has a symbolic meaning for physicians, which was revealed in the several places where we gathered information about physicians' perceptions of income, as reported in Chapter 4. In addition to this symbolic meaning, income is a more complex variable simply in terms of trying to estimate it, as we discovered when attempting to compare our findings to other results in the literature. As when investigating supply, we discovered many areas in which noncomparable estimates are being used.

The following four specific suggestions will help make research on income more comparable. First, income information should be reported and analyzed in similar ways. Net or unadjusted income figures are most appropriate for cross-sectional studies, and most economists agree that median incomes are a much more appropriate measure of central tendency than mean incomes, although many health services researchers continue to use mean incomes. Use of medians is most appropriate when income data are gathered exactly, rather than in categories, as we did. It appears that physicians are not as reluctant to report exact information on income as we feared.

Second, it is important to collect all financial information carefully—and independently from the organizational structure of the practice arrangement. Although, previously, practice patterns provided an ac-ceptable proxy estimate of financial arrangements, that is no longer true. Physicians are paid in a variety of ways, and it is important to assess them carefully. We were not able to collect as much detailed information as would be necessary to do a more systematic analysis.

Third, there are two important sources of income that need to be identified separately: on-call hours and income from medical invest-ments. When asking for net income, some physicians will include these in their estimates and some will not. It is important to delineate whether these should be included or not.

Finally, for income of physicians to be relevant, it should be set in the context of their professional activities. We gathered information on professional activities of physicians in a similar fashion to the AMA. As is true nationwide, the proportion of time spent in direct care ac-tivities by western Massachusetts physicians is high—about 85 percent.

Setting income in the context of professional activities will allow income-generating hours to be considered separately from other professional hours. We used these hours to explore the relationship between productivity and income, a relationship that needs to be explored more carefully. As with supply, using only direct-care hours—the income-generating activities—is probably most appropriate.

Gender

There seems to be widespread acceptance of the notion that men and women practice medicine differently, although the assumption has not been thoroughly examined in the context of the medical care system of the 1990s. Most of the research supporting the different ways in which men and women practice medicine is based on studies conducted when women constituted only 5–7 percent of all practicing physicians in the United States. Current investigations mostly continue to build upon these early findings.

Analysis of the findings from research on women in medicine leads to consideration of three possible explanations. The first is to agree that there are inherent differences between the way in which males and females practice medicine; this conclusion is usually supported by citing various descriptive research studies that indicate differences in practice patterns, specialty choice, and productivity. An alternative is to agree that there seem to be systematic differences between male and female physicians, but these differences may not be inherent; rather, they may be due to a variety of barriers experienced by women as they progress through the medical education system toward active practice. The third alternative is that perhaps women once did practice differently, but the differences are rapidly diminishing. This convergence theory considers both the possibility that women are becoming more similar to men and that male physicians are becoming more similar to female physicians. Obviously, these theories each produce very different sorts of research efforts.

Our review of the literature—both recent and not-so-recent—as well as our own results, lead us to suggest that continued research should be conducted utilizing either the second or third alternative explanation, but not the first. Using observed differences to prove that there are significant differences between male and female physicians is an example of reification. It is much more enlightening to consider either the reasons for the observed differences or to consider that there are fewer differences currently than previously.

Our research—and other recent research—indicates that, for many important variables, the observed differences between male and female physicians are diminishing. As these differences diminish, so too do the explanations for the income differential between male and female physicians. In western Massachusetts, for example, female physicians seem to work about 10 percent less than male physicians, but they earn only 62 percent of what male physicians do.

Three suggestions arise from our experience in examining women in medicine. First, it is crucial to acknowledge the importance of time: the medical world and American society of the 1990s is very different from the social environment of the 1950s and 1960s. It is inappropriate to use research from this era for anything except setting the historical perspective. As noted in Chapter 5, it is also important to reframe the major research questions in order to develop more meaningful insights into the health care world of the 1990s.

Second, research should focus on female physicians who are in active practice, which seems to be a smaller percentage of total female physicians than the male equivalent. Currently, research efforts suffer from an inadequate definition of which female physicians are being studied and compared to male physicians. Although women currently make up almost one-third of all medical school classes, they still only represent at most 15 percent of all practicing physicians.

The final suggestion that arises directly from our study concerns a methodological issue. Actively practicing female physicians are more likely to be younger (as a group) than actively practicing male physicians. Both age and years of professional experience seem to be related to income, practice arrangements, and, perhaps, productivity. We controlled for this bias as best we could, given the sample size limitations. A larger sample size would enable the most appropriate comparison to be used, which is to compare male and female physicians under age 45, with ten or fewer years of professional experience.

The acknowledged objective of this section is to share some of the methodological lessons that we have learned from this study. One of the most important of the many "methodological lessons" learned is that physicians will respond at high rates to primary surveys. Additionally, they will also provide details about specific aspects pertaining to their medical practices, their opinions about related personal practices, and the health care delivery system itself.

Satisfaction

Interest in what provides satisfaction to physicians is steadily increasing, although the ability to measure satisfaction is still fairly primitive. Satisfaction is an example of a research area that experiences both conceptual and operational ambiguity.

Our research has led to two recommendations. The first is to use the conceptual framework of satisfaction rather than dissatisfaction or stress. The second recommendation concerns the development of a measurement for physician satisfaction. Although it is very desirable to have one unified scale, our results lead us to believe that using several separate indexes provides a far more useful and sensitive measure than one summed scale. In Chapter 6, the value of this approach is repeatedly demonstrated. Physician satisfaction is multidimensional and complex; using separate indexes to measure each facet separately provides more information.

Although some research has been done on attempting to discover the relationship between satisfaction and other variables, the most serious need in this area is the development of a measure of satisfaction that is conceptually sound, statistically valid, and well accepted by other researchers. Without this, all other research is arguable.

From Research to Policy

Research in health and human services is frequently used to justify health policies and specific regulations, as well as suggesting more systematic reform of the health care system. Our experience in this regional research project indicates that there are several important areas in which more research needs to be done before the transition from research to policy occurs. This section will summarize three content areas in which basic descriptive research needs to be accomplished and three policy-related areas in which further research is needed, to help to identify options and consequences of possible reforms.

Content-based research

Is what we know still true? There is a wealth of descriptive information about the medical field, but in our extensive review of the literature on several different topics, we discovered that these descriptions may no longer be true. The passage of time always limits generalizations arising from research, but we believe that it is an even more serious limitation currently. There are many areas in which more descriptive information is needed. Perhaps the most important is the elaboration of the many different ways in which physicians may practice and the ways in which they are paid. What used to be known about money and physicians is not good enough any more. This information needs to be gathered using actively practicing physicians, the societal resource in which there is the most interest.

Although new descriptive information is needed, it is also important to go beyond mere description to attempt to understand the process or the function of the variable in medical practice. A good example is specialization, a variable well known for its high level of influence. Much less well known is the process of decision making with respect to specialization, or the functional relationship between postgraduate medical training and actual medical practice. More basic knowledge is needed about how and why physicians change their functional specialty practice patterns. It is very important to develop and consistently use standardized nomenclature and operational definitions; the failure to do so is currently a serious limitation.

Women in medicine. In some ways, examining women in medicine provides a microcosm for research in the medical profession, although there are some unique characteristics as well. Women seem to be entering medical schools in ever greater numbers, but they still are not a strong presence in the actual practice of medicine. Very little is known about whether women travel the medical education pipeline at a different rate than men. There is some evidence that the differences between male and female physicians are decreasing, as suggested by the convergence theory. It remains unresolved whether this decrease is due more to women or to men changing their practice patterns. This theory seems to imply that younger physicians are more similar to each other; more research is needed on the under age 45 physician to determine whether this is true. Then, it can be determined whether increasing years of professional experience is accompanied by changes in practice patterns. There is some evidence, for example, that female physicians have a different lifetime profile with respect to productivity than male physicians. Some suggest that productivity differences that exist between male and female physicians may disappear when the whole lifetime employment experience is considered. Along the same lines, more research is needed on women who are practicing in those specialties that seem to be male dominated, especially surgical specialties. Qualitative research is especially appropriate here in order to garner a better understanding of the process by which these women have been able to succeed.

Researchers must be sensitive to how easy it is to incorporate stereotypic assumptions about women physicians into their investigations, as well as into their interpretation of findings. Of the many appropriate examples, perhaps the following is the most instructive to illustrate this point. A trend is slowly emerging in terms of conclusions about income differentials between male and female physicians; increasingly, it is viewed as a "bad news, good news" phenomenon, with the "good news" pertaining to increasing recruitment of female physicians in order to achieve the cost-containment objective. It does not require a feminist perspective to sense the acceptance of the existence of income differentials in this suggestion. Our research—and others'—seems to indicate that between 20 and 30 percent of the income differential between male and female physicians remains unexplained *after* controlling for other variables that are known to affect income, including age, practice pattern, specialty choice, and productivity.

Perceptions of physicians. Research on medical organizations is frequently framed according to the designations of those with administrative or legislative interests. This approach is defensible, but it is also necessary that some research be based on perceptions of physicians themselves. In our research, perception of income was a better predictor of satisfaction than actual income. An interesting tangential analysis related to income and productivity in western Massachusetts respondents is related to the respondents' perception of whether they are at full capacity in their practice, reported in Chapter 4. When perception of whether a physician is operating at full capacity is analyzed by gender, some of the differences observed in productivity disappear (Table D.5, in Appendix D). Whether a physician perceives himself or herself to be at full professional capacity, whether they are satisfied with that status, and what number of hours per week this represents are important areas for further investigations.

Although these examples are qualitative data, physician perceptions may also be addressed by quantitative means. Research in physician perceptions has been limited by not having an acceptable quantitative measure of physician satisfaction. This research project has contributed to the development of such a measure, as reported in Chapter 6. This measure will allow physician perceptions to more easily be incorporated into research.

Policy-based research

Reimbursement issues. Information about income is critical for development of a more successful health policy, and an increasingly important part of income is various sources of reimbursement. In our study, the incomes of physicians did not seem to be affected by having Medicare or Medicaid responsible for at least 25 percent of their practice income, but we were not able to gather enough information about how physicians might balance the various third party payers in their own particular practices.

Several physicians made comments about changes in either the structure of their medical practices or in their own behavior because of specific reimbursement strategies. For example, a typical story is relayed by this comment:

> I joined an HMO after residency due to large debts for my medical education and because I did not wish to add to my debt burden by incurring practice "start-up" costs. When I decided to leave the HMO, I went to work at a federal facility rather than either starting a practice or joining an existing practice due to the many problems with insurance/Medicare/Medicaid reimbursements.

This and many similar anecdotes underscore a general lack of understanding of the consequences of reimbursement patterns on physician behavior.

One consequence of existing reimbursement patterns that needs more investigation is the resultant income differences between specialties. Although the income differentials are largest between primary care specialties and surgical specialties, there are also reimbursement differences between primary care specialties, as this respondent indicated: "One particularly serious burden for family physicians is the lower reimbursement they receive than general internists for the same care rendered through Medicaid/Medicare." This difference may be an example of policy decisions guiding medical care patterns without a clear understanding of the economic and philosophical incentives that are being communicated.

Another possible consequence of current reimbursement patterns is the mix of physicians that currently define the U.S. health care system, the only system that has a much higher percentage of specialists than primary care physicians. There is continuing discussion on this topic, but little knowledge of the role reimbursement and income play in the specialization decision-making process.

Physicians and organizations. Physicians are increasingly working in organizations, whether they be prepaid HMOs, private group practices, or hospitals. Practically nothing is known about physicians as employees, or about the type of physician that decides to join—or leave—an established group. Physicians are viewed by administrators as difficult to manage, but, in reality, there is an inadequate knowledge base about managing highly trained professionals in any organization.

Our study produced intriguing, but somewhat nonintuitive, findings about income, satisfaction, and organization of medical practice. These findings suggest that physicians may trade off income and satisfaction: physicians in HMOs appeared much more satisfied in their relatively low-income practices than physicians in higher-income practices.

The role of female physicians in organizations is a particular area that needs careful investigation. A fairly consistent finding from other research is that women physicians are more likely to be employed by organizations and are more likely to be satisfied with this practice arrangement. This result can obviously be used in several ways, one of which is to keep incomes lower for female physicians. A more equitable use is to identify what male and female physicians find satisfying and dissatisfying about practicing in an organizational setting.

Physician behavior in response to regulatory action. The topic of physicians and regulations is one that is replete with anecdotes, mostly horrible ones, from both physicians and regulators (policymakers or managers). This area has some urgency, since more changes seem imminent during this decade. Despite all the regulatory activity in the health field, there is practically no research that identifies how physicians behave in response to regulations. There is no research that attempts to differentiate between the effects of state and federal regulations. It is common to assume that physicians change their behavior in response to regulatory pressure. For example, in Massachusetts, about 8 percent of the physicians in the western part of the state had left to practice in other states and about 10 percent had stopped practicing medicine. It was "common wisdom" that this was in response to the Massachusetts regulatory climate, but actually it is not known whether these percentages are any different from the normal migration pattern of physicians, an area about which very little is known. Some physicians are explicit about the effect of state regulation, such as the family practitioner who said: "I have made an initial commitment to practice here but would probably leave for a relatively unregulated state (perhaps in the southwest) if things worsen here such that I feel I'm not being paid fairly for the work I do." However, even in this example, the view of what would constitute an "unregulated state" is unknown.

Needless to say, these three areas are closely related to one another, but the nature and direction of the relationship is not understood. For example, some physicians may view organizations as buffers against the regulatory environment; in Massachusetts it was a frequent comment by HMO physicians that several of the state regulatory efforts did not affect them. However, working in an HMO setting clearly implies a level of acceptance of other types of regulation of medical practice. Also, there were several personal comments by physicians that indicated the importance of the reimbursement system in their decision about a practice setting. It is important to address these three related areas separately, but in order to do so, it is necessary to have more descriptive information about medical practice and a better understanding of physician perceptions.

A Final Word

This book has focused on the importance of increasing the understanding about medical practice in general, and physicians in particular. We have presented extensive reviews of the literature for four topics and then used the data from western Massachusetts to compare our findings and to illustrate the problems we have noticed. The four topic areas selected include important national concerns. We chose to report on supply because of the pervasive methodological problems and because research on supply is so quickly translated into policy, perhaps more so than any other area. An analysis of income was selected because most policy analysis assumes that physicians primarily respond to economic incentives. Our research has demonstrated that physician behavior is far more complicated. Gender was selected because an analysis of women in medicine provides a microcosm of medicine as a profession, while also providing insights into an increasingly important resource. Satisfaction was included because so much research now attempts to demonstrate relationships between satisfaction and physician behavior or organizational structure, but there is no acceptable measure for this perception-based variable.

Throughout the presentation of these four topics are three common themes. The first is that research in medical care organization is not precise enough. There are too many variations in conceptual definitions and operational definitions. This lack of standardization presents serious limitations on comparability and generalizability. The second broad theme relates to time. In all four topics, current research is defined by previous understanding. In many cases, both the social environment and the medical care environment have changed significantly, necessitating the revision of even the description of medical care, particularly with respect to financial arrangements. The third theme throughout this volume is the importance of assessing physicians' perceptions about their own practices as well as their profession and the health care system.

Some will debate the importance of this third theme. Knowing physician perceptions is not the same as taking an advocacy position, and it should not be so interpreted. Ignoring physician perceptions increases the chances of negative consequences of health policy, a situation that is simply too familiar.

Physicians have valuable perceptions about the problems facing the health care system. For every physician who responds that the major problem facing the health care system is "the government" or "red tape" or "too much paperwork" is another physician who offers cogent analysis unique because of its perspective. An internist commented to us:

> I feel that the trend in Massachusetts, which I consider to be moderately unfavorable towards physicians, is only slightly in the forefront of a nationwide tendency toward increasing regulation of health care. I believe it represents the inability or unwillingness of our society to invest dwindling economic resources in health care, versus each individual's expectation that maximum medical care will be provided whenever needed.

An anesthesiologist echoed these sentiments:

> Society demands too much from its health care providers. People want maximum coverage, but don't want to pay. People expect the best—first-dollar coverage if possible—but won't pay in higher taxes or with more out-of-pocket expenses. As the population ages, the Medicare patient is going to have to decide whether he/she will help pay through increased tax or be willing to increase their out-of-pocket co-pay; doctors will only take so much. Soon, the best and brightest will stay out of medicine to avoid the regulatory stresses and second-guessing that various non-medical agencies and middle-men [third-party payers and business self-insurers] put on medical providers.

Physicians do not have a common consensus about the major problems facing the health care system, but they all understand it is a balancing of their professional needs, a patient's individual needs, and a group's (society's) willingness or unwillingness to pay.

Physicians also have valuable insights about solutions. Some of the western Massachusetts respondents are politically active, as this family practitioner:

> I am a member of a consumer coalition which is addressing the problem of medical costs in [name of town] and are presently trying to draw up a pilot medical coverage program that will be more accessible to doctors and patients. I, myself, would favor a plan like that in Canada, and change the insurance companies, especially the Blues.

Another respondent shared the following:

> I left my practice at a staff-based, university-affiliated hospital in 1988. I was paid a salary. I left because of my dissatisfaction with medicine in general. I strongly believe in a national health plan. The current system is unfair to patients and confusing with conflict of interest to physicians.

A recent article in the *New England Journal of Medicine* (Himmelstein et al. 1989) describes a national health plan based on a single public insurance system that would pay all health care costs under federal responsibility. The group writing the article—and presenting the proposal—is called "Physicians for a National Plan." Arnold Relman has observed:

Physicians will have to play an active and constructive part in shaping a new health care system, because no comprehensive arrangement is likely to succeed without their cooperation. Now is the time for our profession to make common cause with government and with the major private payers in seeking solutions to a pressing social problem that is not going to solve itself.

Bringing conflicting sides together to attempt to negotiate acceptable conditions is not unprecedented—whether in labor negotiations or in international conflicts. The process is used within organizations to increase productivity and increase morale. If an approach such as total quality management is thought to work in industry, hospitals, and other organizations, why not apply it to a larger arena? The problems are serious within the health care system, involving several interest groups, each with its own agenda. Undoubtedly, none of the interest groups will be able to achieve all it wants. It is a political compromise that will create any sort of revised health care system. Incorporating all the interest groups—including physicians—will provide the best chance for success.

We hope that a major contribution of this volume will be in setting the direction for future research on physicians, with an emphasis on primary surveys eliciting the physicians' world view. This research would provide an in-depth understanding of what motivates and satisfies this important group of health professionals. This type of analysis could produce a better knowledge base for the formulation of health care policy, and that, in turn, could be used to develop a new social compact among physicians, patients, and society.

References

Himmelstein, D. V., S. Woolhandler, and the Writing Committee of the Working Group on Program Design, Physicians for a National Health Program. "A National Health Program for the United States: A Physician's Proposal." *New England Journal of Medicine* 320 (January 1989): 102–108.

Relman, A. S. "Universal Health Insurance: Its Time Has Come." *New England Journal of Medicine* 320 (Jan. 12, 1989): 117–18.

Sager, A. *The Sky Is Falling: The Massachusetts Medical Society Reports on the "Physician Shortage."* Boston, MA, 1988.

Appendix A:
Comparative Analysis of the Validity
of Three Standard Lists of Physicians

One of the more interesting methodological aspects of this research lies in comparing the accuracy of each of the official source lists that attempts to define the population. These lists can be evaluated because, through the survey process, the true population was identified (see Chapter 2). Also, in creating our own list, designated as "UMass list," we identified on which list each individual name appeared.

In order for any particular list to be accurate, it must include everybody who should be included and also exclude all people who should be excluded. This involves an accuracy estimate as well as an error estimate. An example of an accuracy estimate is that all those who should be on a list are indeed included. An error estimate involves those who are on the list but should not be as well as those who are not on the list but should be. The most appropriate way to discuss this concept may be in terms of the traditional statistical view of error: Type I errors are those who are not included on the list but should be; Type II errors are those who are included on the list but who should not be.

Table A.1 shows each of the three lists separately—the Massachusetts Board of Registration, Folio's Directory, and the AMA Masterfile. Additionally, information about each of the five response categories from Table 2.1 is included in this table, as this may add valuable insight for future research.

Type I error includes all those who are not on the list but who should be, which will obviously lead to an underestimate of what is being counted. Type I errors are calculated as a percentage of those known to

Table A.1   Comparison of Completeness of the Lists of Licensed MDs in Western Massachusetts with Actual Number of Practicing Physicians

Massachusetts Board of Registration List

1. Of the 908 who returned questionnaires:
    824 were on the BRM list (accuracy estimate: 91%)
    84 were not on the BRM list (Type I error estimate: 9%)

2. Of the 394 nonrespondents:
    351 were on the BRM list (accuracy estimate: 89%)
    43 were not on the BRM list (Type I error estimate: 11%)

3. Of the 110 who have left western Massachusetts:
    32 are not on BRM list (accuracy estimate: 29%)
    78 are on the BRM list (Type II error estimate: 71%)

4. Of the 183 who are not practicing:
    100 are not on BRM list (accuracy estimate: 55%)
    83 are on the BRM list (Type II error estimate: 45%)

5. Of the 216 who cannot be located:
    88 are not on BRM list (accuracy estimate: 41%)
    128 are on the BRM list (Type II error estimate: 59%)

Total Type I error estimate: 10% (127/1302)

Total Type II error estimate: 20% (289/1464)

Folio's Directory

1. Of the 908 who returned questionnaires:
    873 were on Folio's (accuracy estimate: 96%)
    35 were not on Folio's (Type I error estimate: 4%)

2. Of the 394 nonrespondents:
    375 were on Folio's (accuracy estimate: 95%)
    19 were not on Folio's (Type I error estimate: 5%)

3. Of the 110 who have left western Massachusetts:
    21 are not on Folio's (accuracy estimate: 19%)
    89 are on Folio's (Type II error estimate: 81%)

4. Of the 183 who are not practicing:
    16 are not on Folio's (accuracy estimate: 9%)
    167 are on Folio's (Type II error estimate: 91%)

5. Of the 216 who cannot be located:
    30 are not on Folio's (accuracy estimate: 14%)
    186 are on Folio's (Type II error estimate: 86%)

Continued

Table A.1   Continued

Total Type I error estimate: 4% (54/1302)

Total Type II error estimate: 26% (442/1690)

American Medical Association Master File List

1. Of the 908 who returned questionnaires:
   559 are on AMA list (accuracy estimate: 62%)
   349 are not on AMA list (Type I error estimate: 38%)

2. Of the 394 nonrespondents:
   234 were on AMA list (accuracy estimate: 62%)
   160 were not on AMA list (Type I error estimate: 38%)

3. Of the 110 who have left western Massachusetts:
   58 are not on AMA list (accuracy estimate: 53%)
   52 are on AMA list (Type II error estimate: 47%)

4. Of the 183 who are not practicing:
   131 are not on AMA list (accuracy estimate: 72%)
   52 are on AMA list (Type II error estimate: 28%)

5. Of the 216 who cannot be located:
   130 are not on AMA list (accuracy estimate: 60%)
   86 are on AMA list (Type II error estimate: 42%)

Total Type I error estimate: 39% (509/1302)

Total Type II error estimate: 19% (190/983)

be practicing in western Massachusetts (1,302), since as a result of the survey, 1,302 is verified to be the actual denominator. This figure includes both respondents and nonrespondents. The total Type I error estimate is lowest for Folio's (4 percent), which reinforces the fact that Folio's is the most inclusive of the lists.

Type II errors involve a more common error encountered in identifying physicians, including those on the list who should not be. These errors will lead to an overestimate of what is being counted. Type II errors have been calculated as a percentage, using as a denominator the corrected version of each list, a process involving eliminating duplicate entries and those whose addresses fell outside the study area. The list with the largest number of these internal corrections was Folio's Directory: a total of 324 out of the original 2,014 entries were deleted due to duplicate entries or addresses that fell outside the designated geographic area. The list with the fewest internal corrections was the state Board of Registration list: only 1.5 percent were duplicate listings. The Type II error rate is higher for each list than the Type I error rate; the AMA list and the state Board of Registration list have a smaller Type II error rate than Folio's, which is consistent with the view of Folio's as the most inclusive list.

The point of this exercise is not to cast dispersion upon these lists, but rather to emphasize that one must select the most appropriate list, given the objectives of the research. For example, if one were interested in those physicians who have left a specific geographic area (such as our Group 3 on Table 2.1) the AMA list is by far the most accurate, as Table A.1 shows. In general, Folio's has the highest Type II error rate, especially for physicians in Group 4 (Table 2.1), which means that Folio's fails to note when physicians have stopped practicing. In general, use of Folio's is more likely to produce an overestimate. Whether an undercount or an overcount is a more serious error depends entirely upon the objectives of the research. The BRM list of 1,464 represents an 11 percent overcount of what we have subsequently discovered to be a total of 1,302 physicians. The BRM list contains a total of 289 physicians who are on the list but who should not be, for a total Type II error rate of 20 percent. The Type I error rate is much less, but still important, since 127 physicians are not included on the list who should be. Although this undercount is only 10 percent of the total, it is important, since these may be new physicians who have moved into the area. Folio's contains a total of 442 physicians on the list who should not be, a Type II error rate of 26 percent. The Type I error rate is low, with only 54 physicians not on the list who should be. The AMA Masterfile list is interesting: 190 physicians are on the list who should not be (19 percent Type II error rate). Their Type I error rate is slightly higher, with 509 physicians not on the list who should be which is a 39 percent Type I error rate.

What do these errors mean? Many of them are expected because of the nature of these lists. For example, it is often desirable to have a list that includes all possible physicians. Folio's Directory, for example, is a commercial list used for marketing, and it is therefore more likely to be all inclusive. This inclusivity leads to a high Type II error rate, with physicians on the list who should not be. For our research, having a low Type II error rate is important since we are particularly sensitive to the possibility of overcounting the number of physicians who are actually in practice in western Massachusetts. The AMA Masterfile list had a surprising tendency to undercount physicians, although it is generally viewed as being more inclusive. In our case, we obtained this list from another group in Massachusetts that may have had a more limited definition of practicing physician.

There are two technical notes that should be mentioned here. We did not address which of the 1,302 physicians are *individually* designated on each of the three lists, primarily due to constraints on time and resources. Also, all the calculations noted in Table A.1 are based on the "cleaned up," or corrected, versions of the lists, after the removal of duplications and obvious errors such as addresses outside the geographic area. Presumably, the error estimates would be higher on the original uncorrected lists, and Type II error estimates would be particularly affected by our corrections.

These lists all reveal the very real practical problem of maintaining an accurate list. The BRM list we used was dated April 1988; physicians are required to respond to the BRM every two years and in between are encouraged to provide the BRM with any changes that are relevant to their practice, especially address changes. Without this voluntary updating, the BRM list may be two years out of date for any particular physician. For example, through our survey, we found 127 physicians practicing in western Massachusetts who are not listed on the BRM list. Some physicians may be new to the area within the last two years. Some may have been missing from the BRM list because they gave the BRM a practice address in eastern Massachusetts although our UMass list shows they have a work address also in western Massachusetts. Others may maintain their registration with the BRM because they once worked in Massachusetts or hope to in the future, but are currently not working in the state, a common practice that adds to the overcounting problem.

Folio's and the AMA Masterfile list also depend on voluntary updating as well as obtaining information from a variety of other sources. Voluntary updating by physicians is notoriously and understandably low. Correcting their personal entries on these lists is not of major importance to them. Such corrections may be more important to some categories of physicians than others. For example, AMA members may be more likely to update their listings than nonmembers. As a result, these lists may be more likely to be inaccurate.

However, part of the "error rate" is particular to our research objectives and is specific to the definition of the population, which is physicians who are actually in practice in western Massachusetts, as opposed to those who are licensed to practice in the state. The BRM maintained on its list 78 of the 110 physicians we identified as having left western Massachusetts. Even though these physicians are not included in our definition of the population, they may very well have maintained their license in Massachusetts. This discrepancy is a clear example that even a relatively accurate list like the BRM cannot be used to answer all research questions. The purpose of the BRM is to delineate what we have termed to be a "potential population": physicians who are licensed to practice in Massachusetts.

A final comment or two on the list problem is in order. First of all, in any effort to capture a group as large and as mobile as physicians, one expects a certain degree of inherent error. Our research team was able to document some of our own errors. We believe they were at a minimum, but they were not zero. The biggest problem is not the existence of errors, but the attempt to identify the nature and direction of the errors and then to determine whether they affect the variables of interest. Of particular concern is the inability to track the movement of physicians in and out of a particular geographic area.

Without a second study, our own research falls into this same trap. We believe that our estimated population of 1,302 physicians actually known to be practicing to some degree in western Massachusetts is the most accurate estimate as of summer 1989. However, this survey provides a cross-sectional view, and as soon as we have collected the information, the accuracy of our own UMass list is also affected by the simple passage of time. The only way to successfully avoid this problem is to keep track now of these 1,302 physicians, using our survey as a baseline measure. In this way, the movement—both into and out of the state—of this particular group of physicians can be accurately monitored. An additional record-keeping system is needed to identify all new physicians locating in Massachusetts.

Appendix B:
The Final Questionnaire as
Given to Study Respondents

MEDICAL PRACTICE PATTERNS
IN
WESTERN MASSACHUSETTS

A Physician Survey

University of Massachusetts
at Amherst

Paula Stamps, Ph.D.
School of Health Sciences
Division of Public Health
Arnold House
Amherst, MA 01003

Sponsored by the Massachusetts Medical Society.

Supported by the Medical Societies of
Berkshire, Franklin, Hampden, and Hampshire Counties.

SECTION I - These first two questions give us basic information about your medical practice.

Q-1 Please circle all the items below that are appropriate to your situation. For each item, answer it for the immediate 12 month period.

Circle All That Apply

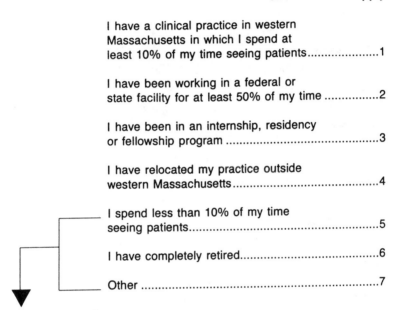

I have a clinical practice in western Massachusetts in which I spend at least 10% of my time seeing patients.....................1

I have been working in a federal or state facility for at least 50% of my time 2

I have been in an internship, residency or fellowship program 3

I have relocated my practice outside western Massachusetts...4

I spend less than 10% of my time seeing patients...5

I have completely retired.......................................6

Other 7

Although you may not currently be involved in an active clinical practice, we need to hear from you. We would appreciate your time in completing all portions of this questionnaire that are relevant to you.

1

Q-2 What is your clinical practice speciality?

	PRIMARY	SECONDARY
	Circle One	Circle One

	PRIMARY	SECONDARY
Allergy and Immunology	1	1
Anesthesiology	2	2
Cardiovascular Disease	3	3
Critical Care Medicine	4	4
Dermatology	5	5
Emergency Medicine	6	6
Family Practice and/or General Practice	7	7
Gastroenterology	8	8
General Surgery	9	9
Gynecology	10	10
Internal Medicine	11	11
Neurology and/or Neurosurgery	12	12
Obstetrics	13	13
Obstetrics and Gynecology	14	14
Oncology	15	15
Ophthalmology	16	16
Orthopedics	17	17
Otolaryngology	18	18
Pathology	19	19
Pediatrics	20	20
Physical Medicine and Rehabilitation	21	21
Psychiatry	22	22
Radiology	23	23
Surgical Specialties	24	24
Urology	25	25
Other	26	26

SECTION II - Questions in this section are intended to gather information about your personal level of satisfaction with your practice.

Q-3 This first set of items includes some of the factors that influence the level of satisfaction with your medical practice. Please respond to each item by circling the response that is closest to your feelings.

REGULATORY FACTORS

		Very Satisfactory	Satisfactory	Not Applicable/Undecided	Unsatisfactory	Very Unsatisfactory
1.	Inpatient reimbursement rates	VS	S	N	U	VU
2.	Utilization reviews	VS	S	N	U	VU
3.	Professional Review Organizations	VS	S	N	U	VU
4.	Tort system of medical malpractice	VS	S	N	U	VU
5.	Mandatory Medicaid participation	VS	S	N	U	VU
6.	Ban on balance billing for Blue Shield	VS	S	N	U	VU
7.	Retroactive medical malpractice premiums	VS	S	N	U	VU
8.	Base medical malpractice premiums	VS	S	N	U	VU

PRACTICE-SPECIFIC FACTORS

9.	Professional interaction with other physicians	VS	S	N	U	VU
10.	Opportunity for regular contact with a medical school	VS	S	N	U	VU
11.	Availability of hospital facilities	VS	S	N	U	VU
12.	Availability of good social welfare, home care, or nursing home services	VS	S	N	U	VU

3

PRACTICE-SPECIFIC FACTORS
(continued)

		Very Satisfactory	Satisfactory	Not Applicable/Undecided	Unsatisfactory	Very Unsatisfactory
13.	Availability of subspecialists for my patients	VS	S	N	U	VU
14.	Income of my practice	VS	S	N	U	VU
15.	My interaction with my patients	VS	S	N	U	VU
16.	High medical need in area	VS	S	N	U	VU
17.	Opportunity to join desirable partnership or group practice	VS	S	N	U	VU

PERSONAL FACTORS

18.	Climate/geographical features	VS	S	N	U	VU
19.	Presence of family and/or friends.	VS	S	N	U	VU
20.	Opportunities for social life	VS	S	N	U	VU
21.	Recreational and sports opportunities	VS	S	N	U	VU
22.	Quality of educational system for children	VS	S	N	U	VU

Q-4 Which three factors from this list have had the greatest impact on your personal practice? Please list the factor numbers.

Factor # _____

Factor # _____

Factor # _____

4

Q-5 This set of items is concerned with how you view your practice. Please circle the response that comes closest to your feelings.

	Strongly Agree	Agree	Undecided	Disagree	Strongly Disagree
1. My current income is satisfactory for the amount of work I do..........	SA	A	UN	D	SD
2. I am generally satisfied with Massachusetts as a place to practice	SA	A	UN	D	SD
3. I am seriously thinking about leaving clinical practice altogether	SA	A	UN	D	SD
4. It is my impression that a lot of physicians are dissatisfied specifically with medical practice in Massachusetts	SA	A	UN	D	SD
5. My professional control over patient treatment decisions has decreased over the last 5 years....	SA	A	UN	D	SD
6. I stay in medicine mainly because I am not sure what else I can do.	SA	A	UN	D	SD
7. It is my impression that a lot of physicians are generally dissatisfied with the practice of medicine today in other parts of the country....................................	SA	A	UN	D	SD
8. I view my practice as being essentially rural.	SA	A	UN	D	SD
9. I don't really think practicing medicine in Massachusetts is any different from practicing medicine anywhere else..............	SA	A	UN	D	SD
10. I wish I had more opportunities to discuss patient care problems with other physicians...................	SA	A	UN	D	SD

5

	Strongly Agree	Agree	Undecided	Disagree	Strongly Disagree
11. I am likely to leave the state of Massachusetts to practice medicine somewhere else	SA	A	UN	D	SD
12. If I had the decision to make all over again, I would still go into medicine.	SA	A	UN	D	SD
13. All things considered I am satisfied with my medical practice	SA	A	UN	D	SD

Q-6 Are you currently practicing at your full professional capacity?

Circle One

Yes...1

No 2

Not applicable 3

If NO, are you:
Satisfied with current level of your practice................................4

Not satisfied with current level of your practice 5

Q-7 Have you ever practiced medicine in any state besides Massachusetts? (including residency experience).

Circle One

No 1

Yes..2

Q-8 Do you personally know any physicians who have moved their medical practice to another state?

Circle One

No 1

Yes..2

If yes, how many? _____

6

SECTION III - **We are particularly interested in whether you have made any changes in your medical practice since 1985. The following series of questions gather information on this. Specific answers may be difficult, since these are recollections over a period of time. Please give us your best estimates.**

Q-9 I have made the following changes in my practice since 1985:

Circle One For Each Item

1. I spend less than 10% of my time seeing patients 1
    I spend 10% or more of my time seeing patients 2

2. The approximate number of patients I see has:
    a. Increased 1
    b. Decreased 2
    c. Stayed about the same 3
    d. Not applicable 4

3. The number of hospital affiliations I have has:
    a. Increased 1
    b. Decreased 2
    c. Stayed about the same 3
    d. Not applicable 4

4. The number of physicians in my practice has:
    a. Increased 1
    b. Decreased 2
    c. Stayed about the same 3
    d. Not applicable 4

5. The number of surgical procedures I do has:
    a. Stopped completely 1
    b. Increased 2
    c. Decreased 3
    d. Stayed about the same 4
    e. Not applicable 5

7

Circle One For Each Item

6. The number of obstetrical patients I see has:
   a. Stopped completely 1
   b. Increased...2
   c. Decreased...3
   d. Stayed about the same....................................4
   e. Not applicable...5

7. My medical malpractice class has:
   a. Increased to a higher risk class.........................1
   b. Decreased to a lower risk class.........................2
   c. Stayed about the same.....................................3
   d. Not applicable...4

8. The limits of coverage of my malpractice policy have:
   a. Increased...1
   b. Decreased 2
   c. Stayed about the same.....................................3
   d. Not applicable...4

9. The proportion of time I spend actually seeing patients has:
   a. Stopped completely 1
   b. Increased...2
   c. Decreased...3
   d. Stayed about the same....................................4
   e. Not applicable...5

10. Other..10

Q-10 What are the major reasons for any of the changes you have indicated here? (Please specify, briefly)

1. _____

2. _____

3. _____

8

SECTION IV - This section gathers information on the characteristics of your practice, including financial aspects and the impact of malpractice premiums. It is important for you to respond to all of these, so that we have complete information on physicians in the western part of the state.

Q-11 How would you classify the primary arrangement of your practice?

Circle One

Solo practice 1	
Dual practice 2	
Group of three or more 3	
Closed panel/staff model HMO 4	
Hospital 5	
Clinic, community, or migrant health center..........................6	
Mental health center 7	
Nursing home or home health agency 8	
School or college 9	
Federal facility providing health care.................................10	
Residential facility for handicapped or disabled 11	
Other...12	

Q-12 The following items pertain to the financial arrangements that characterize your practice. Please circle all that are relevant to you within the last 12 months.

Circle All That Apply

	Always	Partially	Never
I am paid on a fee-for-service basis ....A		S	N
I am paid on a capitation basis...............A		S	N
I am paid on a salary basis....................A		S	N
I have other financial arrangements........A		S	N

9

Q-13 **Below are the most common payer categories of medical care services. Please indicate the categories in which you have at least 25% of your patients. Please circle no more than 4 categories.**

Payer Categories	Circle No More Than Four
Cash	1
Medicare	2
Medicaid	3
Workman's Comp	4
Blue Shield	5
Other commercials	6
Capitated patients	7
Other	8

Q-14 **What is your net annual revenue from your medical practice activities for this past 12 months? (To make this comparable to the AMA Socioeconomic Characteristics Study, please estimate this after all expenses but BEFORE taxes. Be sure to include the value of all fringe benefits that may be paid on your behalf, ie., Keogh Plan.)**

Circle One

less than 40,000	1
41,000 - 60,000	2
61,000 - 80,000	3
81,000 - 100,000	4
101,000 - 120,000	5
121,000 - 140,000	6
141,000 - 160,000	7
over 160,000	8

The following questions are concerned with the impact of malpractice insurance on your practice.

Q-15 What type of policy do you have for this current year?

Circle All That Apply

  a. Occurrence policy (JUA) 1
  b. Claims-made policy (JUA) 2
  c. Non-JUA policy 3
  d. Self-insured...4
  e. Limited practice discount 5
  f. Full-time academic practice 6
  g. Community based discount...7
  h. Not sure..8
  i. None...9
  j. Not applicable..10

Q-16 Has the type of policy changed since 1985?

Circle All That Apply

  a. I have changed from a claims made policy to
     an occurrence policy...1

  b. I have changed from an occurrence policy to
     a claims made policy 2

  c. I am no longer insured through JUA............................3

  d. I have gone from a full practice policy to some
     type of discount policy for a limited practice................4

  e. I have gone from a discount policy for a limited
     practice to a full practice policy 5

  f. I have made no changes 6

  g. I have made other changes 7

Q-17 Who pays for your policy?   **Circle One**

  a. I pay entirely for my own 1
  b. The group practice or HMO for which I work
     pays it entirely 2
  c. The hospital for which I work pays it entirely...............3
  d. I split responsibility for it with the organization
     for which I primarily work..4
  e. Other...5

11

One of the most important parts of this study is our effort to determine how many practicing physicians are generally available to consumers in western Massachusetts. To do this, we need an approximate distribution of your time. We are using the same categories as the AMA Socioeconimic Characteristics of Medical Practice Survey.

Please answer all of the following based on a typical week of practice during the last 12 months. Give us your best estimate to the nearest hour.

Q-18 During a typical week of practice within the last 12 months, about how many hours a week do you spend with:

a. Office-based patients, including
    all offices if your practice involves
    multiple sites.......................................About_____hrs.

b. Surgery patients-time in surgery,
    labor or delivery................................About_____hrs.

c. Hospitalized patients, including
    all hospital rounds ....About_____hrs.

d. Hospital emergency room patients......About_____hrs.

e. Hospital outpatient clinics ....About_____hrs.

f. Patients in nursing or convalescent
    homes, or some other extended
    care facility ....About_____hrs.

g. Telephone conversations with patients
    or their families, consulting with other
    physicians, providing other services to
    patients such as interpreting lab tests and
    X-rays. (Please do not include any other
    time reported in other activities) ....About_____hrs.

h. All other activities related to your professional
    responsibilties including administrative,
    teaching, supervising medical residents,
    medical staff functions, and professional
    reading, writing and research ....About_____hrs.

i. Any other professional activities we
    have left out.......................................About_____hrs.

j. Total number of hours you work in activities
    related to medicine per week..............About_____hrs.

12

SECTION V - A Few Final Items - These last items will help us to complete the profile of physicians in western Massachusetts. Please take one last minute to complete these items.

Q-19 In which county do you have the greatest percentage of your clinical practice?

Circle One

Hampshire 1

Franklin 2

Hampden 3

Berkshire 4

Other, in Massachusetts 5

Other, outside Massachusetts 6

Not currently in clinical practice 7

Q-20 How many years have you been in medical practice in Massachusetts? (Please include the total number of years in active clinical practice, post-training)

Circle One

One year or less 1

1-3 years 2

4-6 years 3

7-10 years 4

11-15 years 5

16-20 years 6

21-25 years 7

26-30 years 8

over 30 years 9

Not applicable 10

13

Q-21 Specify the range which best depicts your age.

Circle One

Less than 30 years old..1
30-44 years old 2
45-54 years old 3
55-64 years old 4
65-74 years old 5
75 and over...6

Q-22 Are you a male or female   Circle One

Male 1
Female 2

Q-23 Are you a member of any of the following?

Circle All That Apply

American Medical Association..1
Massachusetts Medical Society...2
A county medical society 3
A specialty society 4

Q-24 What are two things that you like the most about practicing medicine in the state of Massachusetts?

1. _____

2. _____

Q-25 What are the two things that you like the least about practicing medicine in the state of Massachusetts?

1. _____

2. _____

(Please turn to back page to finish)

14

FINAL NOTE

I would like to thank you for taking the time to respond to this questionnaire. If you have any additional thoughts on this topic, please use this space to note them.

Circle All That Apply

I would prefer that you call me so I can add some comments..1

Telephone Number _____

Best time to call   _____

I would like to see a summary of the results 2

Additional comments below...3

Your response to this survey is very greatly appreciated. If you have any additonal comments, concerns or questions, please call me:

Dr. Paula L. Stamps, Division of Public Health, School of Health Sciences, University of Massachusetts, Amherst, Massachusetts 01002 (413) 545-1313

Appendix C:
Specialty Nomenclature Related
to Physician Supply Estimates

The purpose of this appendix is to demonstrate one of the important methodological problems related to research in the area of physician supply, the nomencature associated with specialty classification. There are several problems related to nomenclature. First is the titles of specialties themselves. One may use board-certification language or more functional titles. For example, we designated a possible 26 different specialties (Q-2, Appendix B), which relies on the more functional titles used by the Massachusetts Board of Registration rather than the formal board-certification titles. A second problem is that physicians may have more than one specialty designation. As can be seen from Q-2, we asked for primary and secondary specialties. However, a physician's actual practice may or may not correspond to his or her specialty certification. The final problem is in making larger categorizations of specialties in order to do analyses, since sample sizes of some specialties may be quite small.

This appendix will focus on this last problem, of combining specialties to create larger categories for analysis purposes. Because of the interest in physician supply in Massachusetts, several studies were available characterizing physician availability. This appendix will compare two specialty categorization techniques, one utilized by the AMA and the other utilized by a Massachusetts-based health research group, which used a more functional categorization method.

Table C.1 shows the frequency distribution in terms of the 26 specialty choices given to the study respondents. As can be seen from this table, the single largest group is internal medicine, which represents almost 16 percent of the active population; family/general practice and pediatrics are the next two largest groups. These three primary care specialties constitute 36 percent of all those responding to this item. There are no significant differences between patient care physicians and the other respondents.

An obvious question that arises from this table is, For a primarily rural/suburban population of 800,000, is it appropriate to have 1,302 patient care physicians, 36 percent of whom are in one of the primary care specialties? How does this compare to other regions of the country? In order to address these questions, we looked at possible comparison studies, both within Massachusetts and at other larger national and regional studies, and were immediately confronted with the problem of variation in creating larger categories of specialties, especially in terms of addressing primary care specialties. Two methods of specialty categorization will be applied to our data to demonstrate. The first method is that used by the AMA; this method regards internal medicine as a medical specialty. The second categorization method is a more functional analysis, in which internal medicine is treated as a primary care specialty. This grouping was utilized by a Massachusetts-based consulting company (Health Data Consortium) for a 1988 study on human resources issues in the state.

As Table C.2 shows, the most important difference in these two methods of categorization concern the primary care specialties. The Health Data Consortium places gynecology, internal medicine, and pediatrics into the primary care category along with family/general practice. The AMA categorizes internal medicine and pediatrics in "medical specialties" and gynecology in "surgical specialties." Table C.3 demonstrates the importance of these different methods of categorization. A common way to summarize physician supply is to describe the percentage of physicians involved in primary care. Using the AMA categorization leads to a much different profile of physicians in the western Massachusetts area.

The Health Data Consortium categories yield what is probably a more accurate functional representation—slightly over one-third of physicians in western Massachusetts are primary care physicians. Estimates for surgical specialties and for that broad category entitled "other" are not so different between these two approaches. The problem lies mainly in the term "primary care" and differentiating it successfully from "medical specialties."

In general, throughout this book we have arranged specialty designations to be similar to those used by the AMA in order to facilitate comparisons to this national data set. We encountered some differences, but they are small since they involve specialties with few physicians. For example, the AMA breaks pediatrics into three groups (pediatrics,

Table C.1 Frequency Distribution of Respondents by Specialty Designation

| | "Active" Respondents | | | | All Respondents | | | |
| | 1st Specialty | | 2nd Specialty | | 1st Specialty | | 2nd Specialty | |
	n	%	n	%	n	%	n	%
1. Allergy and Immunology	4	0.5	9	3.8	5	0.6	9	3.3
2. Anesthesiology	33	4.2	—	—	41	4.6	—	—
3. Cardiovascular Disease	17	2.2	9	3.8	19	2.1	10	3.7
4. Critical Care Medicine	3	0.4	7	3.0	3	0.3	8	2.9
5. Dermatology	11	1.4	—	—	12	1.3	—	—
6. Emergency Medicine	43	5.5	8	3.4	44	4.9	11	4.0
7. Family Practice and/or General Practice	83	10.6	18	7.6	94	10.6	22	8.1
8. Gastroenterology	11	1.4	4	1.7	11	1.2	4	1.5
9. General Surgery	44	5.6	8	3.4	52	5.8	9	3.3
10. Gynecology	7	0.9	3	1.3	7	0.8	4	1.5
11. Internal Medicine	125	15.9	56	23.7	149	16.7	60	22.0
12. Neurology and/or Neurosurgery	14	1.8	2	0.8	14	1.6	2	0.7
13. Obstetrics	1	0.1	—	—	1	0.1	—	—
14. Obstetrics/Gynecology	41	5.2	4	1.7	44	4.9	4	1.5
15. Oncology	12	1.5	6	2.5	13	1.5	6	2.2
16. Ophthalmology	27	3.4	1	0.4	28	3.1	1	0.4
17. Orthopedics	37	4.7	5	2.1	41	4.6	5	1.8
18. Otolaryngology	9	1.1	2	0.8	11	1.2	3	1.1
19. Pathology	15	1.9	3	1.3	27	3.0	4	1.5
20. Pediatrics	74	9.4	13	5.5	78	8.8	15	5.5
21. Physical Medicine and Rehabilitation	4	0.5	2	0.8	5	0.6	3	1.1
22. Psychiatry	59	7.5	6	2.5	67	7.5	6	2.2
23. Radiology	41	5.2	4	1.7	45	5.1	5	1.8
24. Surgical Specialties	23	2.9	13	5.5	26	2.9	15	5.5
25. Urology	16	2.0	—	—	16	1.8	67	24.5
26. Other	30	3.8	53	22.5	37	4.2	—	—
Totals	784		236		890		273	

Table C.2 Comparison of Specialty Designation Categories

American Medical Association Categories	*Health Data Consortium Categories*

1. General and Family Practice
2. Medical Specialties
   Allergy
   Cardiovascular Disease
   Dermatology
   Gastroenterology
   Internal Medicine
   Pediatric Allergy
   Pediatric Cardiology
   Pediatrics
   Pulmonary Disease
 	
3. Surgical Specialties
   General Surgery
   Neurological Surgery
   Obstetrics/Gynecology
   Ophthalmology
   Orthopedic Surgery
   Otorhinolaryngology
   Plastic Surgery
   Colon and Rectal Surgery
   Thoracic Surgery
   Urology
 	
4. Other Specialties
   Aerospace Medicine
   Anesthesiology
   Child Psychiatry
   Neurology
   Occupational Medicine
   Pathology
   Physical Medicine and Rehabilitation
   Psychiatry
   Public Health
   Radiology
   Other
      Critical care medicine
      Oncology
      Emergency medicine
      Unspecified
	1. Primary Care
	   Family/General Practice
	   Gynecology
	   Internal Medicine
	   Pediatrics
	
	2. Medical Specialties
	   Allergy/Immunology
	   Cardiovascular Medicine
	   Dermatology
	   Endocrinology
	   Gastroenterology
	   Hematology
	   Nephrology
	   Oncology
	   Pulmonary Medicine
	   Other
	
	3. Surgical Specialties
	   Obstetrics
	   Ophthalmology
	   Otorhinolaryngology
	   Surgery, Cardiothoracic
	   Surgery, Colon and Rectal
	   Surgery, General
	   Surgery, Neurology
	   Surgery, Orthopedic
	   Surgery, Pediatric
	   Surgery, Plastic
	   Surgery, Vascular
	   Surgery, Other
	   Urology
	
	4. Other Specialties
	   Anesthesiology
	   Emergency Medicine
	   Geriatrics
	   Neonatology
	   Neurology
	   Nuclear Medicine
	   Pathology
	   Psychiatry, Child
	   Radiology, Diagnostic
	   Radiology, Therapeutic
	   Other
	   Physical Medicine and Rehabilitation
	   Psychiatry

Table C.3 Frequency Distribution of Massachusetts Patient Care Physicians in Two Groups of Specialty Categories (All Respondents)

American Medical Association Categories			Health Data Consortium Categories		
	n	%		*n*	%
1. General/Family Practice	83	10.6	1. Primary Care	289	36.9
2. Medical Specialties	242	30.9	2. Medical Specialties	58	7.4
3. Surgical Specialties	219	27.9	3. Surgical Specialties	212	26.9
4. Other	240	30.6	4. Other	225	28.8
Total	784	100.0	Total	784	100.0

pediatric cardiology, and pediatric allergy) while we capture all of these with only one category of pediatrics. The AMA generally uses three specific surgical specialties (plastic surgery, colon and rectal surgery, and thoracic surgery), which we attempted to capture by "surgical specialties." There were five specialty categories we did not use that the AMA utilizes: pulmonary disease (a medical specialty) and aerospace medicine, child psychiatry, occupational medicine, and public health (all under other specialties). We have three specialties they do not have—critical care medicine, emergency medicine, and oncology—which we placed under "other." We very carefully separated into three categories gynecology, obstetrics, and gynecology/obstetrics. The AMA puts them together into one category and includes it under "surgical specialties." Finally, we put into one category neurology and/or neurosurgery, which we placed into "surgical specialties." The AMA has more appropriately separated these two and places one under "surgical specialties" and the other under "other specialties."

Although this specific nomenclature is comparable to AMA information, issues of adequacy of supply involve combining specialty categories and thus the problem of the primary care designation arises. We want to demonstrate the differences that can arise by using our data with AMA categories, the Health Data Consortium categories, and GMENAC categories. Before this comparison can be made, we must adjust our respondents to represent the whole population of western Massachusetts.

The most common way to present these data involves enumerating total number of physicians in a geographic area and presenting that as a ratio to the population. In our case, we have an accurate estimate of the true population (1,302), and we also have complete information on

70 percent of the population. Table C.4 shows the distribution of the 26 specialties among the 88 percent of our respondents who indicated they see patients for at least 10 percent of their time. The distribution of specialties is assumed to be the same among the nonrespondents, and this table shows this frequency adjusted to the population of western Massachusetts, for a total of 1,132 patient care physicians, each of whom spends at least 10 percent of their time seeing patients.

Table C.4   Frequency Distribution of Respondents Adjusted to Whole Population

	Frequency of Active Respondents*	Frequency Adjusted to Whole Population
1. Allergy and Immunology	4	6
2. Anesthesiology	33	48
3. Cardiovascular Disease	17	24
4. Critical Care Medicine	3	4
5. Dermatology	11	16
6. Emergency Medicine	43	62
7. Family Practice and/or General Practice	83	120
8. Gastroenterology	11	16
9. General Surgery	44	64
10. Gynecology	7	10
11. Internal Medicine	125	181
12. Neurology and/or Neurosurgery	14	20
13. Obstetrics	1	1
14. Obstetrics/Gynecology	41	59
15. Oncology	12	17
16. Ophthalmology	27	39
17. Orthopedics	37	53
18. Otolaryngology	9	13
19. Pathology	15	22
20. Pediatrics	74	107
21. Physical Medicine and Rehabilitation	4	6
22. Psychiatry	59	86
23. Radiology	41	59
24. Surgical Specialties	23	33
25. Urology	16	23
26. Other	30	43
Total	784	1132

*1.45 × frequency = adjusted frequency based on 70 percent response rate

Comparison with GMENAC

As can be seen from Table C.5 some specialties seem to be underrepresented in western Massachusetts when we compare our estimates to those of GMENAC. Adult primary care and internal medicine are both markedly underrepresented, even eight years after the estimates were developed. GMENAC suggests that there should be 63/100,000 for each of these, while the numbers based on our population estimates for these two are 37.6/100,000 and 22.6/100,000, respectively. Children's primary care and obstetricians and gynecologists are not far off the GMENAC estimates of what is needed, although it must be noted that the predicted supply for OB/GYN involves family practitioners doing one-third of the deliveries, a factor not included in our data.

In terms of the other specialties, some are very close to the GMENAC estimates of what is needed, including allergy, cardiovascular disease, gastroenterology, neurology, ophthalmology, orthopedics, urology, and radiology. We should note two definitional problems here: neurology in our study includes neurosurgery but these are separate in GMENAC; also our study includes immunology with allergy, while GMENAC includes only allergy.

For only one specialty does there seem to be a higher representation in western Massachusetts: emergency medicine. It should be noted that the GMENAC predictions for emergency medicine are based on visits as well as population while ours is only based on population.

Six other non–primary care specialties may be identified as underrepresented based on the GMENAC report: hematology/oncology, general surgery, otolaryngology, psychiatry, anesthesiology, and pathology. Of these, it should be noted that in our study hematology is not specifically designated to be included with oncology. It is unknown whether hematologists in our study would put themselves into the oncology category or into the "other specialty" category.

Table C.6 shows a slightly different way of looking at the comparison of the western Massachusetts estimate of supply with the GMENAC's projection of what is needed for this same geographic area. The single specialty with the lowest percentage of GMENAC recommendations is otolaryngology (at 47 percent of GMENAC), while emergency medicine is 135 percent of what GMENAC recommends.

Comparison with AMA 1985 Data

AMA Physician Characteristics and Distribution, 1986 edition, gives several overall figures to estimate current physician supply. It gives a nationwide

Table C.5 Physician Supply in Western Massachusetts versus
GMENAC-Recommended Figures

Specialty Categories	Our Figures Adjusted to Population (Actual Numbers)	Our Physician/ Population (Physicians per 100,000)	1980 GMENAC Figures (Physicians per 100,000)
1. Basic Adult Primary Care (includes family and general practice, internal medicine)	301	37.6	63
2. Children's Primary Care (includes 75% pediatricans; 25% family practitioners)	110	13.7	12.4
3. Internal Medicine	181	22.63	63
4. Obstetrics/Gynecology (assumes 1/3 deliveries by family practitioners)	70	8.75	10
5. *Specialties*			
Allergy	6.0	.75	0.8
Cardiovascular	24	3.0	3.3
Dermatology	16	2.0	3.0
Endocrinology	—	—	0.8
Gastroenterology	16	2.0	2.8
Hematology/Oncology	17 (oncology only)	2.13	3.8
Infectious Diseases	—	—	0.9
Nephrology	—	—	1.1
Pulmonary	—	—	1.6
Rheumatology	—	—	0.7
General Surgery	64	8.0	10.1
Neurology	20	2.5	2.4
Ophthalmology	39	4.8	5.0
Orthopedics	53	6.6	6.4
Otorhinolaryngology	13	1.6	3.4
Plastic Surgery	—	—	1.1
Thoracic Surgery	—	—	0.8
Urology	23	2.8	3.3
Psychiatry	86	10.7	16.4
Preventive Medicine	—	—	3.1
Child Psychiatry	—	—	3.8
Emergency	62	7.7	5.7
Anesthesiology	48	6.0	8.9
Pathology	22	2.7	5.7
Radiology	59	7.4	7.7
Nuclear Medicine	—	—	1.7

Table C.6 Physician Supply in Western Massachusetts: Actual Versus GMENAC Recommended for Selected Specialties (Physician/100,000 Population Ratios)

Specialty	Actual Supply	GMENAC Recommended	Percent of GMENAC Recommended
Primary Care			
Family/General Practice			
Internal Medicine			
Pediatrics	51.0	75.4	68
Obstetrics/Gynecology	8.7	10.0	87
Medical Specialties			
Allergy and Immunology	0.8	0.8	100
Cardiovascular Medicine	3.0	3.3	91
Dermatology	2.0	3.0	67
Gastroenterology	2.0	2.8	71
Surgical Specialties			
General Surgery	8.0	10.1	79
Ophthalmology	4.9	5.0	98
Orthopedic Surgery	6.6	6.4	103
Otolaryngology	1.6	3.4	47
Urology	2.9	3.3	88
Other Specialties			
Anesthesiology	6.0	8.9	67
Emergency Medicine	7.7	5.7	135
Pathology	2.7	5.7	47
Psychiatry	10.7	16.4	65
Radiology	7.4	7.7	96

Source: Prepared by the Massachusetts Medical Society based on our data.

ratio of 228/100,000 for all physicians, a ratio of 211/100,000 for what it calls "active" physicians, and a ratio of 205/100,000 for what it defines as "professionally active." Based on these AMA figures, Massachusetts as a state has a total physician/100,000 population ratio of 338.2, a ratio of active physicians of 314.7, and a ratio of physicians who identify their major professional activity as patient care of 263.3. (This approximate figure of 264 was also used in the Health Data Consortium report, which will be described next). This gives Massachusetts the highest physician/population ratio in the whole nation, and is used to support the notion that there is a surplus of physicians in Massachusetts. This may be true for the entire state of Massachusetts, but as Table C.7 shows, the physician surplus is clearly not present in the western part of the state.

Table C.7   Comparison of Our Figures to AMA, 1985

	Our Adjusted-to-Population Frequency Distribution	Our Physician-Population Ratio	AMA Physician-Population Ratio, 1985
General and Family Practice	120	15.0	27.6
Medical Specialties	350	43.7	65.7
Allergy	6	0.7	0.6
Cardiovascular Disease	2.4	3.0	5.4
Dermatology	15	2.0	2.7
Gastroenterology	16	2.0	2.4
Internal Medicine	181	22.6	37.2
Pediatric Allergy ⎤			0.2
Pediatric Cardiology ⎬	107	13.4	0.3
Pediatrics ⎦			14.7
Pulmonary Diseases	—	—	2.1
Surgical Specialties	295	36.8	52.8
General Surgery	64	8.0	15.7
Neurological Surgery	—	—	1.7
Obstetrics/Gynecology	70	8.75	12.7
Ophthalmology	39	4.0	7.1
Orthopedic Surgery	53	6.6	7.1
Otorhinolaryngology	13	1.6	3.0
Plastic Surgery	—	—	1.6
Colon and Rectal Surgery ⎤	33	4.0	0.3
Thoracic Surgery ⎦			0.9
Urology	12	2.8	3.6
Other Specialties	23	2.8	58.6
Aerospace Medicine	—	—	0.3
Anesthesiology	48	6.0	9.1
Child Psychiatry	—	—	1.6
Neurology	20	2.5	3.2
Occupational Medicine	—	—	1.1
Pathology	22	2.7	6.5
Physical Medicine and Rehabilitation	6	0.7	1.3
Psychiatry			13.3
Public Health	—	—	1.2
Radiology	59	7.3	10.4
Other and Unspecified	43	5.4	10.7

When the western Massachusetts physician supply is compared to the AMA national estimates (using our adjusted-to-population figures), for only three specialties is western Massachusetts even close to the AMA-based national figure: allergy, dermatology, and gastroenterology. For four others, western Massachusetts has a slightly lower supply as given by these physician/population ratios: orthopedics, urology, neurology, and physical medicine and rehabilitation. For all other specialties noted in Table C.7, the physician supply in western Massachusetts is far under these national figures of the AMA.

Three technical points should be noted here: the first is to recognize that specialty categorization is still somewhat of a problem here. What the AMA categorizes as two categories—neurology and neurosurgery—we counted as one, so caution is in order for any conclusions related to that particular specialty. Also, we have only one category for pediatrics, while the AMA has three—pediatrics, pediatric allergy, and pediatric cardiology. When those are all added together, the physician/100,000 population ratio is close to 15.0, while ours is 13.4.

Second, in 1985, the AMA revised its categories somewhat to include several subspecialties under general surgery, internal medicine, and pediatrics. The effect of this revision was to increase each of these categories as of 1985. For internal medicine, the effect was particularly large.

Finally, this table does not necessarily mean that the entire state of Massachusetts is represented by these figures. This study has only evaluated the western part of the state, which is decidedly more rural than eastern Massachusetts.

Comparison with Health Data Consortium

Table C.8 compares our adjusted-to-population ratios with the ratios given by the Health Data Consortium study to represent the current physician supply for the whole state of Massachusetts. This table shows many of the same type of results as the AMA table, but also some very interesting differences. The specialties that seem to be particularly underrepresented in western Massachusetts based on these comparisons are the following: gynecology, internal medicine, pediatrics, obstetrics, ophthalmology, general surgery, orthopedic surgery, anesthesiology, neurology, pathology, psychiatry, and radiology. Three specialty categories are slightly lower in western Massachusetts: cardiovascular medicine, dermatology, and urology. Five specialties are roughly the same: allergy, gastroenterology, oncology, otolaryngology, and physical medicine and rehabilitation. As with the AMA study, there seem to be more physicians in emergency medicine than one would expect, based on these figures. According to the Health Data Consortium figures, family and general practitioners are also in higher supply than one would expect in western Massachusetts. This result is almost certainly due to the way the Health Data Consortium categorized specialties: their "primary care" designation includes internal medicine and pediatrics, as well as family and general practice.

Table C.8   Comparisons of Health Data Consortium Estimates with Our Estimates

	Health Data Consortium		Our Estimates	
	1988 Estimates Mass.	Physicians/ 100,000 Population	Physicians (W. Mass.)	Physicians/ 100,000 Population (W. Mass.)
Primary Care Total	5,423	—	(418)	(51.2)
Family/General Practice	791	13.6	120	15.0
Gynecology	217	8.6	10	1.25
Internal Medicine	3,285	56.3	181	22.63
Pediatrics	1,130	73.5	107	13.4
Medical Specialties Total	1,042	—	(79)	(9.9)
Allergy/Immunology	55	0.9	6	0.75
Cardiovascular Medicine	268	4.6	24	3.0
Dermatology	183	3.1	16	2.0
Endocrinology	72	1.2	—	—
Gastroenterology	99	1.7	16	2.0
Hematology	95	1.6	—	—
Nephrology	71	1.2	—	—
Oncology	101	1.7	17	2.13
Pulmonary Medicine	98	1.7	—	—
Other	—	—	—	—
Surgical Specialties Totals	2,847	—	(285)	(35.6)
Obstetrics	467	32.1	60	7.5
Ophthalmology	417	7.1	39	4.9
Otorhinolaryngology	160	2.7	13	1.6
Surgery, Cardiothoracic	25	0.4		
Surgery, Colon and Rectal	9	0.2		
Surgery, General	593	10.2	64	8.0
Surgery, Neurology	59	1.0		
Surgery, Orthopedic	491	8.4	53	6.6
Surgery, Pediatric	24	1.6		
Surgery, Plastic and Reconstructive	103	1.8	33 (all other surgical specialties)	4.1
Surgery, Vascular	83	1.4		
Surgery, Other	214	3.7		
Urology	202	3.5	23	2.9
Other Specialties Total	4,488	—	(303)	(37.9)
Anesthesiology	711	12.2	48	6.0
Emergency Medicine	307	5.3	62	7.7
Geriatrics	19	2.4	—	—
Neonatology	20	24.3	—	—
Neurology	314	5.4	20	2.5
Nuclear Medicine	45	0.8	—	—
Pathology	391	6.7	22	2.7

Continued

Table C.8   Continued

	Health Data Consortium		Our Estimates	
	1988 Estimates Mass.	Physicians/ 100,000 Population	Physicians (W. Mass.)	Physicians/ 100,000 Population (W. Mass.)
Physical Medicine and Rehabilitation	64	1.1	6	0.75
Psychiatry	1,657	28.4	86	10.7
Psychiatry, Child	76	4.9	—	—
Radiology, Diagnostic	621	10.6 ⎫	59	7.84
Radiology, Therapeutic	43	0.7 ⎭		
Other	220	3.8	—	—

There are many more differences between our categories and those used by the Health Data Consortium than with the AMA study. First, gynecology is placed by Health Data Consortium into primary care, and obstetrics into the surgical specialties category. Although we gathered data on gynecology, obstetrics, and gynecology/obstetrics all separately, whether they should be placed in primary care, medical, or surgical is very problematic. The AMA has only one category and puts OB/GYN into medical specialties. Neurology is also a problem here again, primarily because of how we categorized it, in combination with neurosurgery. Perhaps the most problematic is the surgical specialties category—both we and Health Data Consortium have a separate category for general surgery and orthopedic surgery, but we have no further categories while Health Data Consortium has several. Our total for all the surgical specialties is 4.1/100,000 while theirs is 20.7/100,000.

They did not include a physician/population ratio for the total of each category, we have shown this on Table C.8 but we must be very cautious in this interpretation since the specialties that make up the categories are very different.

Tables C.9 and C.10 provide a summary of the comparisons that have been presented here. First of all, it should be noted that on Table C.9, the estimates for only one specialty group indicate a higher number practicing in western Massachusetts than indicated by the other two studies, and higher than indicated as needed by GMENAC: emergency medicine. This interesting finding deserves a closer analysis of practice patterns of emergency physicians. It has been well documented in the literature that this specialty is often a substitute for both adult and pediatric primary care. Also, this particular specialty has seen enormous changes in the medical technology supporting its patient care activities and in the very definition of the specialty itself. Our failure to include the variable of board certification may be particularly important here.

Table C.9   Comparison of Specialty Supply Ratios of Physicians/100,000 Population

	Health Data Consortium (Massachusetts)	AMA (Nation)	GMENAC (Nation)	Our Figures (Western Massachusetts)
Family and General Practice	13.6	27.6	23.2*	15.0
Internal Medicine	56.3	37.2	22.6*	22.6
Pediatrics*	73.5	15.2	9.5*	13.4
Allergy and Immunology	0.9	0.6	0.8	0.75
Cardiovascular Medicine	4.6	5.4	3.3	3.0
Dermatology	3.1	2.7	3.0	2.0
Gastroenterology	1.7	2.4	2.8	2.0
Oncology	1.7	*	3.8*	2.1
Obstetrics/Gynecology*	*	12.7	10	8.75
Ophthalmology	7.1	6.1	5.0	4.9
Otorhinolaryngology	2.7	3.0	3.4	1.6
General Surgery	10.2	15.7	10.1	8.0
Orthopedic Surgery	8.4	7.1	6.4	6.6
Urology	3.5	3.6	3.3	2.9
Anesthesiology	12.2	9.1	8.9	6.0
Emergency Medicine	5.3	—	5.7	7.7
Neurology and/or Neurosurgery*	5.4	4.5*	1.3*	2.5
Pathology	6.7	6.5	5.7	2.7
Physical Medicine and Rehabilitation	1.1	1.3	*	0.75
Psychiatry	28.4	13.3	16.4	10.7
Radiology*	11.3	10.4	7.7	7.4
Other	3.8	10.7	*	5.4
Medical Specialties (totals)	*	65.7	—	43.7
Surgical Specialties (totals)	*	52.8	—	36.8
Other (totals)	*	58.6	—	35.5
Basic Adult Primary Care	—	—	63	37.6
Children's Primary Care	—	—	12.4	13.7

*Coding problems: If a number has an asterisk, it should be compared with caution. An asterisk indicates either a difference in a particular specialty designation or noncomparability of specialty categories (i.e., combinations of particular specialty designations). In some cases, the study did not calculate the ratio at all; these are designated by dashes.

Table C.10   Comparison of Supply by Specialty

Health Data Consortium		*American Medical Association*	
*Higher**	Family/General Practice Emergency Medicine	*Higher*	Emergency Medicine
About the Same	Allergy Gastroenterology Oncology Otolaryngology Physical Medicine and Rehabilitation	*About the Same*	Children's Primary Care Obstetrics/Gynecology Allergy Cardiovascular Disease Gastroenterology Neurology Ophthalmology Orthopedics Urology Radiology
Slightly Lower	Cardiovascular Disease Dermatology Urology	*Slightly Lower*	Oncology General Surgery Otorhinolaryngology Anesthesiology Pathology
Very Much Lower	Gynecology Obstetrics Internal Medicine General Surgery Pediatrics Orthopedic Surgery Ophthalmology Anesthesiology Neurology Pathology Psychiatry Radiology	*Very Much Lower*	Adult Primary Care Internal Medicine Psychiatry

*The rankings (higher, about the same, etc.) compare the results of our study to Health Data Consortium and the AMA. For example, our study has identified relatively more Family and General Practice and Emergency physicians than the Health Data Consortium identified.

For several specialties, our estimate of physician supply in western Massachusetts is very close to that estimated by the Health Data Consortium for the whole state and the AMA for the nation. Those specialties include allergy and immunology, dermatology, gastroenterology, oncology, otolaryngology, orthopedic surgery, urology, and physical medicine and rehabilitation.

There are some particular specialties in which our estimates are markedly lower than other estimates and also markedly lower than what GMENAC suggests are needed: internal medicine, general and family practice (captured by GMENAC as adult primary care), psychiatry, pathology, general surgery, obstetrics/gynecology, anesthesiology, and radiology.

Even after comparing our numbers to AMA figures, GMENAC figures, and another state-based study, it is hard to draw more specific conclusions than those that are represented in Tables C.9 and C.10. Western Massachusetts does not seem to have "too many" doctors on the whole, although there is some indication that there may be a higher representation of emergency medicine than is optimal. Two specialties are

Table C.11   Estimates of Numbers of Physicians Required per 100,000 Population Compared to Numbers Identified in Western Massachusetts, by Specialty

	Range of Estimates		Patient Care Physicians Available in Western Massachusetts
	Low	High	
Primary Care			
General/Family Practice	11.5	55.0	15.0
Internal Medicine	5.0	96.0	22.6
Pediatrics	4.0	37.0	13.4
Medical Specialties			
Allergy	2.0	4.0	0.75
Cardiology	1.0	6.0	3.0
Dermatology	2.0	6.0	2.0
Surgical Specialties			
General Surgery	8.0	15.2	8.0
Ophthalmology	0.5	5.8	4.9
Orthopedic Surgery	1.0	6.3	6.6
Otolaryngology	1.0	23.0	1.6
Urology	1.0	5.0	2.9
Other Specialties			
Anesthesiology	2.0	12.0	6.0
Pathology	1.0	6.9	2.7
Psychiatry	2.0	54.5	10.7
Radiology	3.0	13.0	7.4

Source: Range of Estimates from GMENAC, Vol. III, Geographic Distribution Technical Panel, p. 65. All numbers are estimates of the number of physicians/100,000 population that are needed or required.

clearly lower than would be expected—internal medicine and psychiatry. Other than these observations, it is difficult to characterize either the number or the adequacy of physician supply.

This finding is not new or unexpected; after all, we have been confronted with the problem of enumerating physicians for a long time, and the resultant variability of the several estimates. Table C.11 shows a summary of some 200 studies reviewed by GMENAC as background to their calculations, as well as a comparison with the patient care physicians currently available in western Massachusetts. Two immediate impressions are drawn from this table: The first is the extreme variability across the 200 studies used by GMENAC. The second is the relative inconsistency in comparing the available physicians in western Massachusetts. Allergy is an example of a specialty that was noted in Table C.10 as being about the same using both the Massachusetts study and AMA data. Yet, as can be seen on Table C.11, the supply of allergists in western Massachusetts is far lower than even the low range of estimates. The variation noted in Table C.11, and the variation in characterizing the physician supply in western Massachusetts, supports the use of the more specific physician/population ratio (the DCE physician estimate) and also supports the suggestions made about standardizing specialty nomenclature and categorization. Both may be found in Chapter 3.

Appendix D:
Additional Data Tables

Table D.1 Practice Arrangement by Specialty Group

	Solo Practice		Group of Three or More		Hospital		HMO		Totals Across	
	n	%	n	%	n	%	n	%	n	%
Radiology	—	—	32	78.1	6	14.6	3	7.3	41	100
Surgical										
General	22	57.9	12	31.6	4	10.5	—	—	38	100
Others	47	43.5	55	50.9	5	4.6	1	.9	108	100
Anesthesiology	4	12.5	25	78.1	3	9.4	—	—	32	100
OB/GYN	15	38.4	14	35.9	4	10.3	6	15.4	39	100
Pathology	1	9.1	7	63.6	3	27.3	—	—	11	100
Psychiatry	30	62.5	—	—	15	31.3	3	6.3	48	100
Internal Medicine	27	26.7	47	46.5	8	7.9	19	18.8	101	100
Pediatrics	17	27.4	17	27.4	10	16.1	18	29.0	62	100
General/Family	31	54.4	11	19.3	—	—	15	26.3	57	100
Total	194		220		58		65		537	

Table D.2 Mean and Median Income by Method of Payment

Method of Payment	Always				Partially				Never			
	n	*%*	*Median Income*	*Mean Income*	*n*	*%*	*Median Income*	*Mean Income*	*n*	*%*	*Median Income*	*Mean Income*
Salary	221	44.5	92,780	87,270	112	20.9	107,650	98,670	117	39.4	112,780	103,850
Capitation	4	0.8	90,500	90,500	175	32.6	105,440	97,150	134	45.1	105,370	98,100
Fee-for-Service	271	54.6	121,880	106,510	249	46.5	105,370	97,720	46	15.5	90,500	79,620

Table D.3 Correlations of Financial Arrangements with Income for All Patient Care Physicians

Financial Arrangement That Characterizes Practice	*Pearson Correlation Coefficient†*
Fee-for-Service	−.16*
Capitation	.02
Salary	.18*

* $p \le .001$.
** $p \le .01$.
*** $p \le .05$.
**** $p \le .10$.
†A positive coefficient indicates that income *decreases* as a financial arrangement is used more. A negative coefficient indicates that income *increases* as a financial arrangement is used more.

Table D.4 Income by Payer Category Representing at Least 25 Percent of Patients for Patient Care Physicians

Income Categories	Distribution of All Patient Care Physician Responses		Medicare		Blue Shield		Other Commercials		Medicaid		Capitated		Cash		Workers' Comp		Other	
	n	%	n	%	n	%	n	%	n	%	n	%	n	%	n	%	n	%
Less than 60,000	103	13.9	59	12.1	76	16.2	52	12.4	50	16.7	32	17.2	31	18.7	8	12.7	17	14.2
61,000–100,000	244	32.9	143	29.4	139	29.7	116	27.6	102	34.1	74	39.8	62	37.4	16	25.4	46	38.3
101,000–140,000	210	28.4	144	29.7	136	29.1	119	28.3	87	29.1	49	26.3	40	24.1	14	22.2	41	34.2
141,000–160,000	184	24.8	140	28.8	117	25.0	133	31.7	60	20.1	31	16.7	33	19.8	25	39.7	16	13.3
Total	741	100.0	486	100.0	468	100.0	420	100.0	299	100.0	186	100.0	166	100.0	63	100.0	120	100.0

Table D.5 Relationship of Hours Worked per Week to Perceptions of Being at Full Capacity, by Gender

1. Are you practicing at your full professional capacity?

	At Full Capacity			Not at Full Capacity		
	n	*%*	*Average Hours/Week*	*n*	*%*	*Average Hours/Week*
Males	535	81.3	59.2	123	18.7	54.3
Females	62	60.8	59.3	40	39.2	43.2

2. If *not* at full capacity, are you satisfied?

	Satisfied			Not Satisfied		
	n	*%*	*Average Hours/Week*	*n*	*%*	*Average Hours/Week*
Males	60	45.4	51.7	72	54.6	56.8
Females	33	76.7	42.4	10	22.3	53.3

3. Practice Arrangements: At Full Professional Capacity

	Males			Females			
	n	*%**	*Average Hours/Week*	*n*	*%**	*Average Hours/Week*	*Productivity Difference (%)*
Group of three or more	198	84.6	61.2	13	65	67.7	+10
Hospital	81	88.0	55.4	12	66.7	55.2	0
Solo Practice	141	71.6	60.2	10	52.6	68.1	+12
HMO	44	89.8	56.7	14	60.9	57.5	−0.1

$\chi^2 = 19.8; p < .001$

4. Specialty: At Full Professional Capacity

	Males			Females			
	n	*%**	*Average Hours/Week*	*n*	*%**	*Average Hours/Week*	*Productivity Difference (%)*
General/Family Practice	50	73.5	58.6	8	61.5	54.4	−7
Internal Medicine	88	86.3	62.7	9	45.0	56.0	−11
Pediatrics	45	88.2	60.2	12	54.6	57.1	−5

Continued

Table D.5 Continued

OB/GYN	24 72.7	67.7	11 91.7	66.7	−1
Psychiatry	41 85.4	49.0	3 37.5	56.0	+13
All Others	268 81.2	58.7	14 73.7	58.6	0

$\chi^2 = 35.2; p < .0001$

5. Income: At Full Professional Capacity

	Males			Females		
	n	%*	Average Hours/Week	n	%*	Average Hours/Week	Productivity Difference (%)
$60,000 and less	36	56.3	56.2	15	40.5	61.7	+10
$61,000–100,000	155	80.3	56.8	29	70.7	57.6	+1.0
$101,000–140,000	161	84.3	60.7	13	86.7	64.8	+6.0
$141,000+	144	85.7	61.9	4	66.7	63.8	+3.0

$\chi^2 = 34.67; p < .001$

*The percent figure represents those who perceive themselves to be at their full professional capacity, as opposed to those *not* at their full capacity for that gender and with that practice characteristic.

Table D.6 Relationship of Specialty to Professional Capacity

	Are You Currently Practicing at Full Professional Capacity?				
	Yes		No		
	n	%	n	%	Total
Radiology	36	90.0	4	10.0	40
Surgical					
General	28	66.7	14	33.3	42
Others	86	71.7	34	28.3	120
Anesthesiology	31	96.9	1	3.1	32
OB/GYN	35	77.8	10	22.2	45
Psychiatry	45	78.9	12	21.1	57
Internal Medicine	97	78.8	26	21.2	123
Pediatrics	57	78.1	16	21.9	73
General/Family Practice	58	71.6	23	28.4	81
Total					613

$\chi^2 = 17.248; df = 8; p < .02$

Table D.7 Comparison of Age of Male and Female Physician Respondents

Age	Males		Females		Total	
	n	%	n	%	n	%
30–44	346	50.7	85	81.7	431	54.8
45–54	179	26.2	13	12.5	192	24.4
55+	157	23.0	6	5.8	163	20.7
Totals	682	86.8	104	13.2	786	100.0

χ^2 significant at the .01 level.

Table D.8 Memberships of Active Physicians in Professional Societies

	Males		Females	
	n	%	n	%
American Medical Association member	221	32.4	17	16.3
Massachusetts Medical Society member	492	72.0	53	51.0
County medical society member	472	69.1	50	48.1
Specialty society member	539	79.0	76	73.1

χ^2 signficant at the .01 level.

Table D.9 Percentages of Male and Female Physicians by Specialty Choice

	Males			Females	
Most Common Specialties	Total (%)	Under 35 (%)	Most Common Specialties	Total (%)	Under 35 (%)
1. Internal Medicine	15.8	23.3	1. Internal Medicine	18.4	24.1
2. Family Practice	7.7	10.6	2. Pediatrics	15.1	16.5
3. Pediatrics	4.9	5.8	3. Psychiatry	7.9	5.9
4. General Surgery	7.2	9.2	4. Family Practice	7.7	10.2
5. Psychiatry	5.3	3.7	5. Obstetrics/Gynecology	7.1	8.9
6. Obstetrics/Gynecology	5.2	4.3	6. Anesthesiology	4.5	3.5
7. Anesthesiology	4.2	5.6	7. Pathology	3.6	2.7
8. General Practice	4.3	0.7	8. General Practice	2.4	0.5
9. Orthopedic Surgery	3.6	4.3	9. Diagnostic Radiology	2.3	2.8
10. Pathology	2.4	1.9	10. General Surgery	2.3	3.7
11. Ophthalmology	2.9	2.7	11. Emergency Medicine	1.9	2.1
12. Cardiovascular Disease	2.9	2.6	12. Dermatology	0.1	1.7
Largest Proportionate Increases (%)			Largest Proportionate Increases (%)		
Internal Medicine	29.5		General Surgery	62.6	
Physical Medicine/Rehab	29.3		Neurological Surgery	57.1	
Diagnostic Radiology	29.2		Orthopedic Surgery	54.6	
Family Practice	27.7		Urological Surgery	52.9	
Anesthesiology	27.3		Aerospace Medicine	52.6	
General Surgery	26.0		Family Practice	50.9	
Emergency Medicine	24.6		Internal Medicine	50.2	
Pediatrics	23.8		Otolaryngology	50.3	

Source: Calculated from data presented in Roback, Randolph, and Seidman (1990).

Table D.10   Income of Patient Care Physicians: Males and Females

Income Categories	Patient Care Respondents n	%	Males* n	%	Females* n	%
1. Less than $40,000	33	4.5	23	3.60	10	9.9
2. $41,000–60,000	70	9.4	42	6.57	27	26.73
3. $61,000–80,000	103	13.9	78	12.20	25	24.75
4. $81,000–100,000	141	19.0	123	19.24	18	17.82
5. $101,000–120,000	115	15.5	107	16.74	8	7.92
6. $121,000–140,000	95	12.8	88	13.77	7	6.9
7. $141,000–160,000	54	7.3	49	7.67	5	4.9
8. Over $160,000	130	17.5	129	20.18	1	0.99
Mean income	94,400		103,260		67,208	
Median income	97,500		101,000		61,760	

*A one-way ANOVA shows that gender has a significant effect upon income ($F = 71.51$; $df = 1$; $p = .0001$).

Table D.11 Income by Gender by Specialty Categories

Specialty Categories	Males				Females			
	n	(%)	Mean Income	Median Income	n	(%)	Mean Income	Median Income
1. General/Family Practice	67	(10.9)	69,507	67,270	13	(13.9)	47,769	45,750
2. Internal Medicine	102	(16.7)	83,090	82,330	20	(21.2)	55,250	56,770
3. Pediatrics	47	(7.7)	83,660	81,760	21	(22.3)	48,980	45,750
4. All other medical specialties	40	(6.6)	116,580	118,480	1	(1.1)	81,000	81,000
5. General Surgery	40	(6.6)	113,350	115,820	2	(2.1)	141,000	141,000
6. OB/GYN	35	(5.7)	128,600	134,490	12	(12.7)	81,000	101,000
7. All other surgical specialties	112	(18.3)	128,900	144,040	1	(1.1)	141,000	141,000
8. Radiology	31	(5.0)	141,000	152,970	2	(2.1)	141,000	141,000
9. Anesthesiology	27	(4.4)	126,510	126,320	5	(5.3)	96,200	93,540
10. Pathology	9	(1.5)	123,090	117,530	2	(2.1)	50,500	50,500
11. Psychiatry	50	(8.0)	82,520	81,570	8	(8.6)	63,280	50,500
12. All Others	53	(8.6)	97,340	91,450	7	(7.5)	74,490	75,250
Total	613	(100)			94	(100)		

Table D.12 Correlations of Six Satisfaction Indexes with Productivity

1. Average Direct Hours Worked Each Week†

	0–25 hrs *(n = 47)* r	*26–50 hrs* *(n = 361)* r	*51–74 hrs* *(n = 317)* r	*75+ hrs* *(n = 28)* r
1. Personal	−.063	.044	−.012	−.067
2. Resources	−.080	.049	−.012	−.162
3. Review	−.285	−.051	−.061	.379
4. Sat. with Med.	−.164	.026	−.038	−.179
5. Mass. Reg. Climate	.115	−.005	−.090	.177
6. Mass. Prac.	.157	−.037	−.064	.136

2. Average Total Hours Worked Each Week††

	0–30 hrs *(n = 18)* r	*31–60 hrs* *(n = 365)* r	*61–90 hrs* *(n = 359)* r	*91+ hrs* *(n = 26)* r
1. Personal	.123	−.056	−.094	−.040
2. Resources	.003	.124***	−.024	−.085
3. Review	.088	.085	−.107	.400***
4. Sat. with Med.	.174	−.055	−.109	−.133
5. Mass. Reg. Climate	.041	−.068	−.081	.084
6. Mass. Prac.	.128	−.053	−.181*	−.004

* $p \leq .001$.
** $p \leq .01$.
*** $p \leq .05$.
**** $p \leq .10$.
†Direct hours include the sum of hours spent each week with (a) office-based patients, (b) surgery, (c) hospital patients, (d) emergency room, (e) hospital outpatient clinics, (f) nursing home, and (g) telephone time with matters concerning patients. Based on self-report.
††Total hours include direct hours and all other hours spent in professional activities related to medicine. Based on self-report.

Table D.13 Relationship of Scores on Six Indexes to Responses to Global Satisfaction Item

"All things considered I am satisfied with my medical practice."	Personal Mean Score (range 5-25)	Resources Mean Score (range 5-25)	Review Mean Score (range 2-10)	Satisfaction with Medicine Mean Score (range 5-25)	Massachusetts Regulatory Climate Mean Score (range 5-25)	Massachusetts as a Good Place to Practice Mean Score (range 4-20)
Strongly Agree/Agree						
Total (N = 419)	21.7	19.7	6.0	19.4	9.8	10.8
Male (n = 355)	21.8	19.8	5.9	19.4	9.6	10.8
Female (n = 64)	21.4	18.9	6.1	19.3	10.9	10.9
Undecided						
Total (N = 121)	21.1	18.9	5.3	14.9	8.3	8.6
Male (n = 105)	21.2	19.0	5.3	15.0	8.2	8.5
Female (n = 15)	20.3	17.9	5.4	15.1	8.9	9.1
Disagree/Strongly Disagree						
Total (N = 227)	20.6	18.6	5.2	11.9	7.4	7.2
Male (n = 203)	20.7	18.8	5.2	11.8	7.2	7.1
Female (n = 23)	19.9	17.3	5.4	13.1	8.5	7.9
ANOVA Results						
Total	12.53*	11.15*	13.4*	5.28*	55.28*	172.40*
Male	10.77*	9.86*	11.3*	470.42*	48.39*	157.78*
Female	2.27	2.26	1.72	51.4*	6.22**	13.44*

$*$ $p \leq .001$.
$**$ $p \leq .01$.
$***$ $p \leq .05$.
$****$ $p \leq .10$.

Table D.14 Relationship of Scores on Six Indexes to Responses to General Satisfaction Item Related to Massachusetts

"I am generally satisfied with Massachusetts as a place to practice."	Personal Mean Score (range 5–25)	Resources Mean Score (range 5–25)	Review Mean Score (range 2–10)	Satisfaction with Medicine Mean Score (range 5–25)	Massachusetts Regulatory Climate Mean Score (range 5–25)	Massachusetts Practice Mean Score (range 4–20)
Strongly Agree/Agree						
Total (N = 195)	22.1	19.9	6.2	20.0	11.0	12.9
Male (n = 164)	22.2	20.0	6.2	20.1	11.0	12.9
Female (n = 31)	21.4	19.3	6.2	19.3	11.6	12.8
Undecided						
Total (N = 114)	21.0	19.2	5.7	17.4	9.6	10.4
Male (n = 92)	21.0	19.5	5.7	17.3	9.1	10.3
Female (n = 22)	20.7	18.0	5.9	17.9	12.2	10.6
Disagree/Strongly Disagree						
Total (N = 457)	21.1	19.0	5.4	14.7	7.7	7.6
Male (n = 406)	21.1	19.1	5.4	14.6	7.6	7.6
Female (n = 50)	20.5	18.0	5.7	15.7	8.4	7.9
ANOVA Results						
Total	10.38*	6.29**	12.43*	137.38*	108.15*	623.80*
Male	10.14*	5.52**	11.63*	125.45*	94.47*	535.68*
Female	0.88	1.58	0.69	10.63*	19.36*	81.15*

* $p \leq .001$.
** $p \leq .01$.
*** $p \leq .05$.
**** $p \leq .10$.

Table D.15 Comparison of Nurses' and Physicians' Responses to Selected Satisfaction Items (Percentages)

	Nurses*				Physicians†		
	Agreement (%)	Undecided (%)	Disagreement (%)		Agreement (%)	Undecided (%)	Disagreement (%)
1. My present salary is satisfactory.	38.6	1.2	60.2	1. Income of my practice	61.8	7.4	30.7
2. Considering what is expected of nursing service personnel at this hospital, the pay we get is reasonable.	19.7	2.9	77.4	2. My current income is satisfactory, given the amount of work I do.	46.5	8.2	45.3
3. I have plenty of time and opportunity to discuss patient care problems with other nursing service personnel.	34.4	3.7	61.9	3. Professional interaction with other physicians	92.5	2.0	5.5
4. If I had the decision to make all over again, I would still go into nursing.	59.1	10.8	30.1	4. If I had the decision to make all over again, I would still go into medicine.	59.2	20.3	20.6

Source: Data for nurses from P. L. Stamps and E. B. Piedmonte. *Nurses and Work Satisfaction: An Index for Measurement.* Ann Arbor, MI: Health Administration Press, 1986.

*Nurses study used a seven-point response mode. Agreement includes strongly agree, moderately agree, and agree. Disagreement includes strongly disagree, moderately disagree, and disagree.

†Physicians study used two five-point response modes. Agreement includes strongly agree and agree as well as very satisfactory and satisfactory. Disagreement includes strongly disagree and disagree as well as very unsatisfactory and unsatisfactory.

Index

Age: comparison of male and female physician respondents (Table D.7), 297; distribution of women physicians, 111, 113; income by male and female physicians (Table 5.8), 142; income for men and women physicians, 140, 142; and income for western Massachusetts (Table 4.3), 75; satisfaction, 187, 189–91; satisfaction for male and female physicians (Table 6.3), 189–90

American Association of University Professors: regression analysis to identify salary adjustments for women, 152–53

American Board of Medical Specialties: physician supply, 33–34

American College of Hospital Administrators: physician surplus, 30

American College of Obstetricians and Gynecologists. Massachusetts Chapter: membership survey of medical practice climate, 11

American College of Surgeons. Massachusetts Chapter: membership survey of medical practice climate, 11

American Medical Association: comparison of study figures to (Table C.7), 282; comparisons of physician characteristics and distribution with supply, 279, 281–83; decrease in the number of medical schools, 27; female members, 114; income definition and trends, 64; information about female physicians, 108–9; physicians survey, 5–6; physician supply, 33; speaking for all physicians, 3; specialty designations, 274

American Medical Association. Division of Survey and Data Resources: physician supply, 33–34

American Medical Association Periodic Survey of Physicians: women, 123

American Medical Association Physician Masterfile: list errors, 249, 251–54; mailing lists, 17–18; patient care responsibilities, 36; physician supply, 33–34, 37

American Medical Association Socioeconomic Characteristics Monitoring Survey: characteristics of medical practice, 36; direct

About the Authors

Paula L. Stamps, Ph.D. is a Professor in the Health Policy and Management Program at the University of Massachusetts School of Public Health. Dr. Stamps is best known for her work in developing and standardizing the Stamps-Piedmonte Index of Work Satisfaction, published by Health Administration Press in 1987. This attitude scale measures the level of professional satisfaction of nursing staff: it is now the standard in the field and is currently being used in hundreds of settings nationwide. She is the author of a previous book on the evaluation of ambulatory care, as well as many articles in the field of occupational satisfaction, program evaluation, and family medicine. Her Ph.D. is from the School of Public Health at the University of Oklahoma.

N. Tess Boley Cruz, Ph.D., M.P.H. is a Postdoctoral Fellow at the Institute for Health Promotion and Disease Prevention Research, in the University of Southern California School of Medicine. Dr. Cruz's research interests are in tobacco control, mass communication, and multicultural issues in public health. She holds a doctorate in Community Health Education from the University of Massachusetts School of Public Health.

Other Books Published by
Health Administration Press

▼▼▼▼▼▼▼▼▼▼▼▼▼▼▼▼▼▼▼

PATIENT-CENTERED HOSPITAL CARE: REFORM FROM WITHIN, edited by Kathryn J. McDonagh

An innovative guide to building organizational structures for patient-centered environments. This book explains the benefits of restructuring, defines the concept of work redesign, and illustrates the value of adopting this approach in U.S. hospitals. The art of hospital restructuring is introduced, with an acknowledgment of its significance as a part of the continuous quality improvement (CQI) process. Also explored are other models for implementing and facilitating change, including examples from work redesign programs across the country.

Hardbound, 222 pages, Sept. 1993, $42.00, Order No. 0936, ISBN 1-56793-002-6. An American College of Healthcare Executives Management Series Book.

EVALUATING THE MEDICAL CARE SYSTEM: EFFECTIVENESS, EFFICIENCY AND EQUITY, by LuAnn Aday, Charles E. Begley, David R. Lairson, and Carl H. Slater

This book defines and integrates the fundamental concepts and methods of health services research. The authors provide a solid overview of the field and explain the relationship between health services research and the major objectives of policy research. The authors apply the concepts and methods of epidemiology, economic, sociology, and other disciplines to illustrate the measurement and relevance of the effectiveness, efficiency, and equity criteria in evaluating healthcare system performance.

Softbound, 222 pages, June 1993, $32.00, Order No. 0933, ISBN 0-910701-98-9. An AHSR/HAP Book.

PAYING PHYSICIANS: OPTIONS FOR CONTROLLING COST, VOLUME, AND INTENSITY OF SERVICES, by Mark V. Pauly, John M. Eisenberg, M.D., Margaret Higgins Radany, M. Haim Erder, Roger Feldman, and J. Sanford Schwartz, M.D.

" There is no doubt that this book is a significant contribution to the literature on controlling the costs of physicians' services." John R.C. Wheeler, Associate Professor, The University of Michigan, School of Public Health.

A major healthcare cost-containment strategy involves changing physician behavior by imposing limits on the volume and intensity of physician services. The authors consider the effects of moving from a charge–based payment system to a resource–based relative value scale (RBRVS) and explain the various methods available for controlling the volume and intensity of physician services.

Softbound, 233 pages, 1992, $30.00, Order No. 0920, ISBN 0-910701-87-3. A Health Administration Press Book.

THE NEW GOVERNANCE: STRATEGIES FOR AN ERA OF HEALTH REFORM, by Russell C. Coile, Jr.

THE NEW GOVERNANCE offers information and strategies to healthcare executives and managers, trustees, policymakers, and physicians, charged with facing the future of healthcare and effectively guiding their institutions into the twenty-first century. The author forecasts five trends for the U.S. health system in the next decade, including the need for hospitals to: determine a "preferred future"; adopt an anticipatory management style; ensure customer satisfaction; foster an environment for risk taking; and develop a global outlook. Coile also stresses a new paradigm for hospital governance in this decade and how it will influence tomorrow's health systems.

Hardbound, 241 pages, 1994, $42.00, Order No. 0940, ISBN 1-56793-007-7. An American College of Healthcare Executives Management Series Book.

CREATING NEW HOSPITAL–PHYSICIAN COLLABORATION, by Todd S. Wirth and Seth Allcorn

This book addresses a key strategy for hospital survival in the 1990s–the formation of partnerships between hospitals and physician medical groups. The authors examine integrated relationships and describe in detail methods for effectively managing these new networks. This book begins with a discussion of the economics of medical practice, the healthcare market, and the controls on healthcare delivery, showing motivations for healthcare executives and physicians to work together more closely. The second section concentrates on the management and business operations of medical groups and explores physician behavior, legal and political concerns, and the functioning of group practices. The last section offers specific approaches to hospital–physician affiliations.

Hardbound, 185 pages, May 1993, Order No. 0931, ISBN 0-910701-96-2. An American College of Healthcare Executives Management Series Book.

Also by Paula L. Stamps:

NURSES AND WORK SATISFACTION: An Index for Measurement, by Paula L. Stamps and Eugene B. Piedmonte

This book presents a fully developed and validated survey for measuring nurses' satisfaction with their work. Ready to use and easy to score, the Index of Work Satisfaction is immediately applicable. The results can be used to plan programs leading to job enrichment, lower turnover rates, cost savings in training, greater productivity, and improved patient care.

Winner of a 1987 American Journal of Nursing Books of the Year Award

Softbound, 126 pages, 1986, $33.00, Order No. 0656, ISBN 0-910701-16-4. A Health Administration Press Book.

Journals Published by
Health Administration Press

▼▼▼▼▼▼▼▼▼▼▼▼▼▼▼▼▼▼▼

FRONTIERS OF HEALTH SERVICES MANAGEMENT

The ideal guide for busy executives, each quarterly issue is a collection of forecasts and perspectives on one of today's emerging healthcare topics. Past issues have discussed regional hospital systems, effective governance in the 1990s, universal health insurance, trends in hospital–physician relationships, future health personnel issues, strategic alliance management, and total quality management.

Subscriptions: $60.00/year in the U.S.; $70.00 in Canada and all other countries; $ 16.00/ single issue. ISSN 0748-8157.

HOSPITAL & HEALTH SERVICES ADMINISTRATION

The Official Journal of the American College of Healthcare Executives, this quarterly publication's concise articles explore the myriad facets of healthcare management, from policy to finances. Issues also contain reviews of current, relevant healthcare management books.

Subscriptions: $50.00/year in the U.S.; $60.00 in Canada and all other countries; $12.00/single issue; for ACHE affiliates, paid as part of dues; additional subscriptions to affiliates $35.00. ISSN 8750-3735

Book and Journal ordering information on next page

BOOK ORDERING INFORMATION

All Health Administration Press Publications are sent on a 30-day approval. To order call, (312) 943-0544, ext. 3000 or send your order to The Foundation of the American College of Healthcare Executives, Order Processing Center, Dept ST94, 1951 Cornell Avenue, Melrose Park, IL 60160-1001.

JOURNAL SUBSCRIPTION INFORMATION

Health Administration Press offers a money-back guarantee on all journal subscriptions. If you are not completely satisfied, simply write and cancel your subscription, you will receive a refund on all unmailed issues. Multi-year subscriptions are not available.

Back issues are usually available for single-copy or bulk-copy orders. Orders for back issues in quantities of 10-24 copies sent to one address receive a 15% discoun t from list, quantities of 24–49, a 20% discount.

Please send separate checks payable to the name of the publication for subscriptions. Current rates expire on December 31, 1994. Address orders to: The Foundation of the American College of Healthcare Executives, Order Processing Center, Dept. ST94, 1951 Cornell Avenue, Melrose Park, IL 60160-1001. Or for more information, call: (312) 943-0544, ext. 3000.

▼▼▼▼▼▼▼▼▼▼▼▼▼▼▼▼▼